Frailty and Sarcopenia: Current Issues and Research

Frailty and Sarcopenia: Current Issues and Research

Edited by Kylen Mitchell

STATES
ACADEMIC PRESS
www.statesacademicpress.com

States Academic Press,
109 South 5th Street,
Brooklyn, NY 11249, USA

Visit us on the World Wide Web at:
www.statesacademicpress.com

ISBN: 978-1-63989-219-8

Cataloging-in-Publication Data

Frailty and sarcopenia : current issues and research / edited by Kylen Mitchell.
p. cm.
Includes bibliographical references and index.
ISBN 978-1-63989-219-8
1. Musculoskeletal system--Diseases. 2. Musculoskeletal system--Abnormalities.
3. Musculoskeletal system--Wounds and injuries. I. Mitchell, Kylen.

RC925 .F73 2022
616.74--dc23

Table of Contents

Preface

This book has been an outcome of determined endeavour from a group of educationists in the field. The primary objective was to involve a broad spectrum of professionals from diverse cultural background involved in the field for developing new researches. The book not only targets students but also scholars pursuing higher research for further enhancement of the theoretical and practical applications of the subject.

Frailty is a clinically recognizable syndrome associated with aging and an increased risk of catastrophic decline in the health of elderly people. Muscles start degenerating with age which results in weakness, decreased energy, slowing, lower activity and severe unintended weight loss. Sarcopenia can be a cause of frailty. It is the degenerative loss of skeletal muscle strength, quality and mass with age. The rate of muscle loss depends on several factors such as nutrition, exercise level and co-morbidities. Sarcopenia leads to reduced functional status and can cause significant disability from increased weakness. Muscle loss within this disease occurs due to changes in muscle synthesis signaling pathways. This book provides significant information of this discipline to help develop a good understanding of frailty and sarcopenia. Also included herein is a detailed explanation of the current issues and research on these medical conditions. This book is appropriate for students seeking detailed information in this area as well as for experts.

It was an honour to edit such a profound book and also a challenging task to compile and examine all the relevant data for accuracy and originality. I wish to acknowledge the efforts of the contributors for submitting such brilliant and diverse chapters in the field and for endlessly working for the completion of the book. Last, but not the least; I thank my family for being a constant source of support in all my research endeavours.

Editor

1

Epidemiology of Sarcopenia and Frailty

Harnish P Patel, Esther Clift, Lucy Lewis and
Cyrus Cooper

Abstract

Sarcopenia and frailty are common in older persons and pose particular challenges for health and social care systems especially in the context of global population ageing. Sarcopenia, the loss of skeletal muscle mass, strength and function with age is associated with adverse individual physical and metabolic changes contributing to morbidity and mortality. The health and socioeconomic implications of sarcopenia are also considerable. Sarcopenia is a core component of physical frailty that together impact negatively on an individual's capability to live independently. Frailty is a biological syndrome of low reserve and resistance to stressors resulting from cumulative declines across multiple physiological systems that collectively predispose an individual to adverse outcomes. Frailty develops along a continuum from independence through to death as physiological reserves progressively diminish an individual's capacity to recover from an acute insult or illness. Managing sarcopenia and frailty involves the multidisciplinary led completion of a comprehensive care plan that is patient centred, responsive to the needs of the patient and adaptable therefore enabling an individual to maintain their independence.

Keywords: Sarcopenia, frail, epidemiology, Comprehensive Geriatric Assessment

1. Introduction

Over the past two centuries, there has been a demographic transformation across the world and people are living longer [1]. For the first time in history, people can expect to live beyond their 60th birthday. In fact, survival to age 80 is anticipated to be the norm for all of today's young people. People aged 60 or over are set to increase from 841 million to more than 2 billion between 2013 and 2050. This equates to 21.1% of the world's population [1]. Globally, the number of people aged 80 years or over, the "oldest-old", is growing even faster. In 2000, there were 71 million people aged 80 or over worldwide. Since then, the number of oldest-old has grown by 77% to 125 million in 2015, and it is projected to increase by 61% over the next 15 years, reaching nearly 202 million in 2030. Projections indicate that in 2050 the oldest-old will number 434 million globally, having more than tripled in number since 2015 [2]. These demographic changes are largely due to the advances in public health and modern medicine that have reduced early life mortality, reduced the rate of infectious diseases [3] and have allowed people to live with one or more long-term conditions. Whilst this is a cause for celebration, these cumulative changes pose significant challenges for delivering health and social care to older people in all nations concerned.

The situation within the UK is no different. Medical and technological advances in the treatment of illnesses and diseases have improved mortality rates in the oldest age groups. In 2013–2015, a UK male aged 85 could expect to live to age 90.8 years and a female to 91.8 years. Life expectancy at birth has increased throughout England, Scotland, Wales and Northern Ireland due to improvements in mortality in older age. Life expectancy is highest in England with Scotland having the lowest of the four UK constituent countries (Office of National Statistics 2016, *ONS.gov.uk*).

However, numerous people who are living longer in the UK do so with one or more long-term medical conditions and many are living with frailty. The clinical conditions of sarcopenia and frailty are particularly complex expressions of ageing that impact a range of health and social care settings [4, 5]. Sarcopenia is associated with adverse individual physical and metabolic changes contributing to morbidity and mortality, whilst frailty is defined as a state of increased vulnerability as a consequence of cumulative physiological decline across multiple systems predisposing to poor resolution of homeostasis after a stressor event, which increases the risk of adverse outcomes [4, 6]. In this chapter, we will review the epidemiology, pathogenesis, diagnosis of sarcopenia and frailty as well as give an overview of Comprehensive Geriatric Assessment (CGA) as a method of systematically evaluating an older person's treatment, management and long-term follow-up needs.

2. Skeletal muscle and sarcopenia

Skeletal muscle comprises approximately 40% of total body mass and therefore constitutes one of the largest organ systems of the body [7]. Skeletal muscle plays an essential role in both physical, for example, locomotion and metabolic functioning, for example, thermoregulation, metabolism of glucose and amino acids. Muscle is also a reservoir for proteins and energy that can be utilised in periods of stress or undernutrition, for example, acute deterioration in health and hospitalisation.

2.1. Diagnosing sarcopenia

Sarcopenia has previously been defined based solely on lean mass as a function of height (appendicular lean mass [ALM] is measured by dual-energy X-ray absorptiometry [DXA] divided by height squared) where sarcopenia was diagnosed −1 to −2 SD below gender-specific mean values of a younger control group [8]. However, direct proportionality between loss of muscle mass and impaired strength/function cannot be inferred as longitudinal as well as cross-sectional studies show that younger individuals can be stronger and older individuals are weaker than would be predicted by their muscle mass [9, 10]. Therefore muscle quality or force generated per unit area is important and the definition of sarcopenia now extends to encompass loss of strength and or physical performance [6, 10]. Sarcopenia, is the progressive and generalised loss of skeletal muscle mass, strength and physical performance with age and as such it is a core component of physical frailty [6, 11, 12]. Sarcopenia is associated with a broad array of adverse physical and metabolic outcomes including falls [13], disability, hospitalisation, diabetes [14], osteoporosis [15] and also mortality [16]. The economic costs associated with 'sarcopenia' in the year 2000 were estimated to be $18.5 billion in the USA alone [17].

Recent diagnostic algorithms include those proposed by EWGSOP [6], The International working group (IWG) on sarcopenia [18], The Foundation for the National Health Institutes of Health (FNIH) Sarcopenia Project [11] and the Asian Working Group for Sarcopenia (AWGS) [19]; the later driven by the need to account for ethnic variations in body composition and muscle function in order to further research sarcopenia in the Asian subcontinent.

The EWGSOP definition requires the presence of slower walk speed (<0.8 m/s) [20] or weaker strength (grip <30 kg for men, <20 kg for women) [21] in combination with low muscle mass (defined as ALM/ht^2 ≤7.23 kg/m^2 for men and ≤5.67 kg/m^2 for women). The International Working Group (IWG) on sarcopenia included impaired physical performance in addition to slow walk speed before measuring muscle mass in their working definition for the diagnosis of sarcopenia. The Foundations of National Institutes of Health (FNIH) sarcopenia project based in the USA incorporated clinically relevant cut points of low muscle mass and strength (grip strength <26 kg for men and <16 kg for women and ALM adjusted for BMI <0.789 for men and <0.512 for women) [11]. Similarly, the AWGS included gait speed <0.8 mm/s, ALM/ht^2 <7.0 m^2 in men and <5.4 kg/m^2 in women and grip strength <26 kg for men and <18 kg in women [19] in their working definition of sarcopenia. From a clinical point of view, these algorithms enable case finding for sarcopenia and conceptually identify stages of sarcopenia that allow intervention. For example, the pre-sarcopenia stage is characteristic of low muscle mass without impact on muscle strength or physical performance, the sarcopenia stage is characterised by low muscle mass, low muscle strength or poorer physical performance, whilst severe sarcopenia is when all three criteria within the algorithm are met [6].

2.2. Prevalence of sarcopenia

The prevalence of sarcopenia increases with age but figures are influenced by the diagnostic algorithm used, ethnic population studied, cut-off values for lean mass and function and the health care setting, that is, community versus in hospital [22]. For example, a recent systematic review reported that the prevalence rates differed for community-dwelling older people aged ≥60 years (up to 29%), in long-term care age >70 years (up to 33%) and in an acute care hospitals, age ≥ 65 years (up to 10%) [23].

2.3. Measuring muscle mass

The commonest approach to measuring muscle mass is through bioimpedance analysis (BIA) and where available, dual-energy X-ray absorptiometry (DXA) scanning. Computerised tomography (CT) and magnetic resonance imaging (MRI) can also be used [24]. The approach that is undertaken to measure muscle mass is dependent on feasibility, access, costs and sample size. For example, BIA utilises portable equipment and can be used across a range of health care settings and calculates fat-free mass rather than true muscle mass based on the electrical conductivity of various body tissues. Whole body DXA will enable the calculation of total and appendicular lean mass but may overestimate lean mass values in those with extracellular fluid accumulation. Computerised tomography (CT) and magnetic resonance imaging (MRI) can differentiate fat from muscle, which can be useful to make assumptions on muscle quality. However, high operational costs and radiation, in the case for CT, limits their use in the diagnosis of sarcopenia.

2.4. Measuring muscle strength

Grip strength measured using hand-held dynamometry, has gained wide acceptance as a reliable and valid measure of muscle strength across health care settings and is an integral component in the international diagnostic algorithms for sarcopenia [25–27]. Other methods to measure muscle 'strength' include ascertainment of knee extensor power, isometric knee strength and quadriceps torque but these require static and bulky equipment that are not readily portable and can be impractical in routine clinical practice as well as in epidemiological studies.

2.5. Measuring physical performance

Slower gait speed is associated with risk of future morbidity and mortality and is therefore suitable for inclusion in diagnostic algorithms for sarcopenia [28]. Other objectively measured physical performance measures such as chair rise time; time taken to complete five sit to stand actions and standing balance; and the time for sustaining balance on one leg have also been associated with higher risk of all-cause mortality in older people [16, 29]. Gait speed requires intact coordination, neural and joint control so may not be practical in context of acutely unwell hospitalised older people. Grip strength measurements in this situation may have better predictive value and be more feasible [25–27, 30].

2.6. Questionnaires to aid the diagnosis of sarcopenia

The SARC-F questionnaire was developed to predict poor muscle function [31, 32] and is based on five questions that ascertain how much difficulty an individual has performing the following parameters: ability to rise from a chair, walk assisted or unassisted, climb stairs, carry heavy loads (as a measure of strength) and ascertainment on the number of falls a person has had in the last year.

Each parameter is assigned a score: 0 (none); 1(some) or 2 (a lot); the falls parameter (none = 0, 1–3 = 1, 4 or more = 2). A total score of ≥4 (scale 0–10) suggests that the subject is symptomatic of sarcopenia. The SARC-F questionnaire has been shown to have excellent specificity but poor sensitivity for sarcopenia based on the consensus criteria from the IWG, EWGSOP and AWG. However, it has been shown to predict physical limitation over a four-year follow-up and may be useful for case identification and subsequent diagnostic evaluation for sarcopenia in community based but not hospital or care home-based settings [33].

Despite the recent progress in refining and implementing diagnostic criteria for sarcopenia over the past decade, there is no consensus on global diagnostic criteria for sarcopenia based on cut-off values for skeletal muscle mass indices, grip strength and walking speed. In fact, the variance in the criteria indicate that ethnic, gender and cultural differences dictate population-specific criteria are required in order to account for the genome/environment interactions that contribute to sarcopenia, thus influencing the design of both observational and intervention studies [24, 34].

2.7. Pathogenesis of sarcopenia

In sarcopenic muscle, the rate of muscle injury (from normal contraction) exceeds that of repair and regeneration. There may also be decreased satellite cell (muscle stem cell), proliferative capability and renewal [35, 36] in combination with altered inter- and intracellular environments that favour catabolism. This increase in catabolism is associated with a decrease in growth factors such as circulating insulin, growth hormone and testosterone and muscle-specific IGF-1 levels [37]. Furthermore, the production of reactive oxygen species and oxidative stress can lead to mitochondrial DNA damage and a progressive decline in mitochondrial function and energy depletion [38]. At a tissue level, skeletal muscle is continuously remodelled in response to workload, tension, nutrition and anabolic stimulation. The cues associated with the age-related decline in muscle mass and strength include behavioural (i.e. decrease in physical activity/sedentary lifestyle), extrinsic (i.e. undernutrition) and intrinsic factors (i.e. hormonal changes, inflammation, oxidative stress and denervation) [39] (**Figure 1**).

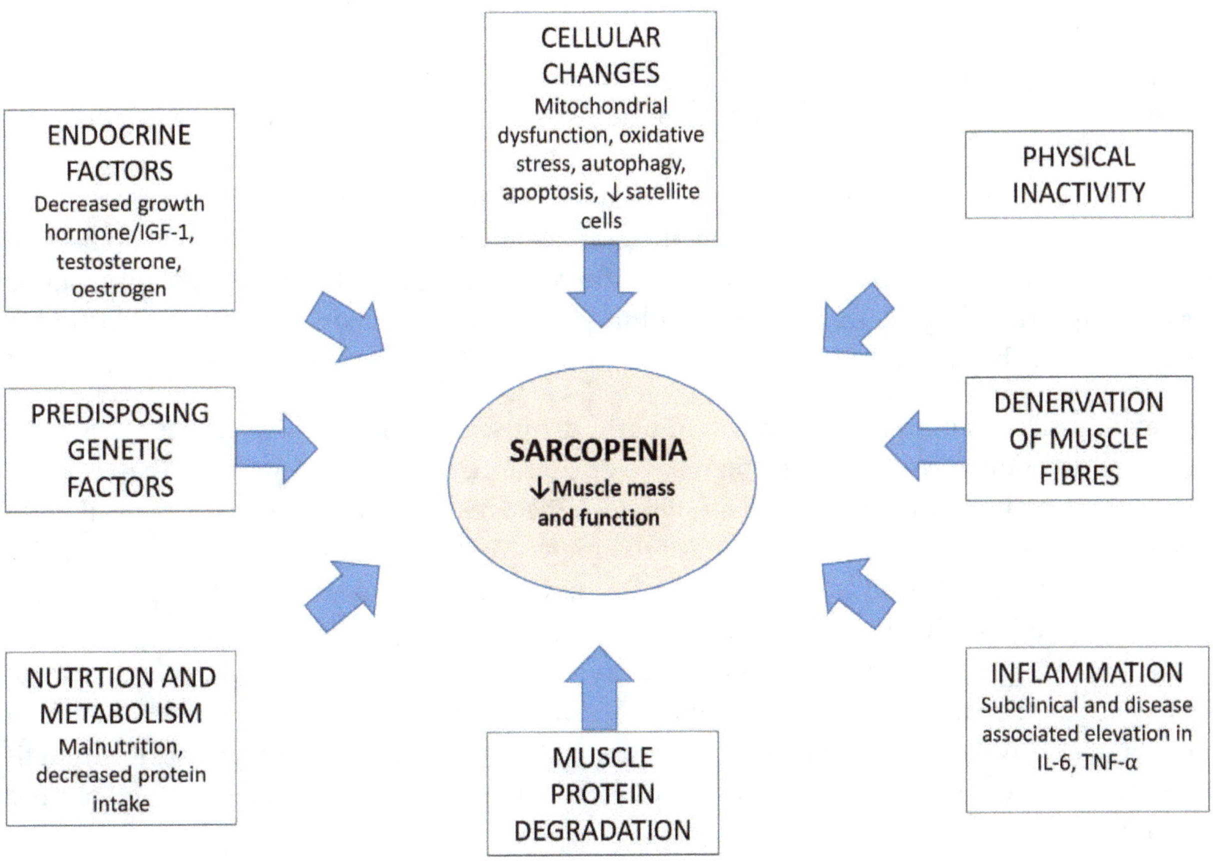

Figure 1. The main mechanisms involved in the aetiology of sarcopenia.

The complex dynamic genome/environment interplay involved in the balancing of muscle synthesis and breakdown is mediated through multiple cell signalling pathways [40] that include IGF-1/AKT/mTOR and NF-κB (nuclear factor-kB). These pathways influence the balance between synthesis and degradation. For example, the IGF-I/AKT/mTOR pathways promote protein synthesis and the maintenance of skeletal muscle mass. By contrast, the activation of NF-kB by inflammatory mediators including tumour necrosis factor (TNF) and interleukin 6 (IL-6) upregulate the E3 ubiquitin ligases MAFbx (atrogin-1) and MURF-1, which signal the muscle atrophic process. Skeletal muscle ageing is also characterised by a continuous cycle of denervation and reinnervation as a consequence of the loss of alpha-motor neurones within the central nervous system (CNS), withdrawal of nerve terminals from the neuromuscular junctions (NMJ) and axonal sprouting from neighbouring neurons collectively giving rise to larger, inefficient motor units.

Remodelling of skeletal muscle tissue through neuropathic, neurohormonal and inflammatory pathways leads to a reduction in muscle cross-sectional area, volume and a reduced rate of force generation. This is characterised by the presence of fewer type I oxidative (slow twitch) and type II glycolytic (fast twitch) myofibres as well as myofibre atrophy. The loss of type II fibres, with concomitant decrease in satellite cells [41], is associated with decreased strength and ability to generate power. Moreover, there is a concurrent increase in non-contractile material within the fascicles that affects muscle quality. Collectively, these processes lead to the reduced muscle functional performance.

2.8. A life course approach to understand the aetiology of sarcopenia

Muscle development in humans begins at 6 weeks of gestation and continues until approximately 24 weeks when the total number of fibres is set. Any subsequent increase in muscle bulk occurs by hypertrophy as evidenced by an increase in fibre cross-sectional area, and not by hyperplasia. Therefore, the number of muscle fibres formed prenatally influences the potential for postnatal hypertrophy [42]. Muscle mass increases during childhood and adolescence until adult muscle cross-sectional areas are reached shortly after puberty. Muscle mass then remains relatively constant in early adulthood until the later part of the 4th decade of life when a decline begins [43].

Skeletal muscle strength is determined, in part, by muscle mass, which is a function of myofibre size and number. On average, men have greater muscle mass and strength than women at any given point in the life course [44]. Between the ages of 20 and 80 years, total lean body mass has been reported to decline by approximately 18% in males and by 27% in females [45]. Therefore, the 'health' of skeletal muscle in an older person is a function of the peak levels attained in early life and the extrinsic and intrinsic changes operating through middle years into old age, for example, physical activity, nutrition, disease and disuse and hormonal changes. There is also robust epidemiological evidence suggesting that low birth weight, a marker of an adverse early intrauterine environment, is associated with a poorer grip strength in older adults and that the mechanism may be driven by myofibre development and number [46, 47].

3. Frailty

Frailty is a common clinical syndrome, which is often seen in older adults, especially in women compared to men and younger aged adults [48–50]. Frailty is distinct from disability and comorbidity and independently carries a high risk for poor health outcomes such as falls, hospitalisation, disability and mortality [51, 52]. Whilst, sarcopenia contributes to and is a core component of physical frailty, the syndrome of frailty is comprised of several interlinked domains that impact on an older person's independence, quality of life and medium- to long-term outcomes. Cognitive frailty refers to progressive cognitive decline in absence of a diagnosis of dementia, social frailty refers to loneliness and the lack of robust social networks as well as poor income whilst psychological frailty refers to the inherent traits in an individual that may predispose an individual to adversity, for example, bereavement, low mood, lack of motivation and labile emotions [53, 54]. Multimorbidity, defined by the UK National Institute for Health and Care Excellence (NICE, guidance 56), is the presence of two or more distinct long-term conditions, is also associated with a higher risk of developing frailty [54, 55]. This conceptual model illustrates that assessing and managing a patient who is living with frailty requires a more holistic approach to manage the cause, or combination of causes that have precipitated acute decompensation [5] (**Figure 2**).

Frailty is best understood as a multisystem disorder, with perhaps both independent and linked mechanisms operating across organ or physiological systems. Accumulating dysregulation across multiple systems can negatively affect previous normal functional homeostatic mechanisms accelerating the development and progression of frailty. This is relevant not only for improved understanding of this syndrome but also because a key implication of loss of reserve across multiple systems is that therapeutic intervention of any single system, that is, endocrine, brain, immune/inflammatory or indeed an individual domain, that is, social, physical or cognitive, is unlikely to ameliorate the abnormal health state of frailty. For those living with frailty, even a minor insult such as a minor infection or change in medication can lead to a large disproportionate change in an individual's health and social care state that inevitably results in an acute hospital admission (**Figure 2**).

Older people living with frailty do so as a consequence of accelerated loss of biological reserves across multiple systems over a lifetime and individuals experience frequent transitions between frailty states over time. Using the life course approach to conceptualise frailty is worth considering as this broadens the window of opportunity to identify markers and mechanisms contributing to frailty with a view to intervention [56] (**Figure 2**). For example, the presence of weight loss or weakness earlier in the life course, that is, slow walk speed and exhaustion may identify people at especially high risk of rapid decline [57].

3.1. Identification of frailty

Detection of frailty should be an essential part of assessment of older people and the identification of reliable tools to determine frailty within acute and community settings is currently a research and clinical priority. Recognising and identifying people who are living with frailty not only enables clinicians and health care professionals to respond quickly and

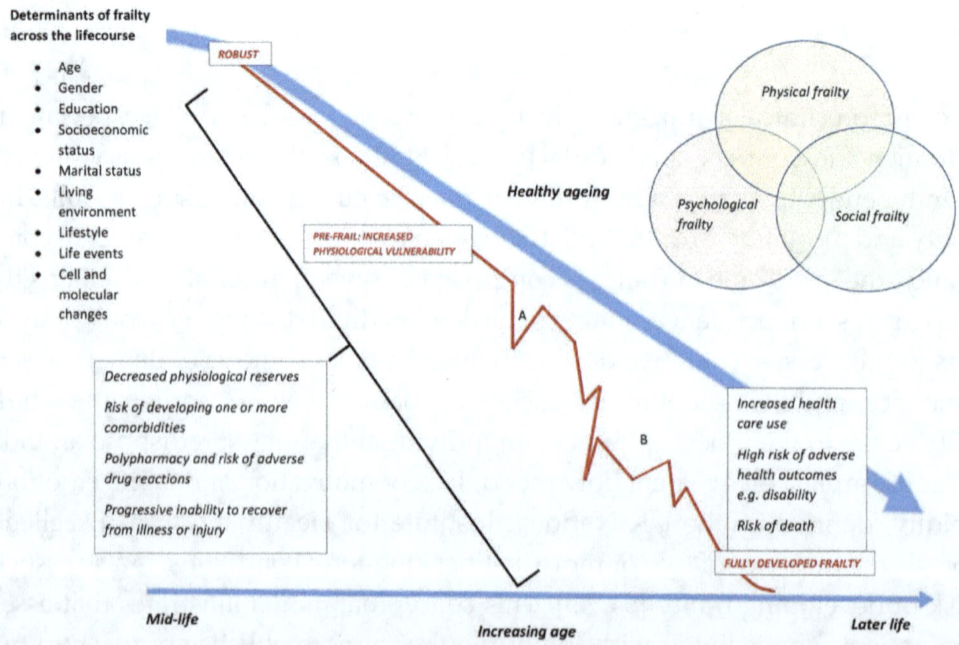

Figure 2. Healthy ageing is depicted by the blue solid line. Frailty (red line) develops as a continuum from being physiologically robust and independent to being at high risk of hospitalisation, institutionalisation and death. In more physiologically robust individuals, full recovery is likely after an insult, for example, infection (A), but later in the time course, moderate to severe frailty predisposes to recurrent hospital admissions as a consequence of a disproportionate deterioration in health and social and/or psychological health from a relatively minor insult or stress (B). The recovery from subsequent insults takes longer as physiological reserves are depleted until the individual cannot compensate adequately, and the ability to perform daily activities diminishes leading to dependency and disability.

appropriately to minimise exposures that may not be beneficial or could be harmful, that is, polypharmacy, invasive investigations, but also anticipate and prevent functional decline and potentially reverse the state of frailty with appropriate interventions.

The two established international models of frailty are the phenotype model and the cumulative deficit model. The phenotype model developed by Fried identifies frailty by the presence of at least three of five physical characteristics: weight loss, exhaustion, low energy expenditure, slow walking speed and low handgrip strength [51]. The cumulative deficit model developed by Rockwood et al. identifies frailty on the basis of the accumulation of a range of 'deficits', which can be symptoms, sensory deficits, clinical signs, diseases, disabilities and abnormal laboratory test results that then allow an index to be calculated. The frailty index is a function of the number of deficits present in an individual divided by the total number of deficits possible within the population sample [58]. The number of deficits measures accumulated vulnerability, which is related to adverse outcomes. In this regard, a frailty index will range from 0 to 1, with values over 0.67 identifying a level of frailty beyond which accumulation of further deficits is not sustainable with life [59]. Despite the difference in approaches to measuring frailty, both tools are able to predict adverse outcome, which provides support for the notion of frailty as a unified construct [60]. In clinical practice, identification of frailty using the Clinical Frailty Scale (CFS), a visual tool based on a comprehensive clinical assessment of a patient, enables assignment of a frailty category [58]. There are seven CFS categories ranging from 1 (fit) to 7 (severe frailty) and increasing CFS frailty has been demonstrated to have predictive validity for adverse outcomes of institutionalisation and mortality. In outpatient settings, The PRISMA-7 questionnaire, can be used to identify persons who are living with frailty and disability. These questions are:

1. Are you more than 85 years? Yes = 1 point
2. Male? Yes = 1 point
3. In general, do you have any health problems that require you to limit your activities? Yes = 1 point
4. Do you need someone to help you on a regular basis? Yes = 1 point
5. In general, do you have any health problems that require you to stay at home? Yes = 1 point
6. In case of need, can you count on someone close to you? No = 1 point
7. Do you regularly use a stick, walker or wheelchair to get about? Yes = 1 point

A score of > 3 can be used to identify frailty.

A further important concept of frailty as a syndrome is that individuals may have previously unrecognised and inadequately addressed conditions that do not characteristically fall into a single organ category but can have a major impact on quality of life. Identification of these 'frailty syndromes' can help health care professionals manage and potentially delay their complications. These, often inter-related syndromes, include but are not limited to falls, delirium, weight loss and malnutrition, fluctuating disability, polypharmacy, social isolation, fragility fracture(s) and recurrent hospital admissions (**Figure 3**).

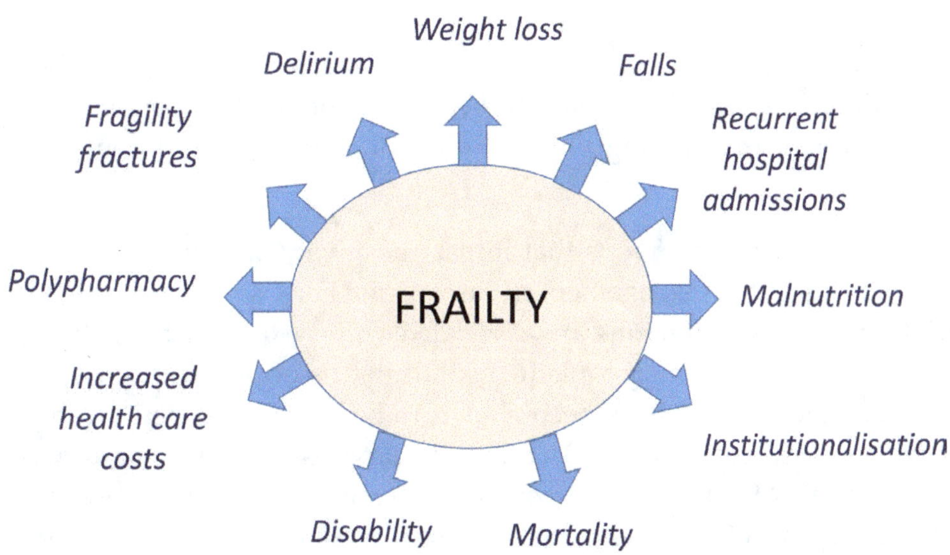

Figure 3. Consequences of living with frailty.

3.2. Prevalence of frailty

Given poor outcomes relating to morbidity, mortality and disability, it is useful to understand the prevalence of frailty to inform the provision of appropriate health and social care interventions. Prevalence figures have been well documented in many OECD (Convention of the Organisation for Economic Cooperation and Development) countries such a USA, Canada, Netherlands and the UK but data on relative incidence in developing countries is sparse [49]. Prevalence estimates based on 21 cohorts of 61,500 community-dwelling older adults across mainly developed countries estimated frailty prevalence between 4 and 59% and varied according to the operational definitions, for example, the physical phenotype versus frailty index-based models. However, there was general agreement that frailty increases with age and is higher in women than in men. In populations aged 80–84, the pooled prevalence rate was reported to be 15.7% whilst in those over 85 the prevalence increased to 26% [49]. This figure may be substantially higher in institutionalised older people. In an analysis of the Study on health, Ageing and Retirement in Europe, SHARE (n = 18,566) and Study on global AGEing and adult health, SAGE (n = 161,542), two large international data sets of adults over 50 years in which a frailty index was calculated, more women were classed as frail and frailty as a syndrome was distributed along the socioeconomic gradient amongst both higher and lower income countries such that individuals with less education and monetary income were more likely to be frail [48]. Recently, a study of 5450 older people aged 60 and over participating in the English Longitudinal Study of Ageing (ELSA) reported that the prevalence of frailty using the physical frailty phenotype rose from 6.5% in those aged 60–69 to 65% in those over the age of 90, with frail individuals reporting decreased physical function and difficulties in performing activities of daily living [50].

3.3. Interventions for individuals living with sarcopenia and frailty

A multi-dimensional approach to managing sarcopenia and indeed frailty involves promoting physical activity, optimising nutrition/prevention of malnutrition, minimising polypharmacy and attending to and individual's social and psychological aspects of health, that is, care support and home adaptations. Management goals for an older person with sarcopenia or frailty revolve around improving physical function and maintaining independence and well-being.

Exercise and nutritional interventions that impact positively on muscle mass and function play a significant role in the management of sarcopenia. For example, combination physical activity and nutritional interventions are associated with better function, strength and less inflammation in older sarcopenic people [61, 62]. In terms of physical activity, progressive resistance and aerobic exercise have been shown to be the most beneficial for the prevention and 'treatment' of sarcopenia [23, 63–65]. Whilst progressive resistance exercise improves lean mass, strength and function [66], optimising exercise capacity through aerobic activity improves metabolic control, reduces oxidative stress, insulin sensitivity and can stimulate a hypertrophic response on muscle fibres. Despite being shown to be safe and effective in older people [63, 67, 68], implementing progressive exercise in clinical practice is not always readily achievable.

Falls are serious and sometimes fatal complications of sarcopenia. In this regard, a multi-component approach that addresses balance and gait, flexibility and endurance, lower limb strengthening exercises is required to manage fallers. Such approaches are associated with improved reaction time, gait, balance, strength coordination and physical and cognitive function [69, 70]. Group and home-based exercise programmes, which incorporate safety interventions, may reduce the rate and risk of falling [71]. Moreover, targeted home-based or group-based exercise interventions can also improve mobility and functional outcomes for older people with frailty [72, 73].

Intervening earlier in the life course before the onset of sarcopenia may have immense benefits for later skeletal muscle health. For example, increased levels of leisure time physical activity in mid-life were associated with stronger grip strength in both men and women at age 60–64. This is consistent with optimising peak strength earlier in the life course, therefore reducing the impact of sarcopenia. Therefore, regular physical activity in adolescence and adulthood may prevent steep decline in muscle strength in early old age [74].

The synthesis of muscle fibres requires adequate protein substrates. Physiological changes in the gastrointestinal system occur with age and result in older people eating less, having early satiety, losing their sense of taste and having a blunted anabolic response to ingested proteins [75]. As such, older people may require more protein to counteract the inflammatory and catabolic effects of co-existent co morbidities and their exacerbations [76]. Protein supplements vary in their composition and evidence from trials at present is inconstant to develop evidence-based recommendations for protein supplementation in sarcopenia [77]. However, observational evidence suggests essential amino acids, that is, leucine, beta-hydroxy-beta-methylbutyrate (HMB), a bioactive metabolite of leucine, stimulates muscle protein synthesis more than non-essential amino acids and may be useful for maintain lean body mass and improving muscle function [78–82]. A recent consensus statement from the multinational PROT-AGE group recommends protein intake in older people of at least 1.2–1.5 g of protein per body weight (kg) a day to maintain muscle homeostatsis [83]. Nutritional interventions in sarcopenia are covered in more detail elsewhere in this book.

3.4. Possible targets for pharmacological treatment

Observational studies indicate the potential beneficial effects of testosterone on muscle mass and function given the associated anabolic and satellite cell stimulatory activity. Randomised controlled trials of testosterone have not demonstrated benefits on muscle function because of adverse cardiovascular outcomes [34]. Studies of growth hormone (GH) supplementation have shown more harm than benefit in older patients; whilst GH therapy may increase muscle mass, it has not always increased muscle strength or functional performance. Moreover, unwanted side effects precludes GH as a treatment for sarcopenia. These include arthralgia, paraesthesia, fatigue, carpal tunnel syndrome and mortality in some observational human studies [84, 85].

There has been interest in selective androgen receptor modulators (SARMS) for sarcopenia treatment, which stems from the observed anabolic effect of testosterone. SARMS are androgen receptor ligands that display selective activation of androgen signalling in target tissues, for example, skeletal muscle. However, none are in clinical use and trials will be needed on the safety and efficacy of SARMS in improving physical function in older people with sarcopenia [34, 86].

Myostatin, a member of the TGF-β superfamily, is a negative regulator of skeletal muscle growth and is upregulated in many muscle wasting disorders [87]. Based on these observations, myostatin and its receptor activin type IIb pose attractive targets for therapeutic intervention. Though there are currently no anti-myostatin drugs used in clinical practice, myostatin receptor antibodies are currently under review with the focus on older people with lower lean mass [34].

Angiotensin-converting enzyme inhibitor (ACEi), for example, perindopril, use was associated with improvement in 6-m walk tests in older persons with functional impairment but did not show increased benefit with additional exercise training. Whilst ACEi use may have beneficial effects on muscle function [88], a recent meta-analysis of four trials concluded that ACEi did not improve walk distance or age-related strength decline in older people therefore, further evidence from clinical trials are needed [89].

3.5. Comprehensive Geriatric Assessment (CGA)

Frailty is a dynamic process that predisposes an individual to a spiral of decline that leads to increasing frailty and risk of worsening disability, predisposition to falls, hospital as well as care home admission and death [51, 58]. Although current screening for frailty identifies individuals at risk, validated tools do not recommend intervention. It is imperative that when managing frailty, assessments should not only seek to determine and treat specific illnesses, but that they should endeavour to maintain and where possible, improve quality of life. It is clear that older person's needs are more complex and that they often have co-existent functional, psychological and social needs. This predisposes an individual to atypical clinical presentations that can often be misunderstood and which often require a different approach to care that diverts away from an organ specific diagnosis towards a holistic and integrated view of their problems.

Older people and their caregivers should purposefully be involved in making informed decisions relating to health and social care needs as well as advanced care planning. A useful method for planning the care of those living with moderate to severe frailty through a process of assessment, summation, conversation, planning, intervention, monitoring and review is Comprehensive Geriatric Assessment (CGA). CGA is a process, which is patient centred, responsive, adaptable and most effective when disseminated amongst key professionals working across the acute and community sectors. CGA is defined as a *'multidimensional interdisciplinary diagnostic process focused on determining a frail older person's medical, psychological and functional capability in order to develop a coordinated and integrated plan for treatment and long term follow up'* [90].

The purpose of CGA is to improve diagnostic accuracy, optimise treatment and outcomes and crucially, allow effective integrated case management to ensure that the care plan is enacted and remains responsive to the patient's needs over time. CGA requires the systematic evaluation of physical, functional, medical, nutritional, cognitive and social components that influences an older person's health that can also extend to financial, spiritual, psychological and palliative needs (**Figure 4**). How CGA is delivered is variable and very much depends on the care setting, for example, home, hospital, clinic or nursing home but, to be effective, often requires coordination of several inter-professional services that can include clinicians, community nursing, therapy, social services, pharmacy, nutrition and dietetics, optometry and audiology. There are no set universal criteria to identify patients in need for a CGA however, patients who are 'too well' or are 'too sick' are less likely to derive benefit from the process. CGA becomes important for patients who are identified as living with frailty through the use of validated instruments or have one or more of the 'frailty syndromes' previously mentioned. There is evidence from multiple meta-analyses that CGA delivered to patients within the hospital setting as well as in the community is associated with better function and cognition, decrease in mortality, less likelihood of being institutionalised, less likelihood of patients experiencing deterioration in their health [90–93].

A critical component of CGA is a medication review and the STOPP/START approach to polypharmacy is a useful evidence-based tool [94]. The well-being components of the CGA may include the promotion of regular physical activity and exercise delivered through home-based plans [95] or external activity classes, social engagement through day centres and community networks, adaptations to the home environment to assist with falls prevention, caregiver support and nutritional optimisation. By undertaking a CGA with the person and those closest to them, if they wish, individuals are able to identify their own personal goals therefore reclaiming some of the lost independence they may have encountered as a result of living with frailty. Equally, the process will enable appropriate advanced care planning discussions for individuals with severe frailty in conjunction with palliative care support for those who may be entering the terminal phase of their life.

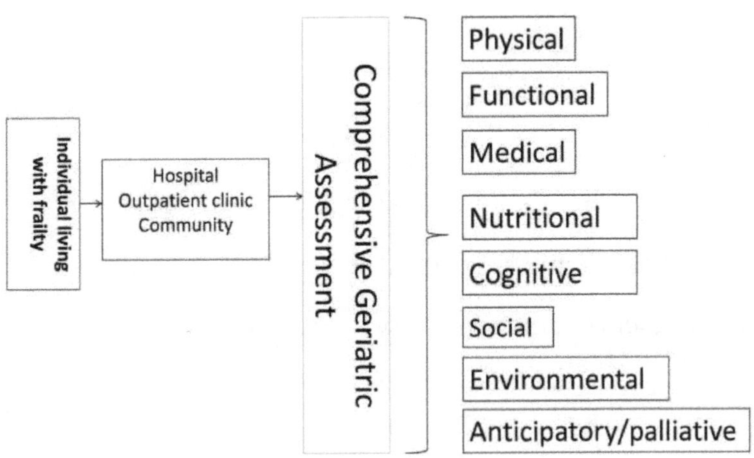

Figure 4. Core components of an inter-professional Comprehensive Geriatric Assessment. The process involves data gathering, multidisciplinary team discussions, development of the plan with the patient and their caregiver, implementation, monitoring and revision of the plan so that it remains responsive to the needs of the patient.

4. Conclusions

Sarcopenia and frailty are inter-related conditions that are common in older age and identify people who have an increased risk of a range of adverse outcomes. Sarcopenia has a complex aetiology involving neurohormonal, immunological and nutritional mechanisms. Frailty is a multisystem disorder, which commonly includes sarcopenia as a core component. Whilst there are clear physiological and pathophysiological explanations for the development and definition of frailty, there is need to understand that frailty as a term can be perceived as a state of dependency, subjugation or defeat; the appearance of being weak in later life. Not all older people are frail. These connotations and negative perceptions need to be challenged through education and training.

There is robust evidence to support the implementation of exercise and activity programmes for older people with sarcopenia and frailty, and that the adverse health trajectories of frailty may be modified through a range of interventions through the process of Comprehensive Geriatric Assessment. Better identification of sarcopenia and frailty in older age enables pro-active targeting of interventions to improve outcomes and modify future health trajectories that benefit older people as well as their caregivers.

Acknowledgements

This work was supported by the NIHR Southampton Biomedical Research Centre, Nutrition, the MRC Lifecourse Epidemiology Unit and the University of Southampton. This report is independent research by the NIHR BRC Funding Scheme. The views expressed in this publication are those of the authors and not necessarily those of the NHS, the NIHR or the Department of Health. HPP is supported by the NIHR Southampton Biomedical Research Centre Nutrition, EC and LL are supported by Health Education England Wessex Consultant Practitioner Trainee scheme. All authors declare they have no conflict of interest.

Author details

Harnish P Patel[1,2,3,4*], Esther Clift[5], Lucy Lewis[5] and Cyrus Cooper[4,6]

*Address all correspondence to: hp@mrc.soton.ac.uk

1 Academic Geriatric Medicine, University Hospital Southampton, UK

2 Department of Medicine for Older People, University Hospital Southampton, UK

3 NIHR Biomedical Research Centre, Southampton, UK

4 MRC Lifecourse Epidemiology Unit, University of Southampton, Southampton, UK

5 Health Education England, Wessex, UK

6 University of Oxford, Oxford, UK

References

[1] Chatterji S, Byles J, Cutler D, Seeman T, Verdes E. Health, functioning, and disability in older adults—present status and future implications. Lancet. 2015;**385**(9967):563-575. DOI: 10.1016/s0140-6736(14)61462-8

[2] World population ageing. United Nations, Department of Economic and Social Affairs, Population Division; 2015. World Population Ageing, United Nations (ST/ESA/SER.A/390)

[3] Willcox DC, Willcox BJ, Poon LW. Centenarian studies: Important contributors to our understanding of the aging process and longevity. Current Gerontology and Geriatrics Research. 2010;**2010**:484529. DOI: 10.1155/2010/484529

[4] Clegg A, Young J, Iliffe S, Rikkert MO, Rockwood K. Frailty in elderly people. Lancet. 2013;**381**(9868):752-762. DOI: 10.1016/s0140-6736(12)62167-9

[5] Turner G, Clegg A. Best practice guidelines for the management of frailty: A British Geriatrics Society, Age UK and Royal College of General Practitioners report. Age and Ageing. 2014;**43**(6):744-747. DOI: 10.1093/ageing/afu138

[6] Cruz-Jentoft AJ, Baeyens JP, Bauer JM, Boirie Y, Cederholm T, Landi F et al. Sarcopenia: European consensus on definition and diagnosis: Report of the European Working Group on Sarcopenia in Older People. Age and Ageing. 2010;**39**(4):412-423

[7] Sender R, Fuchs S, Milo R. Revised estimates for the number of human and bacteria cells in the body. PLoS Biology. 2016;**14**(8):e1002533. DOI: 10.1371/journal.pbio.1002533

[8] Delmonico MJ, Harris TB, Lee JS, Visser M, Nevitt M, Kritchevsky SB et al. Alternative definitions of sarcopenia, lower extremity performance, and functional impairment with aging in older men and women. Journal of the American Geriatrics Society. 2007;**55**(5):769-774. DOI: 10.1111/j.1532-5415.2007.01140.x

[9] Kallman DA, Plato CC, Tobin JD. The role of muscle loss in the age-related decline of grip strength: Cross-sectional and longitudinal perspectives. Journal of Gerontology. 1990;**45**(3):M82-M88

[10] Newman A B, et al. Strength, but not muscle mass is associated with mortality in the health aging and body composition study cohort. Journal of Gerontology: Medical Science. 2006;**61A**(1):72-77

[11] Studenski SA, Peters KW, Alley DE, Cawthon PM, McLean RR, Harris TB et al. The FNIH sarcopenia project: Rationale, study description, conference recommendations, and final estimates. The Journals of Gerontology. Series A, Biological Sciences and Medical Sciences. 2014;**69**(5):547-558. DOI: 10.1093/gerona/glu010

[12] Sayer AA, Robinson SM, Patel HP, Shavlakadze T, Cooper C, Grounds MD. New horizons in the pathogenesis, diagnosis and management of sarcopenia. Age and Ageing. 2013;**42**

[13] Landi F, Liperoti R, Russo A, Giovannini S, Tosato M, Capoluongo E et al. Sarcopenia as a risk factor for falls in elderly individuals: Results from the ilSIRENTE study. Clinical nutrition (Edinburgh, Scotland). 2012;**31**(5):652-658. DOI: 10.1016/j.clnu.2012.02.007

[14] Sayer AA, Dennison EM, Syddall HE, Gilbody HJ, Phillips DI, Cooper C. Type 2 diabetes, muscle strength, and impaired physical function: The tip of the iceberg? Diabetes Care. 2005;**28**(10):2541-2542

[15] Di Monaco M, Vallero F, Di Monaco R, Tappero R. Prevalence of sarcopenia and its association with osteoporosis in 313 older women following a hip fracture. Archives of Gerontology and Geriatrics. 2011;**52**(1):71-74

[16] Cooper R, Kuh D, Hardy R. Objectively measured physical capability levels and mortality: Systematic review and meta-analysis. BMJ. 2010;**341**:c4467. DOI: 10.1136/bmj.c4467

[17] Janssen I, Shepard DS, Katzmarzyk PT, Roubenoff R. The healthcare costs of sarcopenia in the United States. Journal of the American Geriatrics Society. 2004;**52**(1):80-85

[18] Fielding RA, Vellas B, Evans WJ, Bhasin S, Morley JE, Newman AB et al. Sarcopenia: An undiagnosed condition in older adults. Current consensus definition: prevalence, etiology, and consequences. International working group on sarcopenia. Journal of the American Medical Directors Association. 2011;**12**(4):249-256. DOI: 10.1016/j.jamda.2011.01.003

[19] Chen LK, Liu LK, Woo J, Assantachai P, Auyeung TW, Bahyah KS et al. Sarcopenia in Asia: Consensus report of the Asian Working Group for Sarcopenia. Journal of the American Medical Directors Association. 2014;**15**(2):95-101. DOI: 10.1016/j.jamda.2013.11.025

[20] Abellan van Kan G, Rolland Y, Andrieu S, Bauer J, Beauchet O, Bonnefoy M et al. Gait speed at usual pace as a predictor of adverse outcomes in community-dwelling older people an International Academy on Nutrition and Aging (IANA) Task Force. The Journal of Nutrition, Health & Aging. 2009;**13**(10):881-889

[21] Lauretani F, Russo CR, Bandinelli S, Bartali B, Cavazzini C, Di Iorio A et al. Age-associated changes in skeletal muscles and their effect on mobility: An operational diagnosis of sarcopenia. Journal of Applied Physiology. 2003;**95**(5):1851-1860

[22] Patel HP, Syddall HE, Jameson K, Robinson S, Denison H, Roberts HC et al. Prevalence of sarcopenia in community-dwelling older people in the UK using the European Working Group on Sarcopenia in Older People (EWGSOP) definition: Findings from the Hertfordshire Cohort Study (HCS). Age and Ageing. 2013;**42**. Epub ahead of print

[23] Cruz-Jentoft AJ, Landi F, Schneider SM, Zuniga C, Arai H, Boirie Y et al. Prevalence of and interventions for sarcopenia in ageing adults: A systematic review. Report of the International Sarcopenia Initiative (EWGSOP and IWGS). Age and Ageing. 2014;**43**(6):748-759. DOI: 10.1093/ageing/afu115

[24] Cooper C, Dere W, Evans W, Kanis JA, Rizzoli R, Sayer AA et al. Frailty and sarcopenia: definitions and outcome parameters. Osteoporosis International: A Journal Established

As Result of Cooperation Between the European Foundation for Osteoporosis and the National Osteoporosis Foundation of the USA. 2012;**23**(7):1839-1848. DOI: 10.1007/s00198-012-1913-1

[25] Roberts HC, Denison HJ, Martin HJ, Patel HP, Syddall H, Cooper C et al. A review of the measurement of grip strength in clinical and epidemiological studies: Towards a standardised approach. Age and Ageing. 2011;**40**(4):423-429

[26] Roberts HC, Syddall HE, Cooper C, Aihie Sayer A. Is grip strength associated with length of stay in hospitalised older patients admitted for rehabilitation? Findings from the Southampton grip strength study. Age and Ageing. 2012;**41**(5):641-646. DOI: 10.1093/ageing/afs089

[27] Sayer AA, Kirkwood TB. Grip strength and mortality: A biomarker of ageing? Lancet. 2015;**386**(9990):226-227. DOI: 10.1016/s0140-6736(14)62349-7

[28] Vermeulen J, Neyens JC, van Rossum E, Spreeuwenberg MD, de Witte LP. Predicting ADL disability in community-dwelling elderly people using physical frailty indicators: A systematic review. BMC Geriatrics. 2011;**11**:33. DOI: 10.1186/1471-2318-11-33

[29] Mijnarends DM, Meijers JM, Halfens RJ, ter Borg S, Luiking YC, Verlaan S et al. Validity and reliability of tools to measure muscle mass, strength, and physical performance in community-dwelling older people: A systematic review. Journal of the American Medical Directors Association. 2013;**14**(3):170-178. DOI: 10.1016/j.jamda.2012.10.009

[30] Dodds RM, Syddall HE, Cooper R, Benzeval M, Deary IJ, Dennison EM. Grip strength across the life course: Normative data from twelve British studies. PloS One. 2014;**9**. DOI: 10.1371/journal.pone.0113637

[31] Malmstrom TK, Morley JE. SARC-F: A simple questionnaire to rapidly diagnose sarcopenia. Journal of the American Medical Directors Association. 2013;**14**(8):531-532. DOI: 10.1016/j.jamda.2013.05.018

[32] Cao L, Chen S, Zou C, Ding X, Gao L, Liao Z et al. A pilot study of the SARC-F scale on screening sarcopenia and physical disability in the Chinese older people. The Journal of Nutrition, Health & Aging. 2014;**18**(3):277-283. DOI: 10.1007/s12603-013-0410-3

[33] Woo J, Leung J, Morley JE. Validating the SARC-F: A suitable community screening tool for sarcopenia? Journal of the American Medical Directors Association. 2014;**15**(9):630-634. DOI: 10.1016/j.jamda.2014.04.021

[34] Cesari M, Fielding R, Benichou O, Bernabei R, Bhasin S, Guralnik JM et al. Pharmacological interventions in frailty and sarcopenia: Report by the international conference on frailty and sarcopenia research task force. The Journal of Frailty & Aging. 2015;**4**(3):114-120. DOI: 10.14283/jfa.2015.64

[35] Zammit PS, Partridge TA, Yablonka-Reuveni Z. The skeletal muscle satellite cell: The stem cell that came in from the cold. Journal of Histochemistry and Cytochemistry. 2006;**54**(11):1177-1191

[36] Patel HP, White MC, Westbury L, Syddall HE, Stephens PJ, Clough GF et al. Skeletal muscle morphology in sarcopenia defined using the EWGSOP criteria: Findings from the Hertfordshire Sarcopenia Study (HSS). BMC Geriatrics. 2015;**15**:171. DOI: 10.1186/s12877-015-0171-4

[37] Evans WJ, Paolisso G, Abbatecola AM, Corsonello A, Bustacchini S, Strollo F et al. Frailty and muscle metabolism dysregulation in the elderly. Biogerontology. 2010;**11**(5):527-536. DOI: 10.1007/s10522-010-9297-0

[38] Arthur PG, Grounds MD, Shavlakadze T. Oxidative stress as a therapeutic target during muscle wasting: Considering the complex interactions. Current Opinion in Clinical Nutrition and Metabolic Care. 2008;**11**(4):408-416. DOI: 10.1097/MCO.0b013e328302f3fe

[39] Morley JE. Pharmacologic options for the treatment of sarcopenia. Calcif Tissue Int. 2016 Apr;**98**(4):319-33. DOI: 10.1007/s00223-015-0022-5. Epub 2015 Jun 23

[40] Goodman CA, Mayhew DL, Hornberger TA. Recent progress toward understanding the molecular mechanisms that regulate skeletal muscle mass. Cell Signal. 2011;**23**

[41] Verdijk LB, Koopman R, Schaart G, Meijer K, Savelberg HH, van Loon LJ. Satellite cell content is specifically reduced in type II skeletal muscle fibers in the elderly. American Journal of Physiology Endocrinology and Metabolism. 2007;**292**(1):E151-E157. DOI: 10.1152/ajpendo.00278.2006

[42] Maltin CA, Delday MI, Sinclair KD, Steven J, Sneddon AA. Impact of manipulations of myogenesis in utero on the performance of adult skeletal muscle. Reproduction. 2001;**122**(3):359-374

[43] Janssen I. The epidemiology of sarcopenia. Clinics in Geriatric Medicine. 2011;**27**(3):355-363. DOI: 10.1016/j.cger.2011.03.004

[44] Samson MM, Meeuwsen IB, Crowe A, Dessens JA, Duursma SA, Verhaar HJ. Relationships between physical performance measures, age, height and body weight in healthy adults. Age and Ageing. 2000;**29**(3):235-242

[45] Janssen I, Heymsfield SB, Wang ZM, Ross R. Skeletal muscle mass and distribution in 468 men and women aged 18-88 yr. Journal of Applied Physiology. 2000;**89**(1):81-88

[46] Patel HP, Jameson KA, Syddall HE, Martin HJ, Stewart CE, Cooper C et al. Developmental influences, muscle morphology, and sarcopenia in community-dwelling older men. The Journal of Gerontology. Series A, Biological Science and Medical Science. 2012;**67**(1):82-87

[47] Dodds R, Denison HJ, Ntani G, Cooper R, Cooper C, Sayer AA et al. Birth weight and muscle strength: A systematic review and meta-analysis. The Journal of Nutrition, Health & Aging. 2012;**16**(7):609-615

[48] Harttgen K, Kowal P, Strulik H, Chatterji S, Vollmer S. Patterns of frailty in older adults: Comparing results from higher and lower income countries using the Survey of Health, Ageing and Retirement in Europe (SHARE) and the Study on Global AGEing and Adult Health (SAGE). PloS One. 2013;**8**(10):e75847. DOI: 10.1371/journal.pone.0075847

[49] Collard RM, Boter H, Schoevers RA, Oude Voshaar RC. Prevalence of frailty in community-dwelling older persons: A systematic review. Journal of the American Geriatrics Society. 2012;**60**(8):1487-1492. DOI: 10.1111/j.1532-5415.2012.04054.x

[50] Gale CR, Cooper C, Sayer AA. Prevalence of frailty and disability: Findings from the English Longitudinal Study of Ageing. Age and Ageing. 2015;**44**(1):162-165. DOI: 10.1093/ageing/afu148

[51] Fried LP, Tangen CM, Walston J, Newman AB, Hirsch C, Gottdiener J et al. Frailty in older adults: Evidence for a phenotype. The Journal of Gerontology. Series A, Biological Science and Medical Science. 2001;**56**(3):M146-M156

[52] Gill TM, Gahbauer EA, Han L, Allore HG. The relationship between intervening hospitalizations and transitions between frailty states. The Journals of Gerontology. Series A, Biological Sciences and Medical Sciences 2011;**66**(11):1238-1243. DOI: 10.1093/gerona/glr142

[53] Kelaiditi E, Cesari M, Canevelli M, van Kan GA, Ousset PJ, Gillette-Guyonnet S et al. Cognitive frailty: Rational and definition from an (I.A.N.A./I.A.G.G.) international consensus group. The Journal of Nutrition, Health & Aging. 2013;**17**(9):726-734. DOI: 10.1007/s12603-013-0367-2

[54] Gobbens RJ, van Assen MA, Luijkx KG, Schols JM. The predictive validity of the Tilburg Frailty Indicator: Disability, health care utilization, and quality of life in a population at risk. The Gerontologist. 2012;**52**(5):619-631. DOI: 10.1093/geront/gnr135

[55] Farmer C, Fenu E, O'Flynn N, Guthrie B. Clinical assessment and management of multimorbidity: Summary of NICE guidance. BMJ. 2016;**354**:i4843. DOI: 10.1136/bmj.i4843

[56] Gill TM, Gahbauer EA, Allore HG, Ham L. Transitions between frailty states among community-living older persons. Archives of Internal Medicine. 2006;**166**. DOI: 10.1001/archinte.166.4.418

[57] Xue QL, Bandeen-Roche K, Varadhan R, Zhou J, Fried LP. Initial manifestations of frailty criteria and the development of frailty phenotype in the Women's Health and Aging Study II. Journal of Gerontology Series A, Biological Science and Medical Science. 2008;**63**(9):984-990. DOI: 63/9/984 [pii]

[58] Rockwood K, Song X, MacKnight C, Bergman H, Hogan DB, McDowell I et al. A global clinical measure of fitness and frailty in elderly people. CMAJ: Canadian Medical Association Journal = Journal de l'Association Medicale Canadienne. 2005;**173**(5):489-495. DOI: 10.1503/cmaj.050051

[59] Rockwood K, Mitnitski A. Limits to deficit accumulation in elderly people. Mechanisms of Ageing and Development. 2006;**127**. DOI: 10.1016/j.mad.2006.01.002

[60] Rockwood K, Andrew M, Mitnitski A. A comparison of two approaches to measuring frailty in elderly people. The Journals of Gerontology. Series A, Biological Sciences and Medical Sciences 2007;**62**(7):738-743

[61] Rondanelli M, Klersy C, Terracol G, Talluri J, Maugeri R, Guido D et al. Whey protein, amino acids, and vitamin D supplementation with physical activity increases fat-free mass and strength, functionality, and quality of life and decreases inflammation in sarcopenic elderly. The American Journal of Clinical Nutrition. 2016;**103**(3):830-840. DOI: 10.3945/ajcn.115.113357

[62] Churchward-Venne TA, Murphy CH, Longland TM, Phillips SM. Role of protein and amino acids in promoting lean mass accretion with resistance exercise and attenuating lean mass loss during energy deficit in humans. Amino Acids. 2013;**45**(2):231-240. DOI: 10.1007/s00726-013-1506-0

[63] Liu CJ, Latham NK. Progressive resistance strength training for improving physical function in older adults. The Cochrane Database Syst Rev. 2009 Jul **8**;(3):CD002759. DOI: 10.1002/14651858.CD002759.pub2

[64] Pahor M, Guralnik JM, Ambrosius WT, Blair S, Bonds DE, Church TS et al. Effect of structured physical activity on prevention of major mobility disability in older adults: The LIFE study randomized clinical trial. JAMA. 2014;**311**(23):2387-2396. DOI: 10.1001/jama.2014.5616

[65] Valenzuela T. Efficacy of progressive resistance training interventions in older adults in nursing homes: A systematic review. Journal of the American Medical Directors Association. 2012;**13**(5):418-428. DOI: 10.1016/j.jamda.2011.11.001

[66] Peterson MD, Sen A, Gordon PM. Influence of resistance exercise on lean body mass in aging adults: A meta-analysis. Medicine and Science in Sports and Exercise. 2011;**43**(2):249-258. DOI: 10.1249/MSS.0b013e3181eb6265

[67] Fiatarone MA, O'Neill EF, Ryan ND, Clements KM, Solares GR, Nelson ME et al. Exercise training and nutritional supplementation for physical frailty in very elderly people. The New England Journal of Medicine. 1994;**330**(25):1769-1775

[68] Vincent KR, Braith RW, Feldman RA, Magyari PM, Cutler RB, Persin SA et al. Resistance exercise and physical performance in adults aged 60 to 83. Journal of the American Geriatrics Society. 2002;**50**(6):1100-1107

[69] El-Khoury F, Cassou B, Charles MA, Dargent-Molina P. The effect of fall prevention exercise programmes on fall induced injuries in community dwelling older adults: Systematic review and meta-analysis of randomised controlled trials. BMJ 2013;**347**:f6234. DOI: 10.1136/bmj.f6234

[70] Stubbs B, Brefka S, Denkinger MD. What works to prevent falls in community-dwelling older adults? Umbrella review of meta-analyses of randomized controlled trials. Physical Therapy. 2015;**95**(8):1095-1110. DOI: 10.2522/ptj.20140461

[71] Robertson MC, Gillespie LD. Fall prevention in community-dwelling older adults. JAMA. 2013;**309**(13):1406-1407. DOI: 10.1001/jama.2013.3130

[72] Clegg A, Barber S, Young J, Forster A, Iliffe S. Do home-based exercise interventions improve outcomes for frail older people? Findings from a systematic review. Reviews in Clinical Gerontology. 2012;**22**(1):68-78

[73] Theou O, Stathokostas L, Roland KP, Jakobi JM, Patterson C, Vandervoort AA et al. The effectiveness of exercise interventions for the management of frailty: A systematic review. Journal of Aging Research. 2011;**2011**:569194. DOI: 10.4061/2011/569194

[74] Dodds R, Kuh D, Aihie Sayer A, Cooper R. Physical activity levels across adult life and grip strength in early old age: Updating findings from a British birth cohort. Age and Ageing. 2013;**42**(6):794-798. DOI: 10.1093/ageing/aft124

[75] Robinson S, Cooper C, Aihie SA. Nutrition and sarcopenia: A review of the evidence and implications for preventive strategies. Journal of Aging Research. 2012;**2012**:510801. Epub;%2012 Mar 15.:510801

[76] Wandrag L, Brett SJ, Frost G, Hickson M. Impact of supplementation with amino acids or their metabolites on muscle wasting in patients with critical illness or other muscle wasting illness: a systematic review. Journal of Human Nutrition and Dietetics: The Official Journal of the British Dietetic Association. 2015;**28**(4):313-330. DOI: 10.1111/jhn.12238

[77] Hickson M. Nutritional interventions in sarcopenia: A critical review. The Proceedings of the Nutrition Society. 2015;**74**(4):378-386. DOI: 10.1017/s0029665115002049

[78] Deutz NE, Pereira SL, Hays NP, Oliver JS, Edens NK, Evans CM et al. Effect of beta-hydroxy-beta-methylbutyrate (HMB) on lean body mass during 10 days of bed rest in older adults. Clinical Nutrition (Edinburgh, Scotland). 2013;**32**(5):704-712. DOI: 10.1016/j.clnu.2013.02.011

[79] Paddon-Jones D, Sheffield-Moore M, Zhang XJ, Volpi E, Wolf SE, Aarsland A et al. Amino acid ingestion improves muscle protein synthesis in the young and elderly. American Journal of Physiology Endocrinology and Metabolism. 2004;**286**(3):E321-E328

[80] Wu H, Xia Y, Jiang J, Du H, Guo X, Liu X et al. Effect of beta-hydroxy-beta-methylbutyrate supplementation on muscle loss in older adults: A systematic review and meta-analysis. Archives of Gerontology and Geriatrics. 2015;**61**(2):168-175. DOI: 10.1016/j.archger.2015.06.020

[81] Flakoll P, Sharp R, Baier S, Levenhagen D, Carr C, Nissen S. Effect of beta-hydroxy-beta-methylbutyrate, arginine, and lysine supplementation on strength, functionality, body composition, and protein metabolism in elderly women. Nutrition. 2004;**20**(5):445-451. DOI: 10.1016/j.nut.2004.01.009

[82] Stout JR, Smith-Ryan AE, Fukuda DH, Kendall KL, Moon JR, Hoffman JR et al. Effect of calcium beta-hydroxy-beta-methylbutyrate (CaHMB) with and without resistance training in men and women 65+yrs: A randomized, double-blind pilot trial. Experimental Gerontology. 2013;**48**(11):1303-1310. DOI: 10.1016/j.exger.2013.08.007

[83] Bauer J, Biolo G, Cederholm T, Cesari M, Cruz-Jentoft AJ, Morley JE et al. Evidence-based recommendations for optimal dietary protein intake in older people: A position paper from the PROT-AGE Study Group. Journal of the American Medical Directors Association. 2013;**14**(8):542-559. DOI: 10.1016/j.jamda.2013.05.021

[84] Ali S, Garcia JM. Sarcopenia, cachexia and aging: Diagnosis, mechanisms and therapeutic options - a mini-review. Gerontology. 2014;**60**(4):294-305. DOI: 10.1159/000356760

[85] Giannoulis MG, Martin FC, Nair KS, Umpleby AM, Sonksen P. Hormone replacement therapy and physical function in healthy older men. Time to talk hormones? Endocrine Reviews. 2012;**33**(3):314-377. DOI: 10.1210/er.2012-1002

[86] Cohen S, Nathan JA, Goldberg AL. Muscle wasting in disease: Molecular mechanisms and promising therapies. Nature Reviews Drug Discovery. 2015;**14**(1):58-74. DOI: 10.1038/nrd4467

[87] Huang Z, Chen X, Chen D. Myostatin: A novel insight into its role in metabolism, signal pathways, and expression regulation. Cellular Signalling. 2011;**23**(9):1441-1446. DOI: 10.1016/j.cellsig.2011.05.003

[88] Sumukadas D, Witham MD, Struthers AD, McMurdo ME. Ace inhibitors as a therapy for sarcopenia—Evidence and possible mechanisms. The Journal of Nutrition, Health and Aging. 2008;**12**(7):480-485

[89] Zhou LS, Xu LJ, Wang XQ, Huang YH, Xiao Q. Effect of angiotensin-converting enzyme inhibitors on physical function in elderly subjects: A systematic review and meta-analysis. Drugs & Aging. 2015;**32**(9):727-735. DOI: 10.1007/s40266-015-0288-3

[90] Ellis G, Whitehead MA, O'Neill D, Langhorne P, Robinson D. Comprehensive geriatric assessment for older adults admitted to hospital. The Cochrane Database Syst Rev. 2011 Jul **6**;(7):CD006211. DOI: 10.1002/14651858.CD006211.pub2

[91] Stuck AE, Egger M, Hammer A, Minder CE, Beck JC. Home visits to prevent nursing home admission and functional decline in elderly people: Systematic review and meta-regression analysis. JAMA. 2002;**287**(8):1022-1028

[92] Cameron ID, Fairhall N, Langron C, Lockwood K, Monaghan N, Aggar C et al. A multifactorial interdisciplinary intervention reduces frailty in older people: Randomized trial. BMC Medicine. 2013;**11**:65. DOI: 10.1186/1741-7015-11-65

[93] Huss A, Stuck AE, Rubenstein LZ, Egger M, Clough-Gorr KM. Multidimensional preventive home visit programs for community-dwelling older adults: A systematic review and meta-analysis of randomized controlled trials. The Journals of Gerontology. Series A, Biological Sciences and Medical Sciences 2008;**63**(3):298-307

[94] O'Mahony D, O'Sullivan D, Byrne S, O'Connor MN, Ryan C, Gallagher P. STOPP/START criteria for potentially inappropriate prescribing in older people: Version 2. Age and Ageing. 2015;**44**(2):213-218. DOI: 10.1093/ageing/afu145

[95] Clegg A, Barber S, Young J, Iliffe S, Forster A. The Home-based Older People's Exercise (HOPE) trial: A pilot randomised controlled trial of a home-based exercise intervention for older people with frailty. Age and Ageing. 2014;**43**(5):687-695. DOI: 10.1093/ageing/afu033

2

Sarcopenia in the Context of Skeletal Muscle Function Deficit (SMFD)[1]

Rosaly Correa-de-Araujo

Abstract

Evidence shows that not only changes in skeletal muscle mass but changes in strength and other factors underpinning muscle quality play a role in muscle function decline and impaired mobility associated with aging. Changes in both strength and quality may precede loss of muscle mass. Skeletal muscle function deficit (SMFD) is a terminology that embraces this evolving conceptualization of sarcopenia and age-related muscle dysfunctions. This chapter provides a discussion on sarcopenia in the context of SMFD, including operational definitions and methodological challenges associated with their establishment; integration of muscle quality into SMFD; efforts to identify diagnostic cutoff values for low muscle mass and weakness and their predictive validity to mobility disability; need for standardized muscle quality assessment; clinical and public health relevance and research opportunities. Changes in muscle composition, based on excessive levels of inter- and intramuscular or intramyocellular fat are striking features increasingly addressed in the literature, found to affect muscle metabolism and peak force generation. Methods to easily and rapidly assess muscle composition in multiple clinical settings and with minimal patient burden are needed. Further characterization of SMFD should emphasize integration of muscle quality and factors behind changes in quality, as well as associated clinical and research implications.

Keywords: skeletal muscle function deficit, sarcopenia, reduced muscle mass, low muscle mass, low muscle strength, muscle quality, biomarkers, outcomes

[1]The views expressed in this chapter are those of the author and do not necessarily represent the views of the National Institute of Health, National Institute on Aging, the U.S. Department of Health and Human Services (HHS), or the U.S. Federal Government.

1. Introduction

Numerous efforts around the definition of sarcopenia and its better characterization through biomarkers including cutoff values for muscle mass, muscle strength (weakness), and performance measures, as well as the identification of outcomes of clinical and investigational significance have evolved in the past many years and continue to be heavily investigated. Since 1989, when sarcopenia was first defined as an age-related reduction in muscle mass [1] and the association of low muscle mass and functional impairment was demonstrated [2], scientific and technological advances have helped us improve our understanding of the mechanisms underlying age-related alterations in muscle mass, muscle strength, and muscle quality. Substantial attention has also been given to investigate the relationships of these alterations to mobility impairment, disability, fatigue, risk of metabolic disorders, falls, and mortality in older adults [3]. This ongoing work responds to the need to identify preventive and therapeutic interventions that can delay, improve, revert, or eliminate the changes in muscle mass, strength, and quality. The scientific community, including regulatory scientists, and practicing health care professionals recognize that "a more specific definition of sarcopenia may not only be necessary to align it with new scientific advances, but it is highly desirable on practical grounds because specific criteria are critical for identifying candidate patients for clinical trials that test therapies aimed at reversing or alleviating the complications of sarcopenia and its associated manifestations [4]."

It is estimated that by 2050, 2 billion people worldwide will be age ≥65 years. Preserving mobility and quality of life into old age will be a challenge because impaired mobility is often a precursor of functional decline, disability, and loss of independence. Evidence now shows that not only changes in muscle mass, but other factors underpinning muscle quality also play a role in the decline in muscle function and impaired mobility associated with aging. Changes in muscle quality may precede loss of muscle mass. This provides new opportunities for the assessment of muscle mass, strength, and quality particularly to detect who could benefit from interventions to prevent decline or improve muscle function [5].

The purpose of this chapter is to provide basic science, clinical researchers and expert clinicians with a review of the literature on key efforts to establish clinically meaningful diagnostic cutoff values for low muscle mass and low muscle strength, integrate muscle quality into these efforts, discuss the clinical and public health relevance, and highlight research opportunities for sarcopenia in the context of skeletal muscle function deficit. The new terminology "skeletal muscle function deficit" was coined in 2014 to embrace the evolving concepts of sarcopenia and other aging-related muscle dysfunctions that contribute to clinically meaningful mobility impairments [6].

1.1. Terminology and nosology issues: sarcopenia in the context of skeletal muscle function deficit

Sarcopenia is a condition with a complex multifactorial etiology, which is summarized in **Table 1** [7]. Age-related decreases in muscle performance associated with physical impairment are only partially explained by reduction in muscle mass, with many other pathophysiologic factors contributing to age-related impairments in muscle performance. Based on these facts, decreases in muscle performance and in muscle mass require independent evaluation. The importance of assessing muscle quality, currently defined as strength per unit of appendicular skeletal muscle mass, also continues to be highly emphasized.

Although consensus groups noted below have incorporated the criterion of impaired physical and/or muscle performance into their recommended definitions of sarcopenia, they have not addressed the issue of specific diagnostic terminologies. The lack of sufficient specificity resulting from the use of "sarcopenia," an anatomic term currently used to define a functional condition with which it is imperfectly correlated, and for which nonanatomic contributory factors have been identified, generates confusion. Some of this confusion originates from the fact that reduced muscle mass *per se* is a feature of several other conditions in both older and younger people. Adopting a nosology that accommodates the literal concept of sarcopenia—reduced muscle mass—while applying other diagnostic terms for other age-related muscular conditions that contribute to impaired physical performance seems to hold a valuable clinical approach. "Skeletal muscle function deficit" (SMFD) fits this purpose well. The term indicates a shortfall in function that can evolve to more significant impairment and mobility-disability. The diagnostic criteria for "SMFD" can, then, include: (A) Measures of muscle performance and strength that provide effective cutoff values for identifying those whose mobility disability is related to impairments. Muscle performance is the capacity of a muscle or a group of muscles to generate forces to produce, maintain, sustain, and modify postures and movements that are required for functional activity. Strength is the muscle force exerted to overcome resistance under a specific set of circumstances. Power is the work produced per unit of time or the product of strength and speed. (B) Measures of muscle mass (e.g., "sarcopenic SMFD"), and (C) Measures of muscle quality. Factors impacting muscle quality can be described using measures of muscle composition or myosteatosis (fat infiltration of muscles) as these are very relevant to mobility outcomes and to the identification of effective preventative and therapeutic interventions in older adults. Muscle quality is also largely impacted by intricate intramuscular ultrastructure and morphology of contractile tissue, as well as the relationship between structure and function [6, 8].

A variety of known and putative muscular pathologies can be evaluated as their contribution to SMFD, including newly identified contributory pathologies. This approach also specifies other already recognized conditions that can lead to "SMFD" (e.g., diabetic polyneuropathy or secondary malnutrition), which can be distinguished from age-related conditions contributing to "SMFD" with etiology not yet well established. Further, it accommodates future knowledge in diagnostic specificity based on improved understanding of the mechanisms of aging and disease. Specific neurogenic factors, intrinsic muscle factors, or systemic factors may lead to the characterization of specific subtypes of age-related sarcopenia, to methods for diagnosing them, and to the identification of new therapeutic targets. In sum, the broad concept of "SMFD" comprising a variety of contributory etiologies provides a framework for developing diagnostic categories that are useful for both clinical practice and research. This approach has been successfully implemented with conditions that are clinically manifested as impaired physiologic functions (e.g., congestive heart failure, chronic obstructive pulmonary disease) and have multiple contributory factors [6].

Age-related

- Reduced physical activity
- Mitochondrial dysfunction
- Anorexia of aging
- Apoptosis
- Hormones
- Low levels of testosterone
- Low levels of growth hormone
- Low levels of insulin-like growth factor (IGF)-1
- Elevated levels of cortisol
- Low levels of vitamin D

Proinflammatory cytokines

- Interleukin-1
- Interleukin-6
- Tumor necrosis factor (TNF)-alpha
- Neuronal
- Loss of motor endplates
- Peripheral neuropathy

Vascular

- Peripheral vascular disease
- Reduced capillary function

Weight loss

- Dieting
- Malabsorption
- Disease-related

Hormones

- Low levels of testosterone
- Low levels of growth hormone
- Low levels of insulin-like growth factor (IGF)-1
- Elevated levels of cortisol
- Low levels of vitamin D

Neuronal

- Loss of motor endplates
- Peripheral neuropathy

Table 1. Multifactorial etiology for sarcopenia [7].

2. Operational definitions for sarcopenia

Several operational definitions have emphasized that sarcopenia should now be defined as a loss of muscle function associated with a loss of muscle mass [9–18]. This change in definition from the original meaning of sarcopenia [1] is justified by some experts as necessary due to current knowledge that muscle quality and muscle performance do not directly relate to muscle mass [19, 20]. Two very important factors are thought to be responsible for this knowledge: the compromise of neuromuscular junctions in sarcopenia and the myosteatosis accompanying the aging process [21–24]. Below is a brief description of these operational definitions published by key consensus groups. It should be highlighted that a quantitative definition of sarcopenia that characterizes this condition in terms of rationally-defined cutoff values for lean body mass and muscle strength is comparable to the evolution of the operational definition of osteoporosis in terms of bone mineral density to detect individuals at increased risk for fractures. Efforts to identify an operational definition for sarcopenia include those:

- Based on muscle mass in relationship to the range of muscle mass within a reference population;
- Essentially based on expert opinion, but considering muscle mass and performance criteria;
- Essentially based on expert opinion, but considering muscle mass, muscle strength and physical performance; and
- Evidence-based, data-driven, considering muscle mass, muscle strength, and their predictive validity to mobility disability.

Table 2 summarizes in a comparative way, the currently available operational definitions for sarcopenia. While they might involve similar criteria, marked variations in cutoff values exist as alluded below.

Working group/target population	**Screening**	**Operational definition**	
		Muscle mass	**Muscle strength/ function**
EWGSOP – European Working Group on Sarcopenia in Older People [9]*All person ≥ 65 years*	Gait speed. If gait speed is ≤0.8 m/s, proceed to body composition evaluation. If gait speed >0.8 m/s, measure hand grip strength; if low muscle strength (weakness) is detected, proceed to body composition evaluation	Low muscle mass in patients with gait speed ≤0.8 m/s or normal gait speed but low muscle strength.DXA ASM/height^2 ≤7.23 kg/m^2 for men; ≤5.67 kg/m^2 for women	Low grip strength <30 kg for men; <20 kg for womenorgait speed <0.8 m/s
IWGS/IANA - International Working Group on Sarcopenia Task Force/ International Academy on Nutrition and Aging [11] *Persons with clinical declines in physical function, strength, or health status*	Physical function (4-m gait speed). If gait speed < 1.0 m/s, proceed to body composition evaluation	Low appendicular lean mass/height^2 (assessed by DXA):≤7.23 kg/m^2 for men; ≤5.67 kg/m^2 for women	Poor functioning, gait speed

Working group/target population	Screening	Operational definition	
		Muscle mass	Muscle strength/ function
SIG- Special Interest Group: Cachexia-Anorexia in Chronic Wasting Diseases [12]*Older persons*	–	Low muscle mass (≥2 standard deviations below the mean measured in young adults of same sex and ethnic background)	Low usual gait speed (<0.8 m/s in the 4-m walking speed).Gait speed test can be replaced by other physical performance measures
SCWD - Sarcopenia with Limited Mobility [10]*Persons >60 years with clinical declines in physical function, strength, or health status. Exclude specific muscle diseases, peripheral vascular disease with intermittent claudication, central and peripheral nervous system disorders and cachexia*	Distance walked during a 6-min walk test (cutoff value 400 m) or gait speed <1.0 m/s (4- to 6-m track length)	Low appendicular lean mass/height^2 (≥2 standard deviations below the mean measured in healthy persons aged 20–30 years old from the same ethnic group)	Poor functioning, 6-m walk or gait speed
AWGS -Asian Working Group for Sarcopenia [15]*Community-dwelling persons 60 or ≥ 65 years, according to the definitions of elderly in each individual country.Persons with specific clinical conditions in all health care settings.*	Screening in community settings—people aged 60 or ≥65 years (according to definitions of elderly in each individual country) living in communities.Specific clinical conditions in all health care settings—presence of recent functional decline or functional impairment; unintentional body weight loss for over 5% in a month; depressive mood or cognitive impairment; repeated falls; undernutrition; chronic conditions (e.g., chronic heart failure; chronic obstructive pulmonary disease, diabetes mellitus, chronic kidney disease, connective tissue disease, tuberculosis infection, and other chronic wasting conditions)	2-standard deviations below the mean muscle mass of young reference group or the lower quintile as the cutoff value determination.Low appendicular lean mass/ height^2:<7.0 kg/m^2 for men and <5.4 kg/m^2 for women, using DXA.<7.0 kg/m^2 for men and <5.7kg/m^2 for women, using BIA	Gait speed ≤ 0.8 m/s as the cutoff value for low physical performance.Lower 20th percentile of handgrip as strength as cutoff value for low muscle strength before outcome-based data are available.Low handgrip strength is suggested to be defined as < 26 kg for men and < 18 kg for women.
FNIH - Foundation for the National Institutes of Health, Sarcopenia Project [14]	Patient presents with poor physical function. If weakness is present, proceed to evaluate for low muscle mass; if low muscle mass is detected, it is possible it might be the cause of weakness. If weakness is not present or if low muscle mass is not detected, proceed to investigate for other causes of poor physical performance.	Recommended cutoff value:Appendicular lean mass adjusted to BMI (ALM_{BMI}) <0.789 for men and <0.512 for women.Alternate cutoff value:ALM <19.75 kg for men and <15.02 kg for women.	Gait speed < 0.8 m/ sRecommended cutoff value:Grip strength (GS Max) <26 kg for men and <16 kg for women.Alternate cutoff value:GS adjusted to BMI ($GSMax_{BMI}$) <1.0 for men and <0.56 for women.

Table 2. Comparative summary of sarcopenia definitions.

Muscle mass in relationship to the range of muscle mass within a reference population. The first definition of sarcopenia included the relative muscle mass 2 standard deviations (SDs) below the mean of a large sex-specific reference population 18–40 years old [2]. This definition used a measure of relative muscle mass obtained by dividing absolute muscle mass estimated by dual energy x-ray absorptiometry (DXA) by height squared. Following, sarcopenia was classified per its severity as: (1) Class I sarcopenia (skeletal muscle index between 1 and 2 SDs below the young adult values) and (2) Class II sarcopenia (skeletal muscle index above 2 SDs below the young adult reference). Skeletal muscle index was calculated by dividing total muscle mass by total body mass, with muscle mass evaluated by bioelectrical impedance analysis (BIA) [25].

Essentially expert opinion, but considering muscle mass and performance criteria. Numerous recommendations for a definition of sarcopenia consider muscle mass and performance criteria. The European Working Group on Sarcopenia in Older People (EWGSOP) proposed a diagnosis for sarcopenia that requires low muscle mass (estimated by the ratio of appendicular lean mass (ALM) over height squared, ≤7.23 kg/ht^2 for men and ≤5.67 kg/ht^2 for women) accompanied by either low muscle strength (measured by grip strength <30 kg for men and <20 kg for women) or low physical performance (measured by gait speed <0.8 m/s). The group defined three stages for the condition: (1) Presarcopenia (loss of muscle mass); (2) sarcopenia (loss of muscle mass accompanied by either loss of strength or physical performance); and (3) severe sarcopenia, with all three aspects present [9]. The definition of sarcopenia by the International Working Group on Sarcopenia (IWGS)/International Academy on Nutrition and Aging (IANA) [11], the European Society for Clinical Nutrition and Metabolism Special Interest Group on cachexia-anorexia in chronic wasting diseases and nutrition in geriatrics [12], and the Society of Sarcopenia, Cachexia, and Wasting Disorders (SCWA) [10], require that both lean mass and gait speed be included in the diagnostic criteria for the condition.

Essentially expert opinion, but considering muscle mass, muscle strength, and physical performance. The Asian Working Group for Sarcopenia (AWGS) decided to take a similar approach for the diagnosis of sarcopenia, but unlike the EWGSOP, it recommends measuring both muscle strength (handgrip strength) and physical performance (usual gait speed) as the screening test [15]. The group also recommends using 60 or 65 years as the age for sarcopenia diagnosis per the definitions of older adults in each Asian country. The group, though, supports using BIA for sarcopenia diagnosis and evaluation of effects. It recommends: (A) Using 2 standard deviations below the mean muscle mass of young reference groups or lower quintile as the cutoff value determination; height-adjusted skeletal muscle mass; for using DXA, cutoff values include 7kg/m^2 in men and 5.4 kg/m^2 in women; for BIA, cutoff values include 7kg/m^2 in men and 5.7 kg/m^2 in women, defined by appendicular skeletal muscle mass/height^2. (B) Using the lower 20th percentile of handgrip strength of a study population before outcomes data are available; low handgrip strength defined as <26 kg for men and <18kg for women. (C) Using ≤0.8m/s as the cutoff value for low physical performance.

Evidence-based, data-driven, considering muscle mass, muscle strength, and predictive validity to mobility disability. The studies supported by the National Institute on Aging and the Foundation for the National Institutes of Health (FNIH) Sarcopenia Project utilized a data-driven analysis of a large pool of data (>26,000) from studies on aging (epidemiologic and clinical trials) to identify criteria for clinically relevant low muscle strength (weakness) and low lean mass [17]. By addressing the relationship between mobility impairment (defined as gait speed ≤0.8 m/s) and muscle strength (measured by handgrip strength), strength cutoff values (<26 kg for men and <16 kg for women) were determined below where low strength (weakness) is likely to contribute to slow gait [26]. By relating these strength cutoff values to muscle mass (estimated by appendicular lean mass adjusted to body mass index [ALM/BMI]), additional cutoff values were determined (<0.789 for men, <0.512 for women), below which low lean mass is likely to contribute to low muscle strength [27]. The cutoff values resulting from these analyses were also found to have a predictive significance on incident mobility impairment over 3 years of follow-up. This two-step analyses that links a clinical condition (mobility impairment) to a functional test result (weakness), which is in turn linked to a potential therapeutic target (muscle atrophy) is useful for establishing participant selection criteria and outcome measures for trials of pharmaceutical or other interventions [14, 17, 28]. These studies, however, were conducted in relatively heathy community-dwelling older adults. In addition, harmonization of DXA data was not conducted prior to pooling data from all studies for analysis. Therefore, additional research is ongoing to validate the findings above by analysing harmonized pooled data from well-designed observational and interventional studies from populations of older adults with high prevalence of mobility disability (see RFA-AG-15-013 http://grants.nih.gov/grants/guide/rfa-files/RFA-AG-15-013.html). The main goal is to develop and assess differing diagnostic cutoff values with regard to properties such as sensitivity, specificity, and positive predictive value. Because the populations involved display a variety of chronic conditions, it is possible that differing criteria might be needed to identify population subgroups. The extent to which lack of harmonization of DXA data significantly compromised the reliability of previously established cutoff values is to be seen.

2.1. Validation of the different definitions of sarcopenia

Validation of the different definitions of sarcopenia is ongoing. Using the criteria recommended by the IWGS/IANA, the prevalence of sarcopenia was slightly less compared to the EWGSOP criteria [29]. Using the EWGSOP criteria, 4.6% of males and 7.9% of females in Hertfordshire were found to have sarcopenia [30]; Japanese men and women age 65–80 years were found to have sarcopenia at a rate of 21.8 and 22.99%, respectively [31]; among people 80 years and older, sarcopenia was present in 12.5% [32]; and in nursing homes, 32.8% of the residents had sarcopenia [33]. Still using the EWGSOP criteria, sarcopenia was found to be highly predictive of earlier mortality in nursing home residents [34], in community-dwelling older Korean men [35], and in older adults admitted to acute care [36]. Sarcopenia assessed with the EWGSOP criteria has also been associated with a greater increase in falls [37, 38] and has been shown to predict mobility and instrumental activities of daily living disability [39]. Similarly, the SCWD criteria have been found to predict ADL and IADL difficulties, frailty and mortality in a longitudinal study [40].

Because the FNIH criteria were based on developing cutoffs using a variety of large epidemiological studies [14], these criteria are more restrictive with only 1.3% of men and 2.3% of women being defined as having sarcopenia. While a strong negative percent agreement has been reported with EWGSOP, the positive percent concurrences are generally low (5–32%). Additional comparative studies are needed, particularly to evaluate best predictive ability.

2.2. Methodological challenges in establishing diagnostic cutoff values

Analyses of pooled data from large studies on aging with measures of muscle mass, and strength still face numerous challenges including different follow-up intervals, use of more than one brand and/or generation of devices to measure body composition, use of more than one type of handgrip dynamometer, use of more than one distance to calculate gait speed, and data harmonization issues [17]. Cutoff values for measurements of muscle mass, muscle strength, and physical performance for the diagnosis of sarcopenia may also differ across populations due to a series of factors including race and ethnicity, body size, lifestyle, and cultural backgrounds. Cutoff values established for Caucasians may not be applicable to Africans, Asians, or Hispanics. For example, as acknowledged by the AWGS, the Asian continent has a rapidly growing population with a wide range of ethnicities, cultural, social, religious backgrounds, and lifestyles [15]. In addition, Asia's aging population status and economic development varies significantly across Asian countries. Moreover, the age cutoff that defines the population of older adults may differ not only among Asian countries, but also around the world. The lack or paucity of outcomes-based studies is another factor presenting a challenge to the assessment of sarcopenia.

The discussion in this section focuses on key methodological issues associated with the body composition assessment and the need to establish a standardized approach to develop and apply diagnostic cutoff values. Assessments of body composition vary in precision and in the target tissue. The use of anthropometric methods does not allow tissue-specific inferences. BMI, a descriptive index encompassing both the lean and fat mass, is expressed as weight divided by stature squared (kg/m^2). The availability of extensive national reference data and their established relationships with levels of body fat, morbidity, and mortality in adults is an advantage to the use of BMI. However, the use of BMI alone to evaluate athletes and persons with conditions such as sarcopenia where body weight may be altered considerably by changing proportions of muscle and fat masses is cautioned [41].

BIA produces estimates of total body water, fat-free mass, and fat mass by measuring the resistance of the body as a conductor to a very small alternating electrical current. This is not a direct measure of skeletal muscle. Measurements can be easily altered by fluid retention and health status, providing inaccurate results that limit considerably the clinical application. BIA was developed to mainly determine the volume of body fat and muscle mass, but not specific appendicular muscle mass. While validation studies have been reported on BIA's accuracy in the diagnosis of sarcopenia, results also strongly depend on the accuracy of the equation of the equipment and the conditions associated with the assessment (e.g., temperature, humidity, skin condition, and others) [42–45]. New BIA equipment models will likely provide more precise measurements of appendicular muscle mass [24, 46]. Portability, reasonable cost, fast processing, noninvasiveness, radiation-free functions, and convenience of use are advantages to BIA suitability for sarcopenia assessment in the community. Despite recommendations by EWGSOP on the use of BIA validated equations in sarcopenia research, its use has been discouraged by others [10, 47]. Moreover, BIA equipment in Western countries is not derived from populations from other regions of the world and, therefore, results are unlikely to be able to be extrapolated to particular populations [15].

Currently, the precision of devices to measure body composition such as DXA, computed tomography (CT), and magnetic resonance imaging (MRI) has been well recognized [47]. DXA is currently the most widely employed method for muscle mass measurement in sarcopenia research. It is commonly available in both clinical and research settings, is relatively inexpensive, and provides sufficiently precise results [41, 47, 48]. DXA is considered a suitable alternative to distinguish between fat, bone mineral, and lean tissues, it leads to minimal radiation exposure. However, its use in community screening is still challenging. In 2008, the Center for Disease Control and Prevention (CDC), National Center for Health Statistics (NCHS) released a DXA whole body dataset from the National Health and Nutrition Examination Survey (NHANES) population-based sample acquired with modern fan bean scanners in 15 counties across the United States from 1999 through 2004 [49]. The reference dataset was partitioned by gender and ethnicity and DXA whole body measures of %fat, fat mass/height^2, lean mass/height^2, appendicular lean mass/height^2, %fat trunk/%fat legs ratio, trunk/limb fat mass ratio of fat, bone mineral content (BMC), and bone mineral density (BMD) were analysed to provide reference values for subjects 8–85 years old. DXA reference values for adults were normalized to age; reference values for children included total and subtotal whole body results and were normalized to age, height, or lean mass.

The estimation of fat and lean tissue by DXA is based on assumptions regarding levels of hydration, potassium content, or tissue density, and these assumptions vary with manufacturer. Some analytical differences across manufacturers and models, and the risk of generating biased results due to the low differentiation between water and bone-free lean tissue are among limitations with DXA [48]. Estimates of body composition are also affected by differences in software employed, methodological issues, and intra- and intermachine differences. Testing of specific manufacturers and models revealed that overestimations of fat-free mass may occur. DXA systems are currently capable of scanning a very broad range of weights (neonates to morbidly obese). Repeatability is also very high for all reported total body measures, with the percent fat measures typically better than 1% (standard deviation) and 2% (coefficient of variation) for total fat and lean mass measures. Whole-body DXA scans can be subdivided into arms, legs, trunk, head, and android/gynoid soft tissue regions to report all bone and soft tissue measures within a region. While work is ongoing, there is not yet a reliable phantom that can be used to cross-calibrate DXA systems between manufacturers or a standard of accuracy of percent fat. Some success at representing muscle mass as appendicular lean mass in just the legs and arms has been achieved, but it has yet to be shown as a reasonable surrogate of muscle strength or function. Further work with DXA machines will lead to the development of more refined models of visceral and muscle fat [47].

Despite being considered gold standards for the evaluation of body composition, the use of computed tomography (CT) and magnetic resonance imaging/spectroscopy (MRI)/(MRS) has been impacted by their high cost, CT-generated radiation exposure, and inconvenience for use in community screening. Both are techniques relevant to body composition assessment requiring additional time and software to provide whole body quantities of fat and lean tissue. CT can distinguish body tissues based on a technique helpful to assess nonfat tissue or the fatty infiltration of skeletal muscles. It accurately measures a direct physical property of the muscle (e.g., cross-sectional area and volume). It allows the evaluation of muscle density (a parameter related to intramyocellular adipose tissue deposit) as well as subcutaneous and intramuscular adipose tissue deposition [48].

MRI/MRS has been increasingly used to study body composition in related physiological and pathological conditions. MRI can be used for whole body assessment in normal or moderately overweight people (limitations exist in accommodating very obese people) and measure the volume of body components (e.g., fat tissue, skeletal muscle, organs, and bone). Recent advances suggest that fat tissue is not a homogeneous depot but contains distinct components with different metabolic activities. MRI provides similar measures as CT, with the additional capacity of multiple slice acquisition and 3D volumetric estimates, and no radiation exposure. Quantification of subregions of fat depots such as visceral (i.e., omental, mesenteric, and extraperitoneal), intermuscular, and bone marrow is possible with DXA. A single slice in the upper abdomen has been shown not only to provide the best representation of total volume of visceral fat, but also to correlate with health risks even more closely than the traditionally used slice located at the L4–L5 level. When fat infiltration is increased, MRS imaging allows a more accurate measurement of intramyocellular fat [41, 47]. High technical complexity and costs, as well as inapplicability to persons with older models of implanted medical devices (e.g., joint prostheses) are among the limitations associated with MRI.

2.2.1. Harmonization of DXA data from multiple studies

Studies focusing on the development of cutoff values for low muscle mass and low muscle strength frequently use appendicular lean mass (ALM) as a primary independent variable, obtained by DXA. Because these studies generally combine data from many different cohorts to measure ALM, it is critical that DXA measurements be compatible across studies. Owing to the variation between the manufacturers' (Hologic and GE Lunar) designs and systematic improvements in hardware and software instituted over time within each machine type, DXA values obtained for a given individual may vary across machines. It is necessary, therefore, to implement a quantitative adjustment to harmonize or put all measurements on the same theoretical scaling. This harmonization process may require a few steps including the harmonization of DXA values within manufacturer's systems and harmonization between different manufacturers. Studies have been conducted to address standardization and cross-calibration of body composition using GE Healthcare Lunar and Hologic DXA systems. Equations developed are facilitating the combination of results in clinical and epidemiological studies [50–52].

2.3. Sarcopenia diagnosed without measurements

Fracture risk can be determined almost accurately by FRAX questions as by measuring bone mineral density [53]. Because muscle function is more noticeable than bone function, the idea of developing and adopting a simple questionnaire to identify individuals with sarcopenia was realized with the development of the SARC-F scale. This simple and rapid questionnaire to assess the presence of sarcopenia is illustrated in **Table 3** [54]. Robust validation, indicating that SARC-F performed at similar level to the EWSGSOP and AWGS definitions of sarcopenia has been reported, with suggestions that sarcopenia can be screened for without a need to measure muscle mass or to directly measure muscle function [55].

2.4. Sarcopenia and the FY2017 United States Update of the International Statistical Classification of Diseases and Related Health Problems, 10th Revision, Clinical Modifications (ICD-10-CM)

Effective October 1, 2016, the U.S. Department of Health and Human Services (HHS) Centers for Disease Control and Prevention (CDC) has established an ICD-10-CM code for "sarcopenia" (M62.84) for use by the medical community in the United States [56]. For that purpose, sarcopenia is defined as a combination of low muscle mass and weakness in older adults that leads to functional deficits. The new code designation for the condition has the potential to affect the clinical assessment and management of sarcopenia, as well as facilitate data collection and impact sarcopenia research. Because sarcopenia is a condition that can lead to serious adverse outcomes (e.g., mobility impairment, falls, disability, and death) [25, 57–61], the creation of an ICD10-CM code emphasizes the importance of recognizing and treating the condition. The availability of an ICD-10-CM code for sarcopenia has the potential to facilitate recognition of the condition and the future establishment of guidelines for the clinical diagnosis and management of sarcopenia; support requests for tests and referrals, and the development of educational materials targeting potential prevention and management of sarcopenia. It can serve as a stimulus to advance research including new drug development and new indications by the HHS Food and Drug Administration (FDA) for the treatment of sarcopenia. It can certainly contribute to easier access to more reliable data collection on the condition by a variety of system data sources (e.g., electronic medical records, death certificates). Despite these potential advantages, challenges are faced with the need to increase awareness of the availability of such code and, most importantly, how to use it in face of the current lack of a standardized clinical/diagnostic assessment of sarcopenia.

Evaluation component	Questions	Scoring
Strength	How much difficulty do you have in lifting and carrying 10 pounds?	None = 0Some = 1A lot or unable = 2
Assistance with walking	How much difficulty do you have walking across a room?	None = 0Some = 1A lot, use aids, or unable = 2
Rising from a chair	How much difficulty do you have transferring from a chair or bed?	None = 0Some = 1A lot or unable without help = 2
Climbing stairs	How much difficulty do you have climbing a flight of 10 stairs?	None = 0Some = 1A lot or unable = 2
Falls	How many times have you fallen in the past year?	None = 01 to 3 falls = 14 or more falls = 2

Table 3. SARC-F scale: scores of 4 or more indicate sarcopenia [54].

2.5. Biomarkers and outcomes for sarcopenia

The most basic biomarkers (functional, biological, or imaging-related) that can be utilized in clinical trials of sarcopenia and considered the most reliable and promising to evaluate age-related changes of skeletal muscle have been discussed and recommended. **Table 4** summarizes information on these proposed biomarkers for sarcopenia research. In addition, the measurement of motor unit number index, which can be used to assess the number and the size of the motor units is a very important biomarker as loss of motor unit input to muscle is a significant cause of sarcopenia in at least half of older individuals [22, 48, 62].

In view of the molecular mechanisms involved in the pathogenesis of sarcopenia, potential emerging sarcopenia biomarkers have been discussed. Normal muscle mass and function maintenance are thought to be dependent on the dynamic balance between the positive regulators of muscle growth such as bone morphogenetic proteins (BMPs), brain-derived neurotrophic factor (BDNF), follistatin (FST) and irisin, and negative regulators including TGFβ, myostatin, activins A and B, and growth and differentiation factor-15 (GDF-15). The authors hypothesized that the shift in this balance to muscle growth inhibitors, along with increased expression of the C-terminal agrin fragment (CAF) associated with age-dependent neuromuscular junction (NMJ) dysfunction, as well as skeletal muscle-specific troponin T (sTnT), a key component of contractile structure, is a main mechanism underlying sarcopenia pathogenesis. Based on these facts, the molecular elements mentioned above are proposed as emerging sarcopenia biomarkers [63].

As indicated previously the EWGSOP recommends the use of physical performance, muscle strength, and muscle mass as the primary treatment outcome indicators for sarcopenia intervention trials. Activities of daily living, quality of life, metabolic and biochemical markers, inflammatory markers, global impression of change by subject or physician, falls, admission to nursing home or hospital, social support, and mortality are recommended by that group as secondary outcome indicators [9].

The AWGS recommends the following approach in outcome indicators assessment for sarcopenia research. This approach targets the measurement of changes in two ways over a period. The AWGS also recommends the use of fear of falling and incontinence as outcome indicators for sarcopenia research [15]:

a. Static approach: Activities of daily living, quality of life, inflammatory markers, falls, frailty issues, mobility disorders, admission to hospitals, admission to long-term care facilities, and mortality.

b. Dynamic approach: Changes in muscle mass, muscle strength, physical performance, frailty status, instrumental activities of daily living, and activities of daily living.

Finally, the importance of tapping into the patient experience, identifying the linkage between clinical measures and patient reports, and building self-report into submissions for drug

		Inclusion-exclusion criteria	Baseline evaluation	Endpoint assessment
Muscle function	Physical performance measures	+++	+++	+++
	Muscle strength measures	+++	+++	+++
	Disability	+++	+++	+++
Muscle mass	Anthropometry	+	-	-
	Bioelectrical impedance analysis	+	-	-
	Dual energy X-ray absorptiometry	+++	++	++
	Computerized tomography	++	+++	+++
	Magnetic resonance imaging	++	+++	+++
	Echography	++	++	++
	Electrical impedance myography	+	++	++
Biological confounders (mechanisms)	Inflammation	++	++	++
Note:	Oxidative damage	++	++	++
The importance of all these biomarkers in the evaluation of sarcopenia will largely depend on the study hypotheses, the specific aims, and/or the target population	Antioxidants	++	++	++
	Apoptosis	+	++	++
	Nutritional parameters (albumin, hemoglobin, urinary creatinine, others)	+++	++	++
	Hormones (dehydroepiandrosterone, testosterone, insulin-like growth factor-1, others)	++	++	++

- not recommended for this use; + may be of use; but severely limited; ++ suitable for this use; +++ recommended for this use.

Table 4. Potential biomarkers for clinical trials on sarcopenia [48].

approval to the HHS FDA have been a matter of discussion among experts. Work is ongoing with questionnaires focusing on patient-reported outcome measures in sarcopenia, but validation is pending [64]. In addition, the HHS FDA conducted on April 06, 2017, a public meeting on patient-focused drug development for sarcopenia. The HHS FDA is interested in obtaining patient perspectives on the impact of sarcopenia on daily life and patient views on treatment approaches.

3. Integrating muscle quality in efforts to define sarcopenia and muscle quality in the context of skeletal muscle function deficit

Aging is associated with significant changes in body composition, gradual increase in total body fat during adulthood followed by a loss later in life, and remodeling of fat distribution. The latter involves an increase in inter/intramuscular and visceral fat, and a gradual loss of subcutaneous fat. Weight gain and weight loss overtime have been linked with preserved muscle mass and accelerated muscle atrophy, respectively. Both, however, are associated with increased fat infiltration of muscles. Adverse health and functional outcomes including the development of insulin resistance and impaired mechanical muscle function seem to be concurrently or independently associated with the aging changes mentioned above. Evidence suggests that the correlation between "muscle quantity" and "muscle function" (e.g., muscle strength) is relatively weak, and in contrast to muscle strength, muscle mass has been demonstrated to be a poor predictor of functional limitation, gait speed, and even mortality. It is, in fact, becoming increasingly clear that muscle quality (force per unit of muscle mass) and neural function play a key role in the development of mobility disability and that a new endpoint incorporating these aspects in addition to muscle mass and strength might be useful.

3.1. Defining muscle quality: the need for a standardized assessment

Multiple factors are known to underpin muscle quality and determine the changes in muscle function and mobility later in life. Those who conduct sarcopenia-related research have usually used relative force production (ratio of peak force and a measure of body size, regional lean body mass, or cross-sectional area) as the favored approach to characterizing muscle quality [65, 66]. Emerging definitions of muscle quality, however, call for its expansion to include muscle composition, metabolism, aerobic capacity, insulin resistance, fat infiltration, fibrosis, and neural activation [67], all of which easily correlate with the concept of SMFD. The term muscle quality allows investigators to explore aspects of SMFD beyond the construct of age-related decline of lean body mass [6]. While the meaning of muscle quality is linked to the primary functions of the skeletal muscle, it can be expanded to include both physiology and pathophysiology [8]. There is also a need to develop and adopt a standardized assessment of muscle quality. In doing so, it is essential to consider the complexity of the skeletal muscle tissue and its physiologic roles that include not only movement via force production, but also metabolism through its maintenance of glucose/insulin homeostasis and amino acid storage, thermoregulation, and autocrine/paracrine/endocrine signaling via myokine production. This expanded view of muscle quality is essential to improve our understanding of SMFD [8].

A preliminary conceptual model for the assessment of muscle quality has been proposed, built on skeletal muscle primary physiologic functions. This conceptual model is categorized in domains that have both clinical and research applications. The domains are the following: (A) force production; (B) metabolism (endocrine, neurologic, orthopedic); (C) thermoregulation; and (D) signalling/myokine production. No endpoint(s) have been identified as best to establish the quantitative profile of muscle quality. Similarly, no standardized approaches to endpoint measures have been recommended that can be linked to any of the domains above. None have been identified as the most strongly associated with mechanisms controlling muscle function or with predicting mobility status and mortality in older adults. Muscle quality seen under this perspective provides the advantage of going beyond the strict lean body mass-driven assessment approach to sarcopenia research. Ongoing research focusing on the local and systemic effects of fat infiltration of muscles and on the emerging methods to quantify changes in muscle composition and function is reflecting this perspective [8].

3.2. Factors underpinning muscle quality

Below is a brief discussion on the multiple factors underpinning muscle quality, all of which fall under the proposed domains for assessing muscle quality. The concept of muscle quality cannot be represented by a single endpoint measure, but the factors that affect muscle quality are frequent targets of measurement used to characterize skeletal muscle. The discussion provided in this section does not enclose every assessment target, but addresses common examples of factors that may serve as measures for basic, translational, and clinical trials related to muscle quality and sarcopenia or muscle quality in the context of SMFD. Factors intrinsic to skeletal muscles are crucial for function and homeostasis. Factors extrinsic to skeletal muscles considerably impact muscle activity and muscle mass building and maintenance. Both intrinsic and extrinsic factors affect net force production.

3.2.1. *Muscle characteristics/architecture*

Muscle characteristics include size, fiber type, and contractile components. Fiber type and number determine muscle size. Muscle cross-sectional area has a positive relationship with muscle strength in young lean individuals, while smaller and weaker muscles are usually seen in older adults. Muscle cross-sectional area and lower limb skeletal muscle volume are associated with greater fat mass in both men and women [68], likely due to intermuscular lipid or noncontractile components. There are three types of muscle fibers as identified in **Table 5** [68]. The loss of types I and IIb muscle fibers associated with aging is attributed to changes in activity and consequent disuse and denervation. Conflicting literature demonstrates no link at all or a link between advanced age and changes in muscle fiber composition with gradual loss of type IIb muscle fibers [69]. Conflicting limited evidence is also seen in older adults in relation to changes in muscle fiber type, muscle cross-sectional area, and strength. Contractile properties of types I and II muscle fibers at the single fiber level seem to be maintained independent of the presence of mobility limitation [70], but again, evidence is conflicting. It has been suggested that maximal shortening velocity is lower in single fibers from older adults because of changes in myosin heavy chain isoform distribution to a more hybrid pattern. A

Type I	Type IIa	Type IIb
Predominantly generate energy via oxidative pathways for prolonged low force production.Relatively small cross-sectional area compared to type IIb fibers, but have greater oxidative capacity.Recruited during low intensity activities of daily living (e.g., walking)	Capable of generating energy via oxidative and nonoxidative pathways	Predominantly generate energy via nonoxidative pathways for rapid high force production.Recruited during high intensity activity

Table 5. Types and functions of skeletal muscle fibers [68].

lower maximal shortening velocity in myosin heavy chain has been observed in types I and IIa fiber of older adults including those who are very active. The evidence, however, is debatable because of limitations with study power and potential confounding with physical activity. Preservation of single muscle fiber contractile properties with age is thought to imply that differences in skeletal muscle function are related to quantitative changes in muscle fiber size or number rather than qualitative changes in the muscle's contractile properties [68].

Fiber arrangement within a muscle (e.g., parallel or pennation pattern) will determine fascicle length, pennation angle, and cross-sectional area, all of which can change with age. Older adults 70–81 years of age are reported to have smaller fascicle length and pennation angle (compared to younger adults 27–42 years) of the gastrocnemius medialis [71], but several weeks of bed rest have not resulted in changes in the pennation angle of the vastus lateralis muscle. Nevertheless, modest improvements in muscle architecture are reported to be possible with 4–5 weeks of resistance training. Changes in muscle architecture also appear to precede changes in muscle size in young healthy adults.

Cross-sectional assessment of skeletal muscles provides relevant information on muscle function because both individual muscle fiber diameter and cross-sectional diameter of the whole muscle are associated with strength. Force production is related to the architectural characteristics of the skeletal muscle including muscle fiber length and arrangement in relation to the direction of the force produced by the whole muscle. Thus, both cross-sectional and longitudinal orientation of measures of skeletal muscles are valuable in the assessment of the size-strength relationship and the identification of age-related differences in muscle strength per size. Sarcomeric changes in myofibrillar disorder, Z-line streaming, and dilatation in aged skeletal muscle have been observed in electron microscopic analysis. The characteristics/architectural changes highlighted above have been combined in a composite measure—physiological cross-sectional area (PCSA)—to reflect both strength and change in strength in leg extension [8].

Muscle weakness is attributed to changes in muscle composition, muscle contractile quality, and neural activation [72]. However, measures of muscle composition, size, and architecture generally do not consider the neural input into fibers, which dictate contraction potential and force production. Strength measures are an important indicator of muscle performance and show the ability to change in response to a variety of interventions to tackle sarcopenia and frailty in older women with clinically relevant muscle weakness independent of the presence of low muscle mass [73]. Muscle strength and size have been used as a single measure of muscle quality known as "relative strength," reflecting the expression of muscle force production relative to muscle or body size. It has been suggested that strength per unit of muscle tissue may serve as a better indicator of age-related differences in muscle quality prior to changes in lean tissue mass [74]. A novel functional metric–muscle quality index–estimates muscle power from body anthropometrics and timed chair raises; it has been found to have higher reliability and greater responsiveness following a resistance exercise regimen in older adults, compared to other functional measures (e.g., gait speed, grip strength, the get-up and go test, etc.) [75].

3.2.2. *Muscle aerobic capacity*

Muscle quality and function in both middle-aged and older adults are determined by metabolic characteristics of the muscle. Aerobic capacity reflects the maximal ability to use oxygen (cardiovascular adaptation to transport oxygen; within skeletal muscle adaptation to use oxygen) in response to energy demands of physical activity. Evidence shows that aerobic capacity declines at an accelerated rate after age 50, and is a strong predictor of mobility assessed by gait speed in older adults. Evidence from cross-sectional muscle analyses from healthy men and women (18–90 years) reveals that mitochondrial DNA, mRNA abundance, and energy (ATP) production diminishes with age. Both skeletal muscle mitochondrial capacity and efficiency, and whole body peak aerobic capacity have been linked to gait speed [68, 76, 77].

The progressive decline in mitochondrial function observed in aging results in the accumulation of reactive oxygen species (ROS) generated by the incorporation of a single electron to the oxygen molecule. Specifically, ROS negatively impact muscle quality, playing an extremely important role in all muscle functions, muscle aging, contraction, fatigue, dystrophy or waste [78–80]. Mitochondria are the major producers of ROS, which damage DNA, proteins, and lipids. Animal and human studies have typically shown that aging changes in mitochondria can be reflected by increased mutations in mitochondrial DNA, decreased activity of some mitochondrial enzymes, altered respiration with reduced maximal capacity at least in sedentary individuals, and reduced total mitochondrial content with increased morphological changes. With mitochondrial dynamics altered (e.g., fusion and fission rates, mitochondrially induced apoptosis), net muscle fiber loss and age-related sarcopenia may ensue. Strategies such as exercise and caloric restriction that reduce oxidative damage can improve mitochondrial function. While these strategies may not completely prevent the primary effects of aging, they may help to attenuate the rate of decline [81, 82].

It is also well established that contracting muscles produce both ROS and nitrogen species. Although the sources of oxidant production during exercise continue to be debated, growing evidence suggests that mitochondria are not the dominant source [83]. Regardless of the sources of oxidants in contracting muscles, intense and prolonged exercise can result in oxidative damage to both proteins and lipids in the contracting myocytes. Further, oxidants regulate numerous cell signaling pathways and modulate the expression of many genes. There has been much controversy about measurements of mitochondrial energy production. These controversies may be explained by differences in methodological approaches and whether physical activity is controlled for.

Age-related changes in skeletal muscle mass and composition can result in increased insulin resistance and later to reduced capacity for insulin-mediated glucose disposal. Relative muscle mass in healthy nondiabetic older adults is inversely linked to glucose tolerance and insulin resistance [84]. Muscle strength adjusted for BMI, however, has been reported to be negatively associated with insulin resistance in a large population based study of older women, but not men, after adjustment for confounders. No association between muscle leg strength and insulin resistance in men or women >50 years has been observed in an analysis of the National Health and Nutrition Examination Survey (NHANES) [85]. In some studies, gait speed assessments are found to be inversely associated with insulin resistance, suggesting that insulin resistance may serve as an indicator of poor muscle quality underpinning low levels of physical fitness and poor scores on gait speed tests. Improvement in glucose disposal and skeletal muscle metabolism in older overweight or obese men has been observed over 6 months of both regular aerobic and resistance exercise. Fat infiltration of muscles is also associated with insulin resistance.

3.2.3. *Myosteatosis*

Myosteatosis refers to fat infiltration in skeletal muscle that can lead to large negative clinical effects including poor metabolic and skeletal muscle health, accelerated aging, and impaired longevity. This ectopic fat tissue has become an important factor behind muscle quality and may serve as a predictor of muscle function in older adults. Two modalities of myosteatosis are identified: (1) intermuscular fat, which represents the visible extracellular adipose tissue located beneath the muscle and between and within muscle groups; (2) intramuscular fat or intramyocellular lipids, which represents infiltration within myocytes, i.e., the presence of microscopic lipid droplets used as energy within the muscle. This ectopic fat infiltration increases with aging, seems to act synergistically with sarcopenia and is also present in muscular dystrophies. The biological mechanism underlying increases in myosteatosis with aging in humans remain largely under investigated, with the need to identify and better understand regulatory factors including evidence of senescent cells and cultured cells developing into preadipocytes and fat cells. This is an opportunity for future development of therapies to preserve skeletal muscle health [8, 86, 87].

Individuals with comparable thigh circumference may have distinct muscle function due to the proportion of fat infiltration to contractile elements. In older adults with multimorbidity, intermuscular adipose tissue evaluated by MRI was reported as the strongest predictor of mobility, but strength and quadriceps lean tissue explicated some of the variation in mobility in this study [88]. Increased mobility loss, reflected by decreased six-minute walk distance, decreased gait speed, decreased physical performance, difficulty with repeated chair stands, and slower stair descent and timed get-up and go tests have been reported as the result of myosteatosis effects on muscle metabolism and function [8]. In young healthy persons with 30 days of leg disuse by suspension, myosteatosis was found to increase by 15–20% and exceeded the loss of lean muscles (calf and thigh) [89]. Myosteatosis is also known to lead to the transition of muscle fibers from type II to type I, which result in muscles with impaired contractile capacity and decreased power [90, 91]. It is also suggested that myostetatosis may harm muscle and mobility because fat infiltration leads to changes in muscle fiber orientation.

Proinflammatory cytokines secreted by fat tissue in the skeletal muscle microenvironment may also lead to proteolysis and muscle catabolism [8].

Fat storage and infiltration into muscle may be a marker of metabolic profile. In older adults, intermuscular adipose tissue was found to positively correlate with higher fasting plasma glucose and lower glucose tolerance [92]. Myosteatosis has been linked to insulin resistance and an increased risk of developing type-2 diabetes, hypertension, and dyslipidemia, independent of total body adiposity (measured by BMI or DXA whole body fat). Further investigation, however is still needed on the association of myosteatosis and metabolic disease independent of visceral fat. The metabolic consequences of myosteatosis depend on age, race/ethnicity, aerobic conditioning, sensitivity to insulin, amount of physical activity, and anatomic region. Further investigations are necessary to verify whether myosteatosis acts as a marker of metabolic dysfunction or may have an intermediary modifying role in insulin resistance [8].

Physical activity seems to be able to revert intermuscular fat infiltration. In men 60 years old, six months of aerobic exercise and weight loss decreased intermuscular adipose tissue of the leg and improved fasting plasma glucose and glucose tolerance. Four weeks of an imposed decrease in physical activity due to unilateral lower limb suspension resulted in 15–20% increase in the intermuscular adipose tissue in the thigh and calf, respectively. Strength loss was associated with the increase in the intermuscular adipose tissue, after adjustment for loss of muscle mass and considering initial baseline values.

3.2.4. Muscle fibrosis

Impairment in the muscle repair process can lead to muscle fibrosis, which involves the deposition of collagen and extracellular matrix proteins instead of proteins necessary to repair and restore tissue function. Fibrosis is also seen in different tissues because of extra fat accumulation. The presence of fibrosis in the skeletal muscle of older adults is hypothetical at this point, and further studies are needed to investigate how or whether fibrosis is a factor in muscle quality. Evidence, however, is available indicating that progressive intermuscular adipose tissue infiltration in middle aged or older adults may lead to fibrosis and impairment of muscle function and mobility [68].

3.2.5. Motor units and neuromuscular activation

Other potential factors related to muscle quality in middle and old age include components of the neuromuscular system and neuromuscular activation. Skeletal muscle fibers are organized in bundles of motor units. Each motor unit is innervated by a motor nerve, which connects to an alpha motor-neuron in the spinal cord. Across the lifespan, motor units go through remodeling, denervation and reinnervation. These units are reported to be decreased in the tibialis anterior muscle of men 65 years old and those >80 years compared to younger men (25 years), but the reduced motor unit number was only related to strength in men >80 years [93].

Neuromuscular activation has been proposed as another measure of muscle quality. Impairments in neuromuscular activation affect the rate of force development and muscle power needed for dynamic movements. Improvements in neuromuscular activation generally precede increases in muscle mass in response to resistance training. Neuromuscular activity and acceleration was impaired during dynamic leg extensions in mobility-limited older adults compared to mobile older adults [94]. The rate of neuromuscular activation was significantly associated with physical function scores. Among middle-aged and older adults without mobility limitations, no significant differences in measures of neuromuscular activation were detected. However, whether neuromuscular impairment precedes the development of mobility limitations is still unclear.

3.3. Emerging alternative clinical imaging and other measures of muscle quality

Relatively high costs, limitations with access, and the testing burden associated with invasive techniques are barriers to standardized assessment of muscle quality. The use of routine tissue composition analysis is hampered by the need for further demonstration of its diagnostic value and contribution to both diagnostic and therapeutic decision making. The emerging literature on the effects of age-related increases in intramuscular adipose tissue on muscle performance and metabolism, has led to the development of alternative assessment. Methodological approaches ranging from multifrequency electrical impedance analysis to quantitative diagnostic sonography have been used to characterize skeletal muscle mass and quality in older adults and in those with muscle disease [95]. Noninvasive, high precision, imaging modalities such as MRI has been used to diagnose and assess progression of a number of neuromuscular conditions. Quantitative musculoskeletal diagnostic ultrasound has been proposed as a clinically feasible means of characterizing muscle structure. Ultrasound has been shown to be highly reliable for assessing cross-sectional areas of large individual human muscle and particularly useful in mobility-impaired individuals who cannot be easily transported to scanners (CT, MRI) [48].

Electrical impedance myography (EIM) is another promising technique based on the surface application and measurement of a high frequency, low intensity electrical current applied to specific muscles. It detects changes in the conductivity and permittivity of skeletal muscles caused by alterations in muscle composition and structure. It has been found repeatable and sensitive to skeletal muscle changes in persons with amyotrophic lateral sclerosis. Mass isopotomer distribution analysis based on the evaluation of protein and proteome synthesis rate is obtained by heavy water labelling; it is a very promising approach due to the wide spectrum of proteins analysed [48].

The success of emerging alternative imaging measures of muscle quality relies on their easy-to-use in diverse clinical settings and ability to discriminate between older adults with and without sarcopenia, identify those at risk for impaired muscle performance, and those who can benefit from preventive and therapeutic interventions. A symposium report on "The Need for Standardized Assessment of Muscle Quality in Skeletal Muscle Function Deficit and Other Aging-Related Muscle Dysfunctions" provides a good insight on these emerging approaches [8].

4. Conclusion: clinical relevance and research opportunities

Aging muscles and other aging-related muscle dysfunctions present with a functional deficit in one or more elements or components of SMFD involving muscle mass, muscle strength or muscle quality. To further characterize SMFD, additional investigation and understanding of the factors behind changes in muscle quality with aging are needed. The concept of muscle quality is critical and should be expanded beyond muscle strength or power per unit of muscle mass, to encompass muscle aerobic capacity and other key factors which closely relate to mobility and other important activities of daily living. Assessment or diagnostics tools sensitive to small changes within skeletal muscle that precede a decline in mass, strength and function can enable preventative steps to maintain healthy muscles. Diagnostic ultrasound and other assessment methods continue to be developed for characterizing muscle pathology, and enhanced sonography using sensors to provide user feedback and improve reliability is currently the subject of ongoing investigation and development. Measures of relative muscle force (e.g., specific force or grip strength adjusted for body size) have been proposed as methods to assess changes in muscle quality. Performance-based assessments of muscle power via timed tests of function and body size estimates are associated with lower extremity muscle strength and may be responsive to age-related changes in muscle quality. The challenge remains to reach a consensus on diagnostic criteria, tools, and consistent methodological approaches for assessing or measuring components of SMFD that are practical in a community or clinical setting. These should be considered priority for the scientific community and health care providers.

To date, no studies have assessed exclusively and concurrently aging-related changes in muscle mass, muscle strength, muscle function, and muscle quality. Analyses of pooled data from large studies on aging with measures of muscle mass and strength still face numerous methodological challenges. As highlighted by experts in the field, future well-designed large prospective studies of interventions to improve muscle mass, muscle strength, muscle function, and muscle quality can observe age-related changes in skeletal muscles over time and generate the evidence to help identify individuals that will benefit from interventions to prevent or treat these changes.

From the public health perspective, further characterization of SMFD is very relevant to several ongoing therapeutic developments. For example, we already know that resistance exercise is the primary therapeutic strategy to prevent and reverse sarcopenia; aerobic exercise also has a therapeutic role, as demonstrated by the Lifestyle Interventions and Independence for Elders (LIFE); vitamin D has been shown to enhance muscle function in persons with low muscle function; and evidence that leucine-enriched essential amino acid supplementation will increase muscle mass and potentially function. Limited evidence, however, suggests that testosterone increases muscle mass and strength, and potentially function in older adults with hypogonadism, but its safety remains unclear. Drug development efforts with selective androgen receptor modulators (SARMs) are promising in increasing muscle mass and stair climbing. Ongoing research is also investigating numerous antibodies that modulate myostatin and the activin II receptor, as well as ghrelin agonists, which increase food intake and release growth hormone [7].

The potential impact of clearly addressing SMFD and properly integrating muscle mass, muscle strength, and muscle quality is critical to future therapeutic development to help older adults with muscle dysfunctions maintain independence and quality of life.

Author details

Rosaly Correa-de-Araujo

Address all correspondence to: rosaly.correa-de-araujo@nih.gov

Division of Geriatrics and Clinical Gerontology, National Institute on Aging, National Institutes of Health, U.S. Department of Health and Human Services, Bethesda, MD, USA

References

[1] Rosenberg I. Summary comments: Epidemiological and methodological problems in determining nutritional status of older persons. American Journal of Clinical Nutrition. 1989;**50**:1231-1233

[2] Baumgartner RN, Koehler KM, Gallagher D, et al. Epidemiology of sarcopenia among the elderly in New Mexico. American Journal of Epidemiology. 1998;**17**:755-763

[3] Mitchell WK, Williams J, Atherton P, Larvin W, Land J, Narici M. Sarcopenia, dynapenia, and the impact of advancing age on human skeletal muscle size and strength: A quantitative review. Frontiers in Physiology. 2012;**3**:260. DOI: 10.3389/fphys.2012.00260

[4] Roman D, Mahoney K, Mohamadi A. Sarcopenia: What's in a name? Journal of the American Medical Directors Association. 2013;**14**:80-82.

[5] Correa-de-Araujo R. Skeletal muscle function deficit. In Update in Gerontology and Geriatrics. All India Institute of Medical Science (AIIMS). BUKPRINT. New Delhi, India. pp 106-113. 2015.

[6] Correa-de-Araujo R, Hadley E. Skeletal muscle function deficit: A new terminology to embrace the evolving concepts of sarcopenia and age-related muscle dysfunction. Journals of Gerontology. Series A: Biological Sciences and Medical Sciences. 2014;**5**:591-594

[7] Morley JE, Anker SD. Prevalence, incidence, and clinical impact of sarcopenia: Facts, numbers, and epidemiology—Update 2014. Journal of Cachexia, Sarcopenia and Muscle. 2014;**3**:253-259

[8] Correa-De-Araujo R, Harris-Love MO, Miljkovic I, Fragala MS, Anthony BW, Manini TM. The need for standardized assessment of muscle quality in skeletal muscle function deficit and other aging-related muscle dysfunctions: A symposium report. Frontiers in Physiology. 2017;**8**:87. DOI: 10.3389/fphys.2017.00087

[9] Cruz-Jentoft AJ, Baeyens JP, Bauer JM, et al. Sarcopenia: European consensus on definition and diagnosis: Report of the European Working Group on Sarcopenia in Older People. Age Ageing. 2010;**39**:412-423

[10] Morley JE, Abbatecola AM, Argiles JM, et al. Sarcopenia with limited mobility: An international consensus. Journal of the American Medical Directors Association. 2011;**12**:403-409

[11] Fielding RA, Vellas B, Evans WJ, et al. Sarcopenia: An undiagnosed condition in older adults. Current consensus definition: Prevalence, etiology, and consequences. International Working Group on Sarcopenia. Journal of the American Medical Directors Association. 2011;**12**:249-256

[12] Muscaritoli M, Anker SD, Argiles J, et al. Consensus definition of sarcopenia, cachexia and pre-cachexia: Joint document elaborated by Special Interest Groups (SIG) "cachexia-anorexia in chronic wasting diseases" and "nutrition in geriatrics." Clinical Nutrition. 2010;**29**:154-159

[13] Morley JE. Frailty: A time for action. European Geriatric Medicine. 2013;**4**:215-216

[14] Dam TT, Peters KW, Fragala M, Cawthon PM, Harris TB, McLean R, Shardell M,Alley DE, Kenny A, Ferrucci L, Guralnik J, Kiel DP, Kritchevsky S, Vassileva MT, Studenski S. An evidence-based comparison of operational criteria for the presence of sarcopenia. Journals of Gerontology. Series A: Biological Sciences and Medical Sciences. 2014;**69**(5):584-590

[15] Chen LK, Liu LK, Woo J, Assantachai P, Auyeung TW, Bahyah KS, et al. Sarcopenia in Asia: Consensus report of the Asian Working Group for Sarcopenia. Journal of the American Medical Directors Association. 2014;**15**:95-101

[16] Michel JP. Sarcopenia: There is a need for some steps forward. Journal of the American Medical Directors Association. 2014;**15**:379-380

[17] Studenski et al. The FNIH Sarcopenia Project: Rationale, study description, conference recommendations, and final estimates. Journal of Gerontology. Series A: Biological Sciences and Medical. 2014;**5**:547-558

[18] Cederholm T, Morley JE. Sarcopenia: The new definitions. Current Opinion in Clinical Nutrition & Metabolic Care. 2015;**18**:1-4

[19] Barbat-Artigas S, Rolland Y, Vellas B, Aubertin-Leheudre M. Muscle quantity is not synonymous with muscle quality. Journal of the American Medical Directors Association. 2013;**14**:852.e1-852.e7

[20] Morley JE, Cao L. Rapid screening for sarcopenia. Journal of Cachexia, Sarcopenia and Muscle. 2015;**6**:312-314

[21] Alchin DR. Sarcopenia: Describing rather than defining a condition. Journal of Cachexia, Sarcopenia and Muscle. 2014;**5**:265-268

[22] Drey M, Krieger B, Sieber CC, Bauer JM, Hettwer S, Bertsch T, et al. Motoneuron loss is associated with sarcopenia. Journal of the American Medical Directors Association. 2014;**15**:435-439

[23] Barbat-Artigas S, Pion CH, Leduc-Gaudet JP, Rolland Y, Aubertin-Leheudre M. Exploring the role of muscle mass, obesity, and age in the relationship between muscle quality and physical function. Journal of the American Medical Directors Association. 2014;**15:**303.e13-303.e 20

[24] Kim M, Kim H. Accuracy of segmental multi-frequency bioelectrical impedance analysis for assessing whole-body and appendicular fat mass and lean soft tissue mass in frail women aged 75 years and older. European Journal of Clinical Nutrition. 2013;**67**:395e400

[25] Janssen I, Heymsfield SB, Ross R. Low relative skeletal muscle mass (sarcopenia) in older persons is associated with functional impairment and physical disability. Journal of the American Geriatrics Society. 2002;**50**:889-896

[26] Alley DE, Shardell MD, Peters KW, McLean RR, Dam TT, Kenny AM, Fragala MS,Harris TB, Kiel DP, Guralnik JM, Ferrucci L, Kritchevsky SB, Studenski SA,Vassileva MT, Cawthon PM. Grip strength cutpoints for the identification of clinically relevant weakness. Journal of Gerontology. Series A: Biological Sciences and Medical Sciences. 2014;**69**(5):559-566

[27] Cawthon PM, Peters KW, Shardell MD, McLean RR, Dam TT, Kenny AM, Fragala MS,Harris TB, Kiel DP, Guralnik JM, Ferrucci L, Kritchevsky SB, Vassileva MT,Studenski SA, Alley DE. Cutpoints for low appendicular lean mass that identify older adults with clinically significant weakness. Journal of Gerontology. Series A: Biological Sciences and Medical Sciences. 2014;**69**(5):567-575

[28] McLean RR, Shardell MD, Alley DE, et al. Criteria for clinically relevant weakness and low lean mass and their longitudinal association with incident mobility impairment and mortality: The Foundation for the National Institutes of Health (FNIH) Sarcopenia Project. Journal of Gerontology. Series A: Biological Sciences and Medical Sciences. 2014;**5**:576-583

[29] Lee WJ, Liu LK, Peng LN, Lin MH, Chen LK, ILAS Research Group. Comparisons of sarcopenia defined by IWGS and EWGSOP criteria among older people: Results from the I-Lan longitudinal aging study. Journal of the American Medical Directors Association. 2013;**14**:528.e1-528.e7

[30] Patel HP, Al-Shanti N, Davies LC, Barton SJ, Grounds MD, Tellam RL, et al. Lean mass, muscle strength and gene expression in community dwelling older men: Findings from the Hertfordshire sarcopenia study (HSS). Calcified Tissue International. 2014;**95**(4):308-316

[31] Yamada M, Nishiguchi S, Fukutani N, Tanigawa T, Yukutake T, Kayama H, et al. Prevalence of sarcopenia in community-dwelling Japanese older adults. Journal of the American Medical Directors Association. 2013;**14**:911-915

[32] Legrand D, Vaes B, Matheï C, Swine C, Degryse JM. The prevalence of sarcopenia in very old individuals according to the European consensus definition: Insights from the BELFRAIL study. Age Ageing. 2013;**42**:727-734

[33] Landi F, Liperoti R, Fusco D, Mastropaolo S, Quattrociocchi D, Proia A, et al. Prevalence and risk factors of sarcopenia among nursing home older residents. Journals of Gerontology. Series A: Biological Sciences and Medical Sciences. 2012;**67**:48-55

[34] Landi F, Liperoti R, Fusco D, Mastropaolo S, Quattrociocchi D, Proia A, et al. Sarcopenia and mortality among older nursing home residents. Journal of the American Medical Directors Association. 2012;**13**:121-126

[35] Kim JH, Lim S, Choi SH, Kim KM, Yoon JW, Kim KW, et al. Sarcopenia: An independent predictor of mortality in community dwelling older Korean men. Journal of Gerontology. Series A: Biological Sciences and Medical Sciences. 2014;**69**(10):1244-1252

[36] Vetrano DL, Landi F, Volpato S, Corsonello A, Meloni E, Bernabei R, et al. Association of sarcopenia with short- and long-term mortality in older adults admitted to acute care wards: Results from the CRIME study. Journal of Gerontology. Series A: Biological Sciences and Medical Sciences. 2014;**69**:1154-1161

[37] Wu IC, Lin CC, Hsiung CA, et al. Epidemiology of sarcopenia among community-dwelling older adults in Taiwan: A pooled analysis for a broader adoption of sarcopenia assessments. Geriatrics & Gerontology International. 2014;**14**(Suppl 1):52-60

[38] Tanimoto Y, Watanabe M, Sun W, Sugiura Y, Hayashida I, Kusabiraki T, et al. Sarcopenia and falls in community-dwelling elderly subjects in Japan: Defining sarcopenia according to criteria of the European Working Group on Sarcopenia in Older People. Journal of the American Medical Directors Association. 2010;**11**:391-396

[39] Da Silva AT, de Oliveira Duarte YA, Ferreira Santos JL, Wong R, Lebrão ML. Sarcopenia according to the European Working Group on Sarcopenia in Older People (EWGSOP) versus dynapenia as a risk factor for disability in the elderly. The Journal of Nutrition Health and Aging. 2014;**18**:547-553

[40] Malmstrom TK, Miller DK, Herning MM, Morley JE. Low appendicular skeletal muscle mass (ASM) with limited mobility and poor health outcomes in middle-aged African Americans. Journal of Cachexia, Sarcopenia and Muscle. 2013;**4**:179-186

[41] Duren DL, Sherwood RJ, Czerwinski SA, Lee M, Choh AC, Siervogel RM, Chumlea WC. Body composition methods: Comparisons and interpretation. Journal of Diabetes Science and Technology. 2008;**2**(6):1139-1146

[42] Janssen I, Heymsfield SB, Baumgartner RN, Ross R. Estimation of skeletal muscle mass by bioelectrical impedance analysis. Journal of Applied Physiology. 2000;**89**:465e471

[43] Chien MY, Huang TY, Wu YT. Prevalence of sarcopenia estimated using a bioelectrical impedance analysis prediction equation in community-dwelling elderly people in Taiwan. Journal of the American Geriatrics Society. 2008;**56**:1710e1715

[44] Nigam P, Misra A, Colles SL. Comparison of DEXA-derived body fat measurement to two race-specific bioelectrical impedance equations in healthy Indians. Diabetology & Metabolic Syndrome. 2013;**7**:72-77

[45] Mijnarends DM, Meijers JM, Halfens RJ, et al. Validity and reliability of tools tomeasure muscle mass, strength, and physical performance in community dwelling older people: A systematic review. Journal of the American Medical Directors Association. 2013;**14**:170-178

[46] Yamada Y, Watanabe Y, Ikenaga M, et al. Comparison of single- or multi-frequency bioelectrical impedance analysis and spectroscopy for assessment of appendicular skeletal muscle in the elderly. Journal of Applied Physiology. 2013;**115**:812-818

[47] Baracos V, Caserotti P, Earthman CP, Fields D, Gallagher D, Hall KD, Heymsfield SB, Muller MJ, Rose AN, Pichard C, Redman LM, Shen W, Shepherd JA, Thomas D. Advances in the science and application of body composition. Journal of Parenteral and Enteral Nutrition. 2012;**36**(1):96-107

[48] Cesari M, Fielding RA, Pahor M, Goodpaster B, Hellerstein M, van Kan GA, et al. Biomarkers of sarcopenia in clinical trials recommendations from the International Working Group on Sarcopenia. Journal of Cachexia, Sarcopenia and Muscle. 2012;**3**:181-190

[49] Kelly TL, Wilson KER, Heymsfield SB. Dual X-ray absorptiometry body composition reference values from NHANES. PLoS One. 2009;**4**(9):e7038

[50] Shepherd JA, Fan B, Lu Y, Wu XP, Wacker WK, Ergun DL, Levine MA. A multinational study to develop universal standardization of whole-body bone density and composition using GE Healthcare Lunar and Hologic DXA systems. Journal of Bone and Mineral Research. 2012;**27**(10):2208-2216

[51] Malouf J, DiGregorio S, Del Rio L, Torres F, Marin AM, Farrerons J, Herrera S, Domingo P. Fat tissue measurements by dual-energy X-ray absorptiometry: Cross-calibration of 3 different fan-bean instruments. Journal of Clinical Densitometry: Assessment of Musculoskeletal Health. 2013;**16**(2):212-222

[52] Fan B, Shepherd JA, Levine MA, Steinberg D, Wacker W, Barden HS, Ergun D, Wu XP. National Health and Nutrition Examination Survey whole-body dual-energy X-ray absorptiometry reference data for GE lunar systems. Journal of Clinical Densitometry: Assessment of Musculoskeletal Health. 2014;**17**(3):344-377

[53] Kanis JA, McCloskey E, Johansson H, oden A, Leslie WD. FRAX® with and without bone mineral density. Calcified Tissue International. 2012;**90**:1-13

[54] Malmstrom TK, Morley JE. SARC-F: A simple questionnaire to rapidly diagnose sarcopenia. Journal of the American Medical Directors Association. 2013;**14**:531-532

[55] Morley JE, Malmstrom TK. Can sarcopenia be diagnosed without measurements? European Geriatric Medicine. 2014;**5**:291-293

[56] Alliance for Aging Research. Available from: http://aginginmotion.org/news/2388-2/ [Accessed: January 23, 2017]

[57] Rantanen T, Guralnik JM, Foley D, Masaki K, Leveille S, Curb JD, et al. Midlife hand grip strength as a predictor of old age disability. Journal of the American Medical Association. 1999;**281**:558-560

[58] Szulc P, Beck TJ, Marchand F, Delmas PD. Low skeletal muscle mass is associated with poor structural parameters of bone and impaired balance in elderly men—The MINOS study. Journal of Bone and Mineral Research. 2005;**20**:721-721

[59] Ling CH, Taekema D, deCraen AJ, Gussekloo J, Westendorp RG, Maier AB. Handgrip strength and mortality in the oldest old population: The Leiden 85-plus study. Canadian Medical Association Journal. 2010;**182**:429-435

[60] Landi F, Liperoti R, Russo A, Giovannini S, Tosato M, Capoluongo E, et al. Sarcopenia as a risk factor for falls in elderly individuals: Results from the ilSIRENTE study. Clinical Nutrition. 2012;**31**:652-658

[61] Landi F, Cruz-Jentoft AJ, Liperoti R, Russo A, Giovannini S, Tosato M, et al. Sarcopenia and mortality risk in frail older persons aged 80 years and older: Results from ilSIRENTE study. Age Ageing. 2013;**42**:203-209

[62] Scharf G, Heineke J. Finding good biomarkers for sarcopenia. Journal of Cachexia, Sarcopenia and Muscle. 2012;**3**:145-148

[63] Kalinkovich A, Livshits G. Sarcopenia—The search for emerging biomarkers. Ageing Research Reviews. 2015;**22**:58-71

[64] Evans CJ, Chiou CF, Fitzgerald KA, William WJ, Ferral BR, Dale W, et al. Development of a new patient-reported outcome measure in sarcopenia. Journal of the American Medical Directors Association. 2011;**12**:226-233

[65] Cawthon PM, Fox KM, Gandra SR, Delmonico MJ, Chiou C-F, Anthony MS, et al. Do muscle mass, muscle density, strength, and physical function similarly influence risk of hospitalization in older adults? Journal of the American Geriatrics Society. 2009;**57**:1411-1419. DOI: 10.1111/j.1532-5415.2009.02366.x

[66] Kennis E, Verschueren S, Van Roie E, Thomis M, Lefevre J, Delecluse C. Longitudinal impact of aging on muscle quality in middle-aged men. Age **(Dordrecht, Netherlands)**. 2014;**36**:9689. DOI: 10.1007/s11357-014-9689-1

[67] Lafortuna Cl, Tresoldi D, Rizzo G. Influence of body adiposity on structural characteristics of skeletal muscle in men and women. Clinical Physiology and Functional Imaging. 2014;**34**:47-55

[68] McGregor RA, Cameron-Smith D, Poppitt SD. It is not just muscle mass: A review of muscle quality, composition and metabolism during ageing as determinants of muscle function and mobility later in life. Longevity & Healthspan. 2014;**3**:9

[69] Verdjik LB, Snijders T, Beelen M, Savelberg HHCM, Meijer K, Kuipers H, Van Loon LIC. Characteristics of muscle fiber type are predictive of skeletal muscle mass and strength in elderly men. Journal of the American Geriatrics Society. 2010;**58**:2069-2075

[70] Reid KF, Pasha E, Doros G, Clark DI, Patten C, Phillips EM, Frontera WH, Fielding RA. Longitudinal decline of lower extremity muscle power in healthy and mobility limited older adults: Influence of muscle mass, strength, composition, neuromuscular activation and single fiber contractile properties. European Journal of Applied Physiology. 2014;**114**:29-39

[71] Stenroth L, Peitonen J, Cronin NJ, Sipila S, Finni T. Age-related differences in Achilles tendon properties and triceps surae muscle architecture in vivo. Journal of Applied Physiology. 2012;**113**:1537-1544

[72] Clark BC, Manini TM. Functional consequences of sarcopenia and dynapenia in the elderly. Current Opinion in Clinical Nutrition & Metabolic Care. 2010;**13**:271-276. DOI: 10.1097/MCO.0b013e328337819e

[73] Fragala MS, Dam TTL,Barber V, Judge JO, Studenski SA, Cawthon PM et al. Strength and function response to clinical interventions of older women categorized by weakness and low lean mass using classifications from the Foundation for the National Institutes of Health sarcopenia project. The Journal of Gerontology. Series A, Biological Sciences and Medical Sciences. 2015;**70**:202-209. DOI: 10.1093/Gerona/glu110

[74] Francis P, Toomey C, McCormack W, Lyons M, Jakeman P. Measurement of maximal isometric torque and muscle quality of the knee extensors and flexors in healthy 50-70-year-old women. Clinical Physiology and Functional Imaging. 2016 Jan 7. doi:10.1111/cpf.12332. [Epub ahead of print] PubMed PMID: 26749301

[75] Fragala MS, Fukuda DH, Stout JR, Townsend JR, Emerson NS, Boone CH et al. Muscle quality index improves with resistance exercise training in older adults. Experimental Gerontology. 2014;**53**:1-6. DOI: 10.1016/j.exger.2014.01.037

[76] Fiser WM, Hays NP, Rogers SC, Kajkenowa O, Williams AE, Evans CM, Evan WJ. Energetics of walking in elderly people: Factors related to gait speed. The Journal of Gerontology. Series A, Biological Sciences and Medical Sciences. 2010;**65**:1332-1337

[77] Coen PM, Jubrias SA, Distefano G, Amati F, Mackey DC, Glynn NW, Manini TM, Wohigemuth SE, Leeuwenburgh C, Cummings SR, Newman AB, Ferruci L, Toledo FGS, Shankland E, Conley KE, Goodpaster BH. Skeletal muscle mitochondrial energetics are associated with maximal aerobic capacity and walking speed in older adults. The Journal of Gerontology. Series A, Biological Sciences and Medical Sciences. 2013;**68**:447-455

[78] Zuo L, Hallman AH, Yousif M K, Chien MT. Oxidative stress, respiratory muscle dysfunction, and potential therapeutics in chronic obstructive pulmonary disease. Frontiers in Biology. 2012;7:506-513. DOI: 10.1007/s11515-012-1251-x

[79] Zuo L, Shiah A, Roberts WJ, Chien MT, Wagner PD, Hogan MC. Low PO_2 conditions induce reactive oxygen species formation during contractions in single skeletal muscle fibers. AJP Regulatory Integrative and Comparative Physiology. 2013;**304**:R1009-R1016. DOI: 10.1152/ajpregu.00563.2012

[80] Zuo L, Best T M, Roberts W J, Diaz PT, Wagner PD. Characterization of reactive oxygen species in diaphragm. Acta Physiology. 2015;**213**:700-710. doi:10.1111/apha.12410.

[81] Seo SY, Lee SR, Kim N, Ko KS, Rhee BD, Han J. Age-related changes in skeletal muscle mitochondria: The role of exercise. Integrative Medicine Research. 2016;**5**:182-186

[82] Peterson CM, Johansen DL, Ravussin E. Skeletal muscle mitochondria and aging: A review. Journal of Aging Research. 2012. article ID 194821, DOI: 10.1155/2012/194821

[83] Powers SK, Ji LL, Kavaziz AN, Jackson MJ. Reactive oxygen species: Impact on skeletal muscle. Comprehensive Physiology. 2011;**1**(2):941-969

[84] Bijlsma AY, Meskers CGM, van Heemst D, Westendorp RGJ, de Craen AJM, Maier AB. Diagnostic criteria for sarcopenia relate differently to insulin resistance. Age. 2013;**35**:2367-2375

[85] Kuo C-K, Lin L-Y, Yu Y-H, Wu K-H, Kuo H-K. Inverse association between insulin resistance and gait speed in nondiabetic older men: Results from the U.S. National Health and Nutrition Examination Survey (NHANES) 1999-2002. BMC Geriatrics. 2009;**9**:49

[86] Miljkovic I, Zmuda JM. Epidemiology of myosteatosis. Current Opinion in Clinical Nutrition & Metabolic Care. 2010;**13**:260-264. DOI: 10.1097/MCO.0b013e328337d826

[87] Beavers KM, Beavers DP, Houston DK, Harris TB, Hue TF, Koster A, Newman AB, Simonsick EM, Studenski SA, Nicklas BJ, Kritchevsky SB. Associations between body composition and gait-speed decline: Results from the health, aging, and body composition study. American Journal of Clinical Nutrition. 2013;**97**:552-560

[88] Marcus RL, Addison O, Dibble LE, Foreman KB, Morrell G, Lastayo P. Intramuscular adipose tissue, sarcopenia, and mobility function in older individuals. Journal of Aging Research. 2012;629-637

[89] Manini TM, Clark BC, Nalls MA, Goodpaster BH, Ploutz-Snyder LL, Harris TB. Reduced physical activity increases intermuscular adipose tissue in healthy young adults. American Journal of Clinical Nutrition. 2007;**85**:377-384

[90] Mastrocola R, Collino M, Nigro D, Chiazza F, D'Antona G, Aragno M, et al. Accumulation of advanced glycation end-products and activation of the SCAP/SREBP Lipogenetic pathway occur in diet-induced obese mouse skeletal muscle. PLoS One. 2015;**10**:e0119587. DOI: 10.1371/journal.pone.0119587

[91] Reid KF, Fielding RA. Skeletal muscle power: A critical determinant of physical functioning in older adults. Exerc. Sport Sciences Reviews. 2012;**40**:4-12. DOI: 10.1097/JES.0b013e31823b5f13

[92] Prior SJ, Joseph LJ, Brandauer J, Katzel LI, Hagberg JM, Ryan AS. Reduction in midthigh low-density muscle with aerobic exercise training and weight loss impacts glucose tolerance in older men. The Journal of Clinical Endocrinology & Metabolism. 2007;**92**:880-886

[93] McNeil CJ, Doherty TJ, Stashuk DW, Rice CL. Motor unit number estimates in the tibialis anterior muscle of young, old, and very old men. Muscle Nerve. 2005;**31**:461-467

[94] Clark DJ, Pojednic RM, Reid KF, Patten C, Pasha EP, Phillips EM, Fielding RA. Longitudinal decline of neuromuscular activation and power in healthy older adults. The Journal of Gerontology. Series A, Biological Sciences and Medical Sciences. 2013;**68**:1419-1425

[95] Harris-Love MO, Monfaredi R, Ismail C, Blackman MR, Cleary K. Quantitative ultrasound: Measurement considerations for the assessment of muscular dystrophy and sarcopenia. Frontiers in Aging Neuroscience. 2014;**6**:1-4. DOI: 10.3389/fnagi.2014.00172

3

From Sarcopenia to Frailty: The Pathophysiological Basis and Potential Target Molecules of Intervention

Zhuowei Yu, Qingwei Ruan, Grazia D'Onofrio and
Antonio Greco

Abstract

Skeletal muscle is not only an endocrine organ but also one of core components of musculoskeletal system. Sarcopenia refers to a decline in the skeletal muscle mass and function. The former involves the size and number of changes in two types of myofibers, lower satellite cell density, and regeneration ability. The latter shows a loss of muscle strength. Frailty is a geriatric syndrome with multisystem impairment associated with increased vulnerability to stressors. Sarcopenia increases the risk of frailty and may be one of the major causes of physical frailty phenotype. Sarcopenia is also potentially associated with cognitive frailty phenotype. Aging might be the common underlying pathophysiology of sarcopenia and frailty. Therefore, there are some potential target molecules in aging-related signaling pathways that might be associated with sarcopenia and frailty. Nevertheless, sarcopenia can mediate metabolism and promote accelerate systemic aging, frailty, and age-related diseases by myokines in an endocrine manner. Lifestyle interventions (resistance exercise and dietary restriction) of gerontoscience are effective in the prevention of sarcopenia. Some pharmacological agents are registered in different phases of clinical trials for sarcopenia intervention. Phytochemicals, mTOR inhibitors, metformin and acarbose, NAD precursors, and sirtuin activators demonstrated that multiple target antiaging effects might also have preventive and therapeutic perspectives on sarcopenia and frailty.

Keywords: sarcopenia, physical frailty, cognitive frailty, aging

1. Introduction

Sarcopenia and frailty are two common geriatric conditions that may co-occur within a single individual with aging. Frailty is a heterogeneous clinical condition depended on different domains.

Definitions of frailty includes fried physical frailty phenotype (weight loss, exhaustion, physical inactivity, handgrip strength, and walk time) [1] and frailty index (use of walking aid, activities of daily living, incontinence, cognitive impairment, and multiple other components) [2]. Cognition performance decline is considered as a domain in Frailty index, but as "cognitive frailty" phenotype when physical frailty and potentially reversible cognitive impairment simultaneously occur [3]. Sarcopenia refers to decline in skeletal muscle mass and function, which includes primary sarcopenia, or age-related loss of muscle mass and function decline, and secondary sarcopenia resulting from nutrition, activity, and disease-related loss of muscle mass [4]. Sarcopenia is different from cachexia, which combines the loss of both muscle and fat. Obviously, physical frailty and sarcopenia share the core components, physical function impairment (weakness, slow walking speed, and balance problems), and sarcopenia is considered as the biological substrate and the pathway of physical frailty development [5, 6].

Although it is a controversy, sarcopenia and frailty are two separate conditions based on their definitions, and outpatients with sarcopenia were more likely to be more frail than frail outpatients to be sarcopenic [7]. Skeletal muscle is not only a component of muscloskeletal system but also an endocrine organ. Two components of sarcopenia also obviously contribute to frailty, a geriatric syndrome that has been defined as a multisystem impairment characterized by decreased reserve associated with increased vulnerability to stressors. First, the loss of muscle mass plays a critical role in unintentional weight loss of frailty in the elderly. Second, age-related loss of muscle strength, commonly referred as dynapenia, was associated with both sarcopenia and frailty [8]. Sarcopenia and frailty had the sensitivity and specificity for dynapenia of 33 and 89%, 17 and 98%, respectively. A longitudinal aging study with 731 community-dwelling older people demonstrated that dynapenia was related to the cognitive impairment [9]. Thus, dynapenia is also the important factor responsible for frailty. Moreover, muscle cross-talks with other tissues and organs by myokines in an endocrine manner to mediate metabolism and promote aging, diseases, and frailty. Here, we review the epidemiological evidence and pathophysiological basis of skeletal muscle aging, or primary sarcopenia, that result in frailty and potential target molecules of intervention. Particularly, we focus on the pathophysiological basis of sarcopenia, including age-related changes of nutrient and stress sensors, positive and negative regulators of muscle growth, and the maintenance of muscle mass and function. Moreover, we also summarize the underlying mechanisms of sarcopenia accelerating systemic aging, frailty, and age-related diseases. Finally, we looked for the potential target molecules of intervention of sarcopenia according to the pathophysiological basis and relevant signal pathways.

2. From Sarcopenia to frailty: the pathophysiological basis

2.1. From sarcopenia to physical and cognitive frailty: the epidemiological evidence

Frailty is heterogeneous and contains physical and cognitive multiple domains. In this context, the concept of "Cognitive frailty" becomes essential. It refers to simultaneous presence of physical frailty and potentially reversible cognitive impairment but without dementia [3]. Cognitive frailty includes reversible and potentially reversible subtypes [10] and may represent a precursor of neurodegenerative processes [10]. The link between physical function and cognitive decline provides important targets to develop effective preventive strategies in earlier cognitive impairment stages [3, 11, 12].

Epidemiological studies suggested that sarcopenia increases the risks of both physical frailty and cognitive impairment. Loss of muscle mass and strength is associated with increased dependence, frailty, and mortality. Low appendicular lean mass related to body mass index could detect patients at risk for frailty [13]. A cross-sectional study with small subjects, 273 Japanese community-dwelling older women aged >65 years showed that sarcopenia was related only with prefrailty and frailty, and cognitive decline was related to frailty [14]. However, several studies showed an association between sarcopenia parameters and cognitive impairment. Low handgrip strength was shown to correlate with a decrease in Mini Mental State Examination (MMSE) score [15]. Other studies also reported an association between handgrip strength and the risk of Alzheimer disease and the rate of cognitive decline [16–18]. In prospective studies, a decrease in physical performance in relation to future dementia was demonstrated [19, 20]. Subjects aged >65 years who scored low in a physical performance test had a three-times higher risk of developing dementia at a 6-year follow-up [21]. Recently, the new concept of "Motoric Cognitive Risk (MCR) syndrome" was defined as having mild cognitive impairment (MCI) and slow gait, supporting the common underlying mechanism in physical and cognitive impairment [22]. MCR offered further benefit on predicting dementia than MCI or slow gait alone. A recent study demonstrated an association between increased risk of cognitive impairment, mainly MCI, and poor lower extremity function [21].

2.2. Aging promotes sarcopenia and frailty

Factors relating to skeletal muscle mass and strength changes include the loss of motor units innervating muscle, age-related hormone changes, muscle hypoxia resulting from atherosclerosis and chronic proinflammatory status, decreased physical activity and protein intake, age-related insulin resistance, and mitochondrial dysfunction [23]. Aging leads to a preferential reduction of type II myofiber size. There is a significant loss of type II muscle fibers, lower satellite cell density, and lower satellite cell/fiber ratio in older individuals with sarcopenia [24]. The loss of motor units innervating muscle, especially type II myofibers [25], and the decreased blood flow to muscle [26] results in the loss of muscle mass. Meanwhile, many elderly population with insulin resistance who maintains the sensitivity of glucose metabolism, but not protein synthesis, show age-related anabolic resistance, meaning the reduced muscle protein synthesis [27, 28]. However, muscle of older individuals with type 2 diabetes [29] metabolic syndrome [30] demonstrated a significant low proportion of type I fibers that is positively associated with the severity of insulin resistance. Thus, the loss of muscle mass and the alterations of myofiber type proportion due to insulin resistance could potentially affect whole body glucose homeostasis [31]. Age-related hormone changes, for example, the decline of anabolic hormone testosterone leads to the loss of both muscle mass and strength [32]. The decline in both growth hormone and insulin-like growth factor 1 are related to the loss of muscle mass but not muscle strength [33]. Muscle hypoxia results from atherosclerosis and chronic proinflammatory status leads to the loss of both muscle mass and strength [25]. Other factors, decreased physical activity and protein intake, also involve in the loss of muscle mass.

Age-related decline of the levels of 25(OH) vitamin D due to a decreased production of 25(OH) vitamin D in skin or a decline in vitamin D absorption can result in the decline of muscle function [25]. Age-related insulin resistance causes an increase of fat infiltration into muscle and a decline in muscle strength [34]. Mitochondrial dysfunction in aging skeletal muscle causes oxidative damage and the decline of energy generation to maintain function properly [35].

The biological mechanisms underlying the association between sarcopenia and frailty are uncertain [36]. Any plausible explanations are that physical, motor, and cognitive functions are not causally related but are affected by common underlying pathophysiology [37]. Frailty, cognitive impairment, and sarcopenia share many common risk factors, such as immune or inflammatory response, oxidative stress, and hormonal dysregulation [38, 39]. In view of this, frailty, cognitive impairment, and sarcopenia may be highly interrelated [38, 40]. Inflammatory markers such as C-reactive protein and interleukin-6 concentrations are correlated negatively with muscle strength and physical performance [41, 42]. According to the definition of cognitive frailty, physical factors are the potential causes of cognitive impairment. In a study, high levels of these markers are associated with a 66% increase in cognitive impairment risk at 4-year follow-up in elders with metabolic syndrome [43]. Elevated oxidative stress [44], decreased sex steroid levels [45, 46], and insulin resistance [47, 48] are also involved in the association between physical and cognitive dysfunction.

2.3. The maintenance of muscle mass and function

The maintenance of normal muscle mass and function depends on the dynamic balance between positive and negative regulators of muscle growth. Muscle growth promoters include follustatin (FST), bone morphogenetic proteins (BMPs), brian-derived neurotrophic factor (BDNF), and irisin. Muscle growth suppressors contain myostatin, transforming growth factor beta (TGFβ), activins A and B, growth, and differentiation factor-11 and -15 [49, 50]. Age-related changes of these molecules, together with other factors, such as age-related diseases, chronic low-grade systemic inflammation, insulin resistance, endocrine aging, low physical activity, aging-related impairment of neuromuscular junction dysfunction, and contractile insufficiency because of skeletal muscle-specific troponin T leakage from sarcomere, result in imbalance between positive and negative regulators of muscle growth and sarcopenia development [49]. Muscle growth suppressors through the antibody-coupled, T-cell receptor/anaplastic lymphoma kinase 4,5 (ActR/Alk 4,5), or type I and II TGFβ receptor (TβRI and TβRII), phosphorylate mothers against decapentaplegic homolog 2/3 (SMAD 2/3), then combine SMAD 4 and inhibit the activation of an alternative pathway/mammalian target of rapamycin (Alt/mTOR) signal. TGFβ promotes SMAD3 binding to the promoters of both fibronectin type III domain containing 5 (FNDC5) and procaspase-activating compound 1α (PAC-1α), and suppresses the expression of irisin and PAC-1α [51].The elevated growth differentiation factor 11 (GDF11) increases the risk for age-related frailty and comorbidities [50]. Muscle growth promoters through their receptors phosphorylate SMAD 1/5/8 decrease the inhibition of Alt/mTOR signal and maintain muscle mass and strength. Insulin resistance due to aging, obesity, and diabetes results in the suppression of insulin/insulin-like growth factor-1/phosphatidyl Inositol 3-kinase/protein kinase B (IGF 1/PI3K/AKT)/mTOR, and muscle hypotrophy and dysfunction of metabolism;

the less activated Alk fails to block the nuclear translocation of Foxo 3 to enhance the expression of autophagy-related genes and the consequent protein degradation [31, 52].

2.4. Sarcopenia accelerates systemic aging, frailty, and age-related diseases

Skeletal muscle influence systemic aging and lifespan by nutrient and stress sensors and myokines [53]. DNA damage and mutations are particularly prominent in aging skeletal muscle. Overexpression of phosphoenolpyruvate carboxykinase (PEPCK-C) and mitochondrial uncoupling proteins delays reproductive aging and decreases the incidence of several age-related diseases. Nutrient and stress sensors in sarcopenia include decreased sirturin 1 resulting from low nicotinamide adenine dinucleotide (NAD)+ synthesis and high NAD+ consumption and low adenosine monophosphate-dependent protein kinase (AMPK) activity, which results in the decline of the activity of peroxisome proliferator-activated receptor gamma coactivator-1a (PGC-1a) [54, 55]. The overexpression of AMPK and PGC-1a in muscle not only delays the age-related muscle deterioration but also slows the functional decline of other tissues, delay age-related metabolic defects, including systemic low-grade chronic inflammation, insulin resistance, increase in the stress resistance of the organism and extend lifespan. The other two nutrient sensors, insulin/insulin-like growth factor (IIS) and mTOR signaled nutrient abundance (high fat, amino acids, and sugar diet) and anabolic activity, are major accelerators of aging. mTOR inhibition by rapamycin or mTORC1 activity inhibition by genetical modification, and the downregulation of mTORC1/ribosomal protein S6 kinase beta-1 (S6K1) increases lifespan in mammals [55]. The decrease in regenerative capacity and skeletal muscle loss with age coincides with suppression of IIS pathways which is an attempt to promote longevity of the organism and survival within the tissue [56]. Age-related sarcopenia is associated with an increase in abdominal obesity, which refers to sarcopenic obesity [57]. Sarcopenic obesity leads to the infiltration of fat into the muscle and the accumulation of triglycerides within the cell, which impairs the function of the insulin receptor substrate causing insulin resistance, a lower lipid buffering capacity, and anabolic resistance in muscle [23, 58]. Sarcopenic obesity also results in cognitive impairment because of insulin resistance. In a cohort of 1570 older British men, compared with participants in the normal cognitive aging group, those elder men with severe cognitive impairment were more likely to be sarcopenic, with waist circumference >102 cm, BMI >30 kg/m^2 and to be in the upper quintile of total fat mass, central fat mass, peripheral fat mass, and visceral fat level after age-adjusted multinomial logistic regressions [59]. In experiment animal mouse, obesity in combination with sarcopenia exacerbates blood-brain barrier disruption, neuroinflammation, and oxidative stress of hippocampus, which likely contribute to the remarkable cognitive decline [60]. Calorie restriction and exercise increase the concentrations of metabolic effectors NAD+ and AMP but reduce the concentrations of the hormonal effectors IIS and growth hormone. Meanwhile, these interventions also decrease the levels of glucose, amino acids, and lipids, recover downstream activity, such as DNA repair, mitochondrial biogenesis, and function, promote homeostasis, decrease frailty and comorbidities.

Beyond the profound influence on systemic aging and body metabolism, muscle secrete myokines, which act on muscles and other tissues, such as adipose, bones and brain in an autocrine, paracrine, and endocrine fashion [61]. The metabolites released from muscle and the interactions between muscle and nerve also participate in the systemic effects of muscle on the organism's physiology. Exercise can activate PGC-1α/FNDC5 pathway, promote myokine irisin secretion, induce hippocampal BDNF release, and improve cognitive function [62].

3. From sarcopenia to frailty: the potential target molecules of intervention

The major causes of frailty include chronic diseases, such as congestive heart failure, diabetes, chronic obstructive pulmonary disease (COPD), anemia, polymyalgia rheumatic, and endocrine disorder; decreased nutrient intake because of anorexia resulting from social factors, decline in taste and smell, altered fundal compliance, enhanced release of cholecystokinin, increased leptin and cytokines, sarcopenia, and pain [63]. Treating the chronic diseases can reverse the loss of muscle mass and frailty, such as with angiotensin-converting enzyme inhibitors in some patients with congestive heart failure, both erythropoietin and darbepoietin-α in the individuals with anemia, and vitamin B12 supplementation in acrocytic anemia and related cognitive impairment. Lifestyle interventions play critical roles in the prevention of sarcopenia, frailty, and cognitive impairment. Physical exercise, particularly resistance exercise, can improve muscle mass and strength in the elderly [64, 65] and obese elderly [58]. Individuals with higher initial adiposity experience less improvement in both muscle strength and physical function [66]. Moreover, the addition of caloric restriction during resistance training improves mobility and does not compromise other functional adaptations to resistance training [66]. Resistance training also can increase circulating irisin [67] and improve cognitive performance [62]. In addition, physical exercise and caloric restriction can benefit age-related insulin resistance, reduced mitochondrial biogenesis, and failure of autophagy [68]. However, it is undesirable to use caloric restriction alone in sarcopenic elderly, which results in further loss of lean tissue mass. The oldest olds also with anabolic resistance and frailty find it difficult to perform resistance exercise to achieve benefit effects.

Dietary interventions including protein intake, antioxidants, and vitamin D fortification may benefit the conditions of sarcopenia and frailty. Protein supplies the amino acids, especially leucine, which may activate the signaling pathways required for muscle synthesis. Vitamin D deficiency is common in individuals with sarcopenia, frailty, and cognitive impairment. However, the effects of both protein supplementation and vitamin D intervention on muscle strength and physical performance have mixed results [69]. Although individuals with higher overall antioxidant status have better physical function, such as walking speed [70], antioxidant interventions might not attenuate, and even aggravate sarcopenia due to the health-promoting action of reactive oxygen spices [71].

There are no licensed treatments for sarcopenia and frailty. Pharmacological agents proposed and focused by investigators, with potential for treating sarcopenia include the myostatin signaling pathway and hormone replacement therapy (**Table 1**), currently are at various stages of development [72]. Myostatin, the family member of TGF-β, is a skeletal muscle-specific myokine. Myostain binding with activin type IIB receptor inhibits myoblast proliferation, muscle

Mechanism of action	Drug name	Drug developer	Indication sought	Study phase
I. Myostatin antagonists				
Activin receptor trap	ACE-031	Acceleron	Duchenne muscular dystrophy	Phase 3 (trial terminated early)
Myostatin antibody	REGN-1033	Regeneron/Sanofi	Sarcopenia	Phase 2
	LY-2495655	Eli Lilly	Hip arthroplasty Elderly Fallers Cancer cachexia	Phase 2
	PF-06252616	Pfizer	Inclusion body myositis	Phase 1
Activin receptor inhibitor	Bimagrumab (BMY338)	Novartis	Sarcopenia Hip fracture Cancer and COPD cachexia	Phases 2 and 3 Phase 2
II. Selective androgen receptor modulators	Enobasarm (ostarine)	GTx	Cancer cachexia	Phase 3 (did not meet primary endpoint)
III. Skeletal troponin activators	Tirasemtiv CK-2017357	Cytokinetics	Amyotrophic lateral sclerosis myasthenia gravis	Phases 2 and 3

Table 1. Pharmacological agents in development with potential for treating sarcopenia [72].

strength, and mass by negative regulation of mTOR signaling [73]. Myostatin inhibition by activin receptor trap or inhibitor and myostatin antibody might be useful agent for the treatment of human muscle degenerative diseases (**Table 1**) [72]. Testosterone supplementation is another major focus for drug discovery of sarcopenia. Testosterone could increase both muscle mass and strength in men but are linked to adverse cardiovascular events with short durations of therapy [74, 75]. In order to decrease the side effects of testosterone, the selective androgen receptor molecules, including steroids and nonsteroids, have been developed, and some are at phase 3 (**Table 1**). Tirasemtiv is a fast skeletal troponin activator that sensitizes the sarcomere to calcium and amplifies the function of muscle in neuromuscular diseases, such as Amyotrophic Lateral Sclerosis and myasthenia gravis (**Table 1**) [76, 77].

Age is the greatest risk factor for nearly every major cause of mortality in developed nations [78] and the profound effect of aging on sarcopenia, frailty, and cognitive impairment is often overlooked. A number of aging-associated molecular signals might be the potential target in the prevention and treatment of sarcopenia, frailty, and cognitive impairment. Genetic or pharmacological regulation of NAD+/Sirt1, sestrins/AMPK/PGC1α, IGF-1/Akt/mTOR, TGF-β, myostatin, activins, GDFs /SMAD2/3, BMPs/SMAD1/5/8 signal molecules, myokine irisin and FGF21, the antagonist of myokine myostatin propeptide follistatin or follistatin-like 3, and urocortins can not only improve muscle mass and/or function but also delay frailty and age-related diseases [31, 54, 68]. Besides dietary restriction and exercise, geroscience interventions with translational potential include mTOR inhibitors, metformin and acarbose, NAD precursors and sirtuin activators, modifiers of senescence and telomere dysfunction, hormonal and circulating factors, and mitochondrial-targeted therapeutics [78]. Phytochemicals obviously are ideal geroscience interventions with translational potential. They not only have multiple target molecules in many aging-related signalling pathways, such as sestrins/AMPK/PGC1α, IGF-1/Akt/mTOR, against chronic inflammation and oxidative stress but also have systemic influence with low side effects, including skeletal muscle and other domains of frailty [79, 80].

4. Conclusion and perspective

Sarcopenia is one of the important causes of physical frailty. Frailty contains different phenotypes, such as physical frailty and cognitive frailty or multiple domains in frailty index. Skeletal muscle influences body metabolism, systemic aging, accelerates physical frailty, cognitive impairment, and decrease healthy lifespan. Individuals with primary sarcopenia have an increase in the risk for frailty, cognitive impairment, and age-related diseases. Aging might be the common mechanism of sarcopenia, frailty, and cognitive impairment. Cognitive frailty is an important target of the prevention for both physical and cognitive disability [81]. Although some pharmacological agents are registered in different phases of clinical trials for sarcopenia intervention, no drug is really used for the clinical treatment of sarcopenia. Phytochemicals have effects on multiple targets of aging-related signaling pathways, and other targeted aging molecules, such as mTOR inhibitors, metformin and acarbose, NAD precursors, and sirtuin activators [78, 82], have preventive and therapeutic perspectives on sarcopenia, frailty, and age-related diseases.

Acknowledgements

This work was supported by grants from the Shanghai Hospital Development Center (No. SHDC12014221), Shanghai Municipal Commission of Health and Family Planning, Key developing disciplines (2015ZB0501).

Author details

Zhuowei Yu[1,2], Qingwei Ruan[1,2]*, Grazia D'Onofrio[3] and Antonio Greco[3]

*Address all correspondence to: 13661717346@163.com

1 Shanghai Institute of Geriatrics and Gerontology, Shanghai Key Laboratory of Clinical Geriatrics, Huadong Hospital, Shanghai, China

2 Research Center of Aging and Medicine, Shanghai Medical College, Fudan University, Shanghai, China

3 Department of Medical Sciences, Geriatric Unit & Laboratory of Gerontology and Geriatrics, IRCCS "Casa Sollievo della Sofferenza", San Giovanni Rotondo, Foggia, Italy

References

[1] Fried LP, Tangen CM, Walston J, et al. Frailty in older adults evidence for a phenotype. The Journals of Gerontology. Series A, Biological Sciences and Medical Sciences. 2001;**56**:M146eM157

[2] Rockwood K, Stadnyk K, MacKnight C, et al. A brief clinical instrument to classify frailty in elderly people. Lancet. 1999;**353**:205-206

[3] Kelaiditi E, Cesari M, Canevelli M, et al. Cognitive frailty: Rational and definition from an (I.A.N.A./I.A.G.G.) international consensus group. The Journal of Nutrition Health and Aging. 2013;**17**:726-734

[4] Cruz-Jentoft AJ, Baeyens JP, Bauer JM, et al. Sarcopenia: European consensus on definition and diagnosis report of the European working group on sarcopenia in older people. Age Ageing. 2010;**39**:412-423

[5] Bernabei R, Martone AM, Vetrano DL, Calvani R, Landi F, Marzetti E. Frailty, physical frailty, sarcopenia: A new conceptual model. Studies in Health Technology and Informatics. 2014;**203**:78-84

[6] Landi F, Calvani R, Cesari M, Tosato M, Martone AM, Bernabei R, Onder G, Marzetti E. Sarcopenia as the biological substrate of physical frailty. Clinics in Geriatric Medicine. 2015;**31**(3):367-374

[7] Reijnierse EM, Trappenburg MC, Blauw GJ, Verlaan S, de van der Schueren MA, Meskers CG, Maier AB. Common ground? The concordance of sarcopenia and frailty definitions. Journal of American Medical Directors Association. 2016;**17**(4):371.e7-12

[8] Iwamura M, Kanauchi M. A cross-sectional study of the association between dynapenia and higher-level functional capacity in daily living in community-dwelling older adults in Japan. BMC Geriatrics. 2017;**17**:1

[9] Huang CY, Hwang AC, Liu LK, Lee WJ, Chen LY, Peng LN, Lin MH, Chen LK. Association of dynapenia, sarcopenia, and cognitive impairment among community-dwelling older Taiwanese. Rejuvenation Research. 2016;**19**(1):71-78

[10] Ruan Q, Yu Z, Chen M, et al. Cognitive frailty, a novel target for the prevention of elderly dependency. Ageing Research Reviews. 2015;**20**:1-10

[11] Desai AK, Grossberg GT, Chibnall JT. Healthy brain aging: A road map. Clinics in Geriatric Medicine. 2010;**26**:1-16

[12] Ruan Q, D'Onofrio G, Sancarlo D, Greco A, Yu Z. Potential fluid-biomarkers of pathologic brain changes in Alzheimer's disease, implication in the screening of cognitive frailty. Molecular Medicine Report. 2016;**14**(4):3184-3198

[13] Spira D, Buchmann N, Nikolov J, Demuth I, Steinhagen-Thiessen E, Eckardt R, Norman K. Association of low lean mass with frailty and physical performance: A comparison

between two operational definitions of sarcopenia-data from the Berlin Aging Study II (BASE-II). The Journals of Gerontology. Series A, Biological Sciences and Medical Sciences. 2015;**70**(6):779-784

[14] Nishiguchi S, Yamada M, Fukutani N, Adachi D, Tashiro Y, Hotta T, Morino S, Shirooka H, Nozaki Y, Hirata H, Yamaguchi M, Arai H, Tsuboyama T, Aoyama T. Differential association of frailty with cognitive decline and sarcopenia in community-dwelling older adults. Journal of American Medical Directors Association. 2015;**16**(2):120-124

[15] Auyeung TW, Lee JS, Kwok T, Woo J. Physical frailty predicts future cognitive decline- a four-year prospective study in 2737 cognitively normal older adults. The Journal of Nutrition Health and Aging. 2011;**15**:690-769

[16] Alfaro-Acha A, Al Snih S, Raji MA, Kuo YF, Markides KS, Ottenbacher KJ. Handgrip strength and cognitive decline in older Mexican Americans.. The Journals of Gerontology. Series A, Biological Sciences and Medical Sciences. 2006;**61**:859-865

[17] Taekema DG, Gussekloo J, Maier AB, Westendorp RG, de Craen AJ. Handgrip strength as a predictor of functional, psychological and social health. A prospective population-based study among the oldest old. Age Ageing. 2010;**39**:331-337

[18] Boyle PA, Buchman AS, Wilson RS, Leurgans SE, Bennett DA. Association of muscle strength with the risk of Alzheimer disease and the rate of cognitive decline in community-dwelling older persons. Archives of Neurology. 2009;**66**(11):1339-1344

[19] Wang L, Larson EB, Bowen JD, van Belle G. Performance-based physical function and future dementia in older people. Archives of Internal Medicine. 2006;**166**:1115-1120

[20] Camicioli R, Howieson D, Oken B, Sexton G, Kaye J. Motor slowing precedes cognitive impairment in the oldest old. Neurology. 1998;**50**:1496-1498

[21] Moon JH, Moon JH, Kim KM, Choi SH, Lim S, Park KS, Kim KW, Jang HC. Sarcopenia as a predictor of future cognitive impairment in older adults. The Journal of Nutrition Health and Aging. 2016;**20**(5):496-502

[22] Verghese J, Annweiler C, Ayers E, et al. Motoric cognitive risk syndrome: Multicountry prevalence and dementia risk. Neurology. 2014;**83**:718-726

[23] Kalyani RR, Corriere M, Ferrucci L. Age-related and disease-related muscle loss: The effect of diabetes, obesity and other diseases. Lancet Diabetes Endocrinology. 2014;**2**(10):819-829

[24] Purves-Smith FM, Sgarioto N, Hepple RT. Fiber typing in aging muscle. Exercise and Sport Sciences Reviews. 2014;**42**:45-52

[25] Morley JE. Frailty and sarcopenia: The new geriatric giants. Rev Invest Clin. 2016; **68**(2):59-67

[26] Leenders M, Verdijk LB, van der Hoeven L, et al. Patients with type 2 diabetes show a greater decline in muscle mass, muscle strength, and functional capacity with aging. Journal of American Medical Directors Association. 2013;**14**:585-592

[27] Rasmussen BB, Fujita S, Wolfe RR, Mittendorfer B, Roy M, Rowe VL & Volpi E. Insulin resistance of muscle protein metabolism inaging. FASEB Journal. 2006;**20**:768-769

[28] Fujita S, Glynn EL, Timmerman KL, Rasmussen BB & Volpi E. Supraphysiological hyperinsulinaemia is necessary to stimulate skeletal muscle protein anabolism in older adults: Evidence of atrue age-related insulin resistance of muscle protein metabolism. Diabetologia. 2009;**52**:1889-1898

[29] Oberbach A, Bossenz Y, Lehmann S, Niebauer J, Adams V, Paschke R, Schon MR, Bluher M & Punkt K. Altered fiber distribution and fiber-specific glycolytic and oxidative enzyme activity in skeletal muscle of patients with type 2 diabetes. Diabetes Care. 2006;**29**:895-900

[30] Stuart CA, McCurry MP, Marino A, South MA, Howell ME, Layne AS, Ramsey MW & Stone MH. Slow-twitch fiber proportion in skeletal muscle correlates with insulin responsiveness. Journal of Clinical Endocrinology and Metabolism. 2013;**98**:2027-2036

[31] Cleasby ME, Jamieson PM, Atherton PJ. Insulin resistance and sarcopenia: Mechanistic links between common co-morbidities. Journal of Endocrinology. 2016;**229**:R67-R81

[32] Baumgartner RN, Waters DL, Gallagher D, et al. Predictors of skeletal muscle mass in elderly men and women. Mechanisms of Ageing and Development. 1999;**107**:123-136

[33] Morley JE. Scientific overview of hormone treatment used for rejuvenation. Fertility and Sterility. 2013;**99**:1807-1813

[34] Rolland Y, Lauwers-Cances V, Cristini C, et al. Difficulties with physical function associated with obesity, sarcopenia, and sarcopenic-obesity in community-dwelling elderly women: The EPI-DOS study. The American Journal of Clinical Nutrition. 2009;**89**:1895-1900

[35] Hipple RT. Mitochondrial involvement and impact in aging skeletal muscle. Frontiers in Aging Neuroscience. 2014;**6**:211

[36] Clegg A, Young J, Iliffe S, Rikkert, MO, Rockwood K. Frailty in elderly people. Lancet. 2013;**381**(9868):752-762

[37] Hausdorff JM, Buchman AS. What links gait speed and MCI with dementia? A fresh look at the association between motor and cognitive function. The Journals of Gerontology. Series A, Biological Sciences and Medical Sciences. 2013;**68**: 409-411

[38] Fulop T, Larbi A, Witkowski JM, et al. Aging, frailty and age-related diseases. Biogerontology. 2010;**11**(5):547-563

[39] Small GW. The pathogenesis of Alzheimer's disease. Journal of Clinical Psychiatry. 1998;**59**(Suppl 9):7-14

[40] Ruan Q, D'Onofrio G, Sancarlo D, Greco A, Lozupone M, Seripa D, Panza F, Yu Z. Emerging biomarkers and screening for cognitive frailty. Aging Clinical and Experimental Research. 2017. DOI: 10.1007/s40520-017-0741-8 [Epub ahead of print]

[41] Cesari M, Penninx BW, Pahor M, et al. Inflammatory markers and physical performance in older persons: The InCHIANTI study. The Journals of Gerontology. Series A, Biological Sciences and Medical Sciences. 2004;**59**:242-248

[42] Schaap LA, Pluijm SM, Deeg DJ, Visser M. Inflammatory markers and loss of muscle mass (sarcopenia) and strength. American Journal of Medicine. 2006;**119**:526:e529-526. e517

[43] Yaffe K, Kanaya A, Lindquist K, et al. The metabolic syndrome, inflammation, and risk of cognitive decline. Journal of the American Medical Association. 2004;**292**:2237-2242

[44] Berr C, Balansard B, Arnaud J, Roussel A-M, Alpérovitch A. Cognitive decline is associated with systemic oxidative stress: The EVA study. Etude du Vieillissement Arteriel. Journal of American Geriatrics Society. 2000;**48**:1285-1291

[45] Hogervorst E, Bandelow S, Combrinck M, Smith AD. Low free testosterone is an independent risk factor for Alzheimer's disease. Experimental Gerontology. 2004;**39**:1633-1639

[46] Szulc P, Duboeuf F, Marchand F, Delmas PD. Hormonal and lifestyle determinants of appendicular skeletal muscle mass in men: The MINOS study. The American Journal of Clinical Nutrition. 2004;**80**:496-503

[47] Srikanthan P, Karlamangla AS. Relative muscle mass is inversely associated with insulin resistance and pre-diabetes. Findings from the third National Health and Nutrition Examination Survey. The Journal of Clinical Endocrinology & Metabolism. 2011;**96**:2898-2903

[48] Craft S. Insulin resistance and Alzheimer's disease pathogenesis: Potential mechanisms and implications for treatment. Current Alzheimer Research. 2007;**4**:147-152

[49] Kalinkovich A, Livshits G. Sarcopenia—The search for emerging biomarkers. Ageing Research Reviews. 2015;**22**:58-71

[50] Egerman MA, Cadena SM, Gilbert JA, et al. GDF11 increases with age and inhibits skeletal muscle regeneration. Cell Metabolism. 2015;**22**(1):164-174

[51] Tiano JP, Springer DA, Rane SG. SMAD3 negatively regulates serum irisin and skeletal muscle FNDC5 and peroxisome proliferator-activated receptor Y co-activator 1-α during exercise. The Journal of Biological Chemistry. 2015;**290**(12):7671-7684

[52] Sakuma K, Aoi W, Yamaguchi A. Current understanding of sarcopenia: Possible candidates modulating muscle mass. Pflugers Archiv—European Journal of Physiology. 2015;**467**:213-229

[53] Demontis F, Piccirillo R, Goldberg AL, et al. The influence of skeletal muscle on systemic aging and lifespan. Aging Cell. 2013;**12**(6):943-949

[54] Bonkowski MS, Sinclair DA. Slowing ageing by design: The rise of NAD+ and sirtuin-activating compounds. Nature Reviews Molecular Cell Biology. 2016;**17**(11):679-690

[55] López-Otín C, Blasco MA, Partridge L, Serrano M, Kroemer G. The hallmarks of aging. Cell. 2013;**153**(6):1194-1217

[56] Sharples AP, Hughes DC, Deane CS, Saini A, Selman C, Stewart CE. Longevity and skeletal muscle mass: The role of IGF signalling, the sirtuins, dietary restriction and protein intake. Aging Cell. 2015;**14**(4):511-523

[57] Jura M, Kozak LP. Obesity and related consequences to ageing. AGE. 2016;**38**:23

[58] Tardif N, Salles J, Guillet C, Tordjman J, Reggio S, Landrier JF, Giraudet C, Patrac V, Bertrand-Michel J, Migne C, Collin ML, Chardigny JM, Boirie Y, Walrand S. Muscle ectopic fat deposition contributes to anabolic resistance in obese sarcopenic old rats through eIF2α activation. Aging Cell. 2014;**13**(6):1001-1011

[59] Papachristou E, Ramsay SE, Lennon LT, Papacosta O, Iliffe S, Whincup PH, Wannamethee SG. The relationships between body composition characteristics and cognitive functioning in a population-based sample of older British men. BMC Geriatrics. 2015;**15**:172

[60] Tucsek Z, Toth P, Sosnowska D, Gautam T, Mitschelen M, Koller A, Szalai G, Sonntag WE, Ungvari Z, Csiszar A. Obesity in aging exacerbates blood-brain barrier disruption, neuroinflammation, and oxidative stress in the mouse hippocampus: Effects on expression of genes involved in beta-amyloid generation and Alzheimer's disease. The Journals of Gerontology, Series A, Biological Sciences and Medical Sciences. 2014;**69**(10):1212-1226

[61] Ilich JZ, Kelly OJ, Inglis JE, et al. Interrelationship among muscle, fat, and bone: Connecting the dots on cellular, hormonal, and whole body levels. Ageing Research Reviews. 2014;**15**:51-60

[62] Wrann CD, White JP, Salogiannnis J, et al. Exercise induces hippocampal BDNF through a PGC-1α/FNDC5 pathway. Cell Metabolism. 2013;**18**(5):649-659

[63] Sinclair AJ, Morley JE and Vellas B. Pathy's Principles and Practice of Geriatric Medicine. 5th ed. UK: John Wiley & Sons, Ltd; 2012. pp. 1387-1393

[64] Peterson M, Sen A, Gordon P. Influence of resistance exercise on lean body mass in aging adults: A meta-analysis. Medicine & Science in Sports & Exercise. 2012;**43**:249-258

[65] Liu CJ, Latham NK. Progressive resistance strength training for improving physical function in older adults. The Cochrane Database of Systematic Reviews. 2009;(3):CD002759

[66] Nicklas BJ, Chmelo E, Delbono O, Carr JJ, Lyles MF, Marsh AP. Effects of resistance training with and without caloric restriction on physical function and mobility in overweight and obese older adults: A randomized controlled trial. The American Journal of Clinical Nutrition. 2015;**101**(5):991-999

[67] Jedrychowski MP, Wrann CD, Paulo JA, Gerber KK, Szpyt J, Robinson MM, Nair KS, Gygi SP, Spiegelman BM. Detection and quantitation of circulating human irisin by tandem mass spectrometry. Cell Metabolism. 2015;**22**(4):734-740

[68] Sanchis-Gomar F, Pareja-Galeano H, Mayero S, Perez-Quilis C, Lucia A. New molecular targets and lifestyle interventions to delay aging sarcopenia. Front Aging Neuroscience. 2014;**6**:156

[69] Dodds R, Sayer AA. Sarcopenia and frailty: New challenges for clinical practice. Clinical Medicine (London). 2016;**16**(5):455-458

[70] Kaiser M, Bandinelli S, Lunenfeld B. Frailty and the role of nutrition in older people. A review of the current literature. Acta Biomedicine. 2010;**81**(Suppl 1):37-45

[71] Sanchis-Gomar F, and Derbre F. Mitochondrial fission and fusion in human diseases. The New England Journal of Medicine. 2014;**370**:1073-1074

[72] Beaudart C, McCloskey E, Bruyère O, Cesari M, Rolland Y, Rizzoli R, Araujo de Carvalho I, Amuthavalli Thiyagarajan J, Bautmans I, Bertière MC, Brandi ML, Al-Daghri NM, Burlet N, Cavalier E, Cerreta F, Cherubini A, Fielding R, Gielen E, Landi F, Petermans J, Reginster JY, Visser M, Kanis J, Cooper C. Sarcopenia in daily practice: Assessment and management. BMC Geriatrics. 2016;**16**(1):170

[73] Garatachea N, Pinos T, Camara Y, Rodriguez-Romo G, Emanuele E, Ricevuti G, et al. Association of the K153R polymorphism in the myostatin gene and extreme longevity. Age (Dordr). 2013;**35**:2445-2454

[74] Xu L, Freeman G, Cowling BJ, Schooling CM. Testosterone therapy and cardiovascular events among men: A systematic review and meta-analysis of placebo-controlled randomized trials. BMC Medicine. 2013;**11**:108

[75] Wallis CJ, Lo K, Lee Y, Krakowsky Y, Garbens A, Satkunasivam R, Herschorn S, Kodama RT, Cheung P, Narod SA, Nam RK. Survival and cardiovascular events in men treated with testosterone replacement therapy: An intention-to-treat observational cohort study. Lancet Diabetes Endocrinology. 2016;**4**(6):498-506

[76] Sanders DB, Rosenfeld J, Dimachkie MM, Meng L, Malik FI; Tirasemtiv in Myasthenia Gravis Study Group. A double-blinded, randomized, placebo-controlled trial to evaluate efficacy, safety, and tolerability of single doses of tirasemtiv in patients with acetylcholine receptor-binding antibody-positive myasthenia gravis. Neurotherapeutics. 2015;**12**(2):455-460

[77] Russell AJ, Hartman JJ, Hinken AC, Muci AR, Kawas R, Driscoll L, Godinez G, Lee KH, Marquez D, Browne WF 4th, Chen MM, Clarke D, Collibee SE, Garard M, Hansen R, Jia Z, Lu PP, Rodriguez H, Saikali KG, Schaletzky J, Vijayakumar V, Albertus DL, Claflin DR, Morgans DJ, Morgan BP, Malik FI. Activation of fast skeletal muscle troponin as a potential therapeutic approach for treating neuromuscular diseases. Nature Medicine. 2012;**18**(3):452-455

[78] Kaeberlein M, Rabinovitch PS, Martin GM. Healthy aging: The ultimate preventative medicine. Science. 2015;**350**(6265):1191-1193

[79] D'Onofrio G, Sancarlo D, Ruan Q, Yu Z, Panza F, Daniele A, Greco A, Seripa D. Phytochemicals in the treatment of Alzheimer's disease: A systematic review. Current Drug Targets. 2016. [Epub ahead of print]

[80] Corrêa RC, Peralta RM, Haminiuk CW, Maciel GM, Bracht A, Ferreira IC. New phytochemicals as potential human anti-aging compounds: Reality, promise, and challenges. Critical Reviews in Food Science and Nutrition. 2016. [Epub ahead of print]

[81] Panza F, Seripa D, Solfrizzi V, Tortelli R, Greco A, Pilotto A, Logroscino G. Targeting cognitive frailty: Clinical and neurobiological roadmap for a single complex phenotype. Journal of Alzheimer's Disease. 2015;**47**(4):793-813

[82] Verdin E. NAD^+ in aging, metabolism, and neurodegeneration. Science. 2015;**350** (6265):1208-1213

4

Sarcopenia and Malnutrition in the Elderly

Beatriz Lardiés-Sánchez and Alejandro Sanz-París

Abstract

Sarcopenia and malnutrition are both commonly occurring conditions in elderly population. As understood today, sarcopenia is a syndrome characterised by progressive and generalised loss of skeletal muscle mass, physical performance and/or strength, whereas malnutrition has been defined as a condition of an imbalance of energy, protein and other nutrients that can cause measurable negative effects. In many populations, malnutrition and sarcopenia are present simultaneously, and they appear clinically through a combination of decreased body weight and nutrient intake, along with a decrease in muscle mass and function. Moreover, malnutrition is one of the key pathophysiological causes of sarcopenia. Both entities result in numerous and substantial negative outcomes to the patients and the healthcare system, including decreased quality of life and functionality and increased healthcare costs, hospitalisation rates, morbidity and mortality. Early identification of sarcopenia would be of great clinical relevance because the loss of muscle mass and strength with ageing can be largely reversed by proper exercise and nutritional intervention. Clinicians should integrate nutritional assessment with sarcopenia screening for optimal evaluation of these two interrelated issues to help improve clinical outcomes.

Keywords: sarcopenia, malnutrition, muscle, prevalence, elderly people

1. Introduction

The aged population in the developed world is increasing rapidly. Ageing is accompanied by changes in body composition, including a decrease in muscle mass. From the age of 50 years onwards, muscle mass decreases by 1–2% annually and muscle strength is reduced by approximately 1.5% annually between the age of 50 and 60 years [1]. This age-related loss of skeletal muscle mass, resulting in loss of strength and function, is defined as sarcopenia. This geriatric syndrome is associated with an increased risk for adverse outcomes, such as poor quality of life, risk of falls and death. Moreover, it is a major contributing factor of physical disability, frailty and loss of independence in the elderly. It may be thus an important and potentially reversible cause of morbidity and mortality in older persons [2].

On the other hand, malnutrition is described as a chronic or acute condition of the body in which a deficiency or imbalance of energy, protein and other nutrients leads to negative effects on function, clinical outcomes and body composition [3].

Sarcopenia and malnutrition have similar physiological mechanisms and are common and overlapping in older adults. Both entities result in numerous and substantial negative outcomes to the patients and the healthcare system, including decreased quality of life and functionality and increased healthcare costs, hospitalisation rates, morbidity and mortality. Both entities are highly prevalent among population over the age of 65 years and more, especially in those living in nursing homes or hospitalised [4].

Early identification of sarcopenia and malnutrition would seem to be of clinical relevance because the nutritional deficiencies and the loss of muscle mass and strength with ageing can be largely reversed by proper lifelong improvements in nutritional intervention and physical activity. They are probably the most effective intervention to improve physical functioning, prevent falls and disabilities and, consequently, improve the quality of life in the older population. This is especially important given that world is ageing and older adults will utilise healthcare services at an increased rate in the next years [4].

2. Sarcopenia

2.1. Definition, mechanisms, causes and prevalence of sarcopenia

The term sarcopenia is derived from the Greek words 'sarx' (flesh) and 'penia' (loss). Unlike earlier definitions of sarcopenia, focusing on measurements of low muscle mass only, the current definition of sarcopenia according to the European consensus of the EWGSOP (European Working Group on Sarcopenia in Older People) [5] requires the presence of both low muscle mass and low muscle function (muscle strength or physical performance), although they have not achieved consensus on the cut-off points of muscle mass indicating sarcopenia. The International Working Group on Sarcopenia (IWGS) also proposed an operational definition of sarcopenia, which was targeted to individuals with functional decline, mobility-related difficulties, history of recurrent falls, recent unintentional weight loss, post-hospitalisation and chronic conditions [6, 7].

In many older people, sarcopenia is a multifactorial process where several mechanisms can be involved. When the only evident cause of sarcopenia is the ageing, sarcopenia can be considered as primary (or age-related). In fact, malnutrition status is one of the main causes of sarcopenia (protein-poor diet determines a compensatory response characterised by a reduction in lean mass) [8].

Epidemiological data suggest that the prevalence of sarcopenia varies widely, depending on the different populations studied, gender, age, settings, diagnostic criteria used and the cut-off points chosen to define a low muscle mass. In a recent systematic review [9], five European studies were found using EWGSOP criteria to define sarcopenia in ageing people using BIA (bioelectrical impedance analysis) in different settings, with a prevalence of sarcopenia between 7.5 and 77.6%. The highest prevalence was found in people staying in convalescence and rehabilitation units, while community-dwelling older people had the lowest prevalence.

3. Malnutrition

3.1. Definition and aetiology of malnutrition

Malnutrition has been defined as a condition of an imbalance of energy, protein and other nutrients that can cause measurable negative effects on body composition, physical function and clinical outcomes [10].

Older adults are known to be at high risk of malnutrition. Advanced age is an independent risk factor for malnutrition and is associated with a lower body weight, body mass index (BMI) and serum albumin. Malnutrition is not an inevitable side effect of ageing, but many changes associated with the process of ageing can promote a poor nutritional status. The decline in taste acuity and smell, poor dentition and a decreased appetite are some factors that can affect nutrient intake and can lead to malnutrition and its potentially serious consequences. Other factors, such as an increased frequency and severity of acute and chronic medical conditions, multiple medications, social or economic challenges and cognitive decline, all play a role in the aetiology of malnutrition among older adults [11].

3.2. Nutritional assessment in the elderly

The best validated and most widely used test to measure nutritional status of older people is the Mini Nutritional Assessment (MNA). This includes 18 questions regarding weight change, dietary change, gastrointestinal symptoms, mobility, physical assessment and disease and its relationship with nutritional requirements, with a maximum score of 30 points. Patients who score >24 points are considered well nourished, those that score 17–23.5 points are classified as at risk of malnutrition and those who score <17 points are considered malnourished. Using MNA, Guigoz found 5–71% prevalence of malnutrition among 6821 elderly persons after a review of 32 studies and reported that malnutrition risk was higher in those living in nursing homes than in community-dwelling elderly [12].

Another nutritional assessment tool developed for the elderly population is the Nutritional Form for the Elderly (NUFFE). This instrument was designed as a form that contains items that reflect functional, social, nutritional and health-related aspects of nutritional intake [13].

On the other hand, ESPEN (The European Society for Clinical Nutrition and Metabolism) has recently proposed a new consensus definition of malnutrition [14]. According to this definition, individuals identified as 'at risk' of malnutrition proceed in the diagnostic process, with two possible options: body mass index (BMI) <18.5 kg/m² or unintentional weight loss (>10% independent of time or >5% in last 3 months), this last option is always combined with either a low BMI <20 kg/m² (if <70 years old) or <22 kg/m² (if >70 years old) or a low fat-free mass index (FFMI) <15 kg/m² (women) and <17 kg/m² (men).

3.3. Prevalence of malnutrition

Depending on the method or parameters used for the nutritional assessment, prevalence rates of malnutrition among elderly subjects range between 6.5 and 85%. Early identification of older adults at nutritional risk, followed by adequate nutritional intervention, is expected to contribute to conservation of muscle function and muscle strength, and herewith to maintenance the functional independence, the quality of life and possibly to prolong the survival [15].

The prevalence of malnutrition depends on multiple factors, including the definition and the diagnostic criteria used. This prevalence is greater among older adults in healthcare settings. In fact, in hospital settings, malnutrition is approximately 56% in elderly patients [16].

3.4. Malnutrition-sarcopenia syndrome

Malnutrition is common across varying patient populations, particularly in older adults, and sarcopenia prevalence also increases with age. Moreover, malnutrition is regarded as one important contributing factor in the complex aetiology of sarcopenia, and it may be amenable to intervention. In fact, a diagnostic category of malnutrition-related sarcopenia has been proposed [5]. However, usually older people admitted to nursing homes are screened or assessed for either malnutrition or sarcopenia, but rarely for both conditions concurrently. In several populations, malnutrition and sarcopenia are present simultaneously and manifest clinically through a combination of decreased nutrient intake, decreased body weight, along with a decrease in muscle mass, strength and/or physical function [17].

Vanderwoude et al. [4] proposed the term 'malnutrition-sarcopenia syndrome', which embodies the inherent association of both entities, highlighting their combined impact on clinical outcomes, including increased morbidity, infection and complications (as falls and disability), length of hospital stay and rehospitalisation rates, mortality and healthcare costs, apart from decreased quality of life. Malnutrition and sarcopenia are each independently associated with negative health consequences that impact older adults across healthcare settings [18, 19].

There are few published data demonstrating the co-occurrence of malnutrition and sarcopenia in older adults. In a recent study [20], both entities have been studied in a post-acute care geriatric unit, applying the new ESPEN definition of malnutrition and EWGSOP criteria, assessing the potential clinical relationship between them. The prevalence of malnutrition in this population was 19.3%, and the prevalence of sarcopenia was significantly higher in patients with malnutrition: 82.3 versus 45.1% ($p = 0.03$), which means that most patients with sarcopenia fulfilled the ESPEN criteria for diagnosis of malnutrition. On the other hand, in the study of Senior et al. [21], sarcopenia was defined with EWGSOP criteria and nutritional status was assessed with MNA short-form test. According to these criteria, 14.9% of participants with sarcopenia were malnourished and 48.5% were at risk of malnutrition. The prevalence of malnutrition was higher in subjects with low handgrip strength (62.8%) and in participants with severe sarcopenia (60.8%). Moreover, research has shown that reductions in handgrip strength are common in individuals who have sarcopenia as well as in individuals who are malnourished [5, 22].

4. Screening for malnutrition-sarcopenia

Clinicians should integrate nutrition assessment with sarcopenia screening for optimal evaluation of these two interrelated nutritional issues to help improve patients' clinical outcomes [4].

For sarcopenia screening, a simple clinician tool has been suggested by the EWGSOP [5]. This group has developed an algorithm based on gait speed measurement (a cut-off point of >0.8 m/s identifies risk for sarcopenia) as the easiest and most reliable way to begin sarcopenia screening in clinical practice.

Screening tools for malnutrition are intended for the quick identification of patients at risk of malnutrition, for more in-depth nutritional assessment, or for identifying patients at risk of developing complications or even increased risk of mortality. A variety of malnutrition screening tools are available such as the Malnutrition Screening Tool (MST), Malnutrition Universal Screening Tool (MUST) [23], the short form of the Mini Nutritional Assessment (SF-MNA) [24] and Nutrition Risk Screening-2002 (NRS-2002) [25]. Based on the evidence presented, the combination of screening and assessing for malnutrition and sarcopenia is recommended to screen for the presence of malnutrition-sarcopenia syndrome in at-risk patient populations, particularly older adults in clinical settings [4].

Clinicians are urged to screen, assess and treat these conditions currently. By examining aspects of both conditions, clinicians can more fully assess their patients' clinical and nutritional status and can design targeted therapies to meet their needs and improve outcomes [4].

Examining patient's nutritional and functional status through screening and assessment for both malnutrition and sarcopenia will enable clinical practitioners to determine the presence of both entities in their patients and to target interventions to prevent and avoid them [4].

5. Nutritional interventions to prevent sarcopenia

The relationship between muscle mass, strength, physical function and nutritional status has significant clinical implications regarding the therapeutic approaches [26].

Early identification of sarcopenia would be of great clinical relevance because the loss of muscle mass and strength with ageing can be largely reversed by proper exercise programs and nutritional intervention [27]. Of all the therapeutic options available, lifelong improvements in physical activity and diet are probably the most effective public health intervention and the most important treatment option in nursing home residents for this condition, ongoing independence and autonomy in older people. The Society for Sarcopenia, Cachexia and Wasting Disease developed nutritional recommendations for the prevention and management of sarcopenia, which combined exercise with adequate protein and energy intake [28].

On the other hand, adequate caloric intake has to be considered as an essential requisite for any successful therapeutic approach in the institutionalised elderly participants, in terms of prevention and treatment of sarcopenia. Nutrient intake, especially adequate amounts of high-quality protein and amino acids, is the most important anabolic stimulus of skeletal muscle protein synthesis. Epidemiological studies suggest that a low protein intake is associated with sarcopenia. To prevent it, as optimal dietary protein intake, daily 1.0–1.2 g/kg with an optimal repartition over each daily meal or 25–30 g of high-quality protein per meal are recommended. Specifically, the amino acid leucine and meal-induced insulin, both independently stimulate muscle protein synthesis. It has been demonstrated that exercise and amino acid supplementation (3 g of a leucine-enriched balanced essential amino acid mixture twice a day) together may actually be effective in enhancing muscle strength, variables of muscle mass and walking speed in sarcopenic women [29]. Antioxidants and ω 3-polyunsaturated fatty acids may also contribute to the preservation of muscle function. Low 25-hydroxyvitamin D (25(OH)D) serum level in adults is also a potentially modifiable risk factor for sarcopenia [30]. In fact, nutritional interventions combining adequate amounts of vitamin D and proteins are promising strategies to attenuate sarcopenia development [31]. Some studies have shown the effectiveness of other nutritional factors, such as cheese and milk protein and beta-hydroxy-beta-methylbutyrate (HMB), as a potential supplement to improve muscle quality in sarcopenic elderly people [32, 33].

In a recent study [34], Mediterranean dietary pattern (high in olive, low-fat dairy, vegetable, fish, nut and vegetable oil) has demonstrated a favourable role in the prevention of sarcopenia in postmenopausal women, in comparison with a Western pattern (based on high commercial beverage, sugar and dessert, snacks, solid fat, potato, high-fat dairy, legume, organ meat, fast food and sweets). Another study [35] demonstrated that improvements in clinically relevant measures, such as strength and functionality, could be achieved by supplementation with high-quality oral nutritional supplementation.

Other treatments of sarcopenia currently under investigation include testosterone replacement therapy, oestrogens in women, growth hormone and other behavioural and pharmacological strategies. The main limitation of these treatments is the lack of long-term adherence [8].

Author details

Beatriz Lardiés-Sánchez* and Alejandro Sanz-París

*Address all correspondence to: bealardies@gmail.com

Universitary Hospital Miguel Servet, Zaragoza, Spain

References

[1] Buford TW, Anton SD, Judge AR, Marzetti E, Wohlgemuth SE, Carter CS, et al. Models of accelerated sarcopenia: Critical pieces for solving the puzzle of age-related muscle atrophy. Ageing Research Reviews. 2010;**9**(4):369-383. DOI: 10.1016/j.arr.2010.04.004

[2] Serra Rexach JA. Clinical consequences of sarcopenia. Nutrición Hospitalaria. 2006; **21**(3):46-50

[3] García de Lorenzo A, Álvarez-Hernández J, Planas M, Burgos R, Araujo K. The multi-disciplinary consensus work-team on the approach to hospital malnutrition in Spain. Multidisciplinary consensus on the approach to hospital malnutrition in Spain. Nutrición Hospitalaria. 2011;**26**(4):701-710

[4] Vanderwoude MFJ, Alish CJ, Sauer AC, Hegazi RA. Malnutrition-sarcopenia syndrome: Is this the future of nutrition screening and assessment for older adults? Journal of Aging Research. 2012;**2012**:1-8. DOI: 10.1155/2012/651570

[5] Cruz-Jentoft AJ, Baeyens JM, Bauer JM, Boirie Y, Cederholm T, Landi F, et al. Sarcopenia: European consensus on definition and diagnosis: Report of the European Working Group on Sarcopenia in Older People. Age Aging. 2010;**39**:412-423. DOI: 10.1093/ageing/afq034

[6] Fielding RA, Vellas B, Evans WJ, Bhasin S, Morley JE, Newman AB, et al. Sarcopenia: An undiagnosed condition in older adults. Current consensus definition: Prevalence, etiology, and consequences. International Working Group on Sarcopenia. Journal of the American Medical Directors Association. 2011;**12**(4):249-256. DOI: 10.1016/j.jamda.2011.01.003

[7] Visser M, Schaap LA. Consequences of sarcopenia. Clinics in Geriatric Medicine. 2011;**27**:387-399. DOI: 10.1016/j.cger.2011.03.006

[8] Rolland Y, Czerwinski S, Abellan Van Kan G, et al. Sarcopenia: Its assessment, etiology, pathogenesis, consequences and future perspectives. Journal of Nutrition Health and Aging. 2008;**12**:433-450

[9] Lardiés Sánchez B, Sanz-París A, Boj-Carceller D, Cruz-Jentoft AJ. Systematic review: Prevalence of sarcopenia in ageing people using bioelectrical impedance analysis to assess muscle mass. European Geriatric Medicine. 2016;**7**:256-261. DOI: 10.1016/j.eurger.2016.01.014

[10] Sttraton RJ, Green CJ, Elia M. Disease-Related Malnutrition: An Evidence-Based Approach to Treatment. Wallingford, UK; Cambridge, MA: CABI Pub; 2003.

[11] Jensen GL, Mirtallo J, Compher C, Dhaliwal R, Forbes A, Grijalba RF, et al. Adult starvation and disease related malnutrition: A proposal for etiology-based diagnosis in the clinical practice setting from the International Consensus Guideline Committee. Journal of Parenteral and Enteral Nutrition. 2010;**34**(2):156-159

[12] Guigoz Y. The Mini Nutritional Assessment (MNA) review of the literature: What does it tell us? Journal of Nutrition Health and Aging. 2006;**10**(6):466-485

[13] Söderhamn U, Söderhamn O. Reliability and validity of the nutritional form for the elderly (NUFFE). Journal of Advanced Nursing. 2002;**37**(1):28-34

[14] Cederholm T, Bosaeus I, Barazzoni R, Bauer J, Van Gossum A, Klek S, et al. Diagnostic criteria for malnutrition: An ESPEN Consensus Statement Clinical Nutrition. 2015;**34**(3): 335-340. DOI: 10.1016/j.clnu.2015.03.001

[15] Beck AM. Weight loss, mortality and associated potentially modifiable nutritional risk factors among nursing home residents: A Danish follow-up study. Journal of Nutrition Health and Aging. 2015;**19**(1):96-101

[16] Pirlich M, Schütz T, Norman K, et al. The German hospital malnutrition study. Clinical Nutrition. 2006;**25**(4):563-572

[17] Vivanti A, Ward N, Haines T. Nutritional status and associations with falls, balance, mobility and functionality during hospital admission. Journal of Nutrition Health and Aging. 2011;**15**:388-391

[18] Saka B, Ozkaya H, Karisik E, Akin S, Akpinar TS, Tufan F, et al. Malnutrition and sarcopenia are associated with increased mortality rate in nursing home residents: A prospective study. European Geriatric Medicine. 2016;**7**(3):232-238. DOI: 10.1016/j.eurger.2015.12.010

[19] Landi F, Cruz-Jentoft AJ, Liperoti R, Russo A, Giovanni S, Tosato M, et al. Sarcopenia and mortality risk in frail older persons aged 80 years and older: Results from ilSIRENTE study. Age Ageing. 2013;**42**(2):203-209. DOI: 10.1093/ageing/afs194

[20] Sánchez-Rodríguez D, Marco E, Ronquillo-Moreno N, Miralles R, Vázquez-Ibar O, Escalada F. Prevalence of malnutrition and sarcopenia in a post-acute care geriatric unit: Applying the new ESPEN definition and EWGSOP criteria. Clin Nutr. 2016 Sep 9. pii: S0261-5614(16)30233-3. DOI:10.1016/j.clnu.2016.08.024. [Epub ahead of print]

[21] Senior HE, Henwood TR, Beller EM, Mitchell GK, Keogh JW. Prevalence and risk factors of sarcopenia among adults living in nursing homes. Maturitas 2015;**82**(4):418-423. DOI: 10.1016/j.maturitas.2015.08.006

[22] Norman K, Stobäus N, González MC, Schulzke JD, Pirlich M. Hand grip strength: Outcome predictor and marker of nutritional status. Clinical Nutrition. 2006;**30**(2):135-142

[23] Stratton RJ, Hackston A, Longmore D, Dixon R, Price S, Stroud M, King C, Elia M. Malnutrition in hospital outpatients and inpatients: Prevalence, concurrent validity and ease of use of the "malnutrition universal screening tool" (MUST) for adults. British Journal of Nutrition. 2004;**92**(5):799-808

[24] Ranhoff AH, Gjoen AU, Mowé M. Screening for malnutrition in elderly acute medical patients: The usefulness of MNA-SF. Journal of Nutrition Health and Aging. 2005;**9**(4): 221-225

[25] Kondrup J, Rasmussen HH, Hamberg O, Stanga Z, Ad Hoc ESPEN Working Group. Nutritional risk screening (NRS 2002): A new method based on an analysis of controlled clinical trials. Clinical Nutrition. 2003;**22**(3):321-336

[26] Roubenoff R. Sarcopenia: Effects on body composition and function. The Journals of Gerontology. Series A, Biological Sciences and Medical Sciences. 2003;**58**:1012-1017

[27] Malafarina V, Uriz-Otano F, Iniesta R, Gil-Guerrero L. Effectiveness of nutritional supplementation on muscle mass in treatment of sarcopenia in old age: A systematic review. Journal of the American Medical Directors Association. 2013;**14**:10-17. DOI: 10.1016/j.jamda.2012.08.001

[28] Morley JE, Argiles JM, Evans WJ, et al. Nutritional recommendations for the management of sarcopenia. Journal of the American Medical Directors Association. 2010;**11**:391-396

[29] Yanai H. Nutrition for sarcopenia. Journal of Clinical Medicine and Research. 2015;**7**(12): 926-931

[30] Visser M, Deeg DJ, Lips P. Longitudinal Aging Study. Low vitamin D and high parathyroid hormone levels as determinants of loss of muscle strength and muscle mass (sarcopenia): The Longitudinal Aging Study Amsterdam. Journal of Clinical Endocrinology and Metabolism. 2003;**88**(12):5766-5772

[31] Verlaan S, Maier AB, Bauer JM, Bautmans I, Brandt K, Donini LM, et al. Sufficient levels of 25-hydroxyvitamin D and protein intake required to increase muscle mass in sarcopenic older adults: The PROVIDE study. Clinical Nutrition. 2017;**pii:S0261-5614**(17):30010-30019. DOI: 10.1016/j.clnu.2017.01.005

[32] Makanae Y, Fujita S. Role of exercise and nutrition in the prevention of sarcopenia. Journal of Nutritional Science and Vitaminology. 2015;**61**:S125-S127

[33] Kim HK, Sazuki T, Saito K, et al. Effects of exercise and amino acid supplementation on body composition and physical function in community-dwelling elderly Japanese sarcopenic women: A randomized controlled trial. Journal of the American Geriatrics Society. 2012;**60**(1):16-23

[34] Mohseni R, Aliakbar S, Abdollahi A, Yekaninejad MS, Maghbooli Z, Mirzaei K. Relationship between major dietary patterns and sarcopenia among menopausal women. Aging Clin Exp Res. 2017 Feb 21. doi:10.1007/s40520-016-0721-4. [Epub ahead of print]

[35] Cramer JT, Cruz-Jentoft AJ, Landi F, Hickson M, Zamboni M, Pereira SL, et al. Impacts of high-protein oral nutritional supplements among malnourished men and women with sarcopenia: A multicenter, randomized, double-blinded, controlled trial. Journal of the American Medical Directors Association. 2016;**17**(11):1044-1055. DOI: 10.1016/j.jamda.2016.08.009

5

Sarcopenic Dysphagia as a New Concept

Kotomi Sakai and Kunihiro Sakuma

Abstract

Dysphagia (swallowing difficulties) is a serious problem associated with malnutrition, dehydration, aspiration pneumonia, and death. Its well-known causes include stroke, neuromuscular disease, and head and neck cancer, and these affect muscles and sensation during deglutition. In recent years, dysphagia due to sarcopenia (i.e. "sarcopenic dysphagia") has been reported as a new concept. Sarcopenic dysphagia results from low swallowing and general skeletal muscle mass and strength. The characteristic changes in swallowing muscles occur primarily in oral and pharyngeal muscles along with other associated factors. With a rapidly aging population, the number of older adults with sarcopenic dysphagia is expected to increase. Therefore, it is necessary to investigate the pathophysiology and treatment strategies for sarcopenic dysphagia. In this chapter, we summarize previous studies related to sarcopenic dysphagia.

Keywords: sarcopenia, deglutition disorders, rehabilitation

1. Introduction

The term "sarcopenia" was first proposed by Rosenberg [1] to describe age-related decrease in muscle mass. In 2010, the European Working Group on Sarcopenia in Older People (EWGSOP) proposed the sarcopenia consensus on definition and diagnostic criteria. The EWGSOP defined sarcopenia as a geriatric syndrome characterized by progressive and generalized loss of muscle mass and strength. In addition, they proposed diagnostic criteria for sarcopenia [2]. Subsequently, the International Working Group on Sarcopenia (IWGS) proposed similar definitions [3]. In 2014, the Asian Working Group for Sarcopenia (AWGS) proposed diagnostic criteria based on data on Asian populations [4]. In 2016, sarcopenia was recognized as an independent condition by an ICD-10-CM code [5]. Currently, sarcopenia is recognized worldwide.

Since sarcopenia is characterized by generalized loss of muscle mass and function, it can involve a concomitant reduction in swallowing muscles mass and function. Swallowing is defined as "the function of clearing food and drink through the oral cavity, pharynx, and esophagus into the stomach at an appropriate rate and speed" by the International Classification of Functioning, Disability and Health [6]. According to medical terminology, "dysphagia" is the symptom (not a disease) characterized by swallowing problems. Dysphagia has been proposed as a geriatric syndrome such as sarcopenia [7]. In 1992, Veldee and Peth indicated that malnutrition affects swallowing muscles; however, the term "sarcopenia" was not coined [8]. In 2005, Robbins et al. used the term "dysphagia due to sarcopenia" in their study [9]. Since then, studies on dysphagia related to sarcopenia have increased drastically. The term "sarcopenic dysphagia" was first used by kuroda in 2012 [10]. Since then, the term "sarcopenic dysphagia" has been used by mainly Japanese researchers [11]. However, this is not a standard medical term. In 2015, Clave and Shaker, worldwide leading researchers in dysphagia, used the term "sarcopenic dysphagia" in a review article [12], wherein sarcopenic dysphagia was introduced as a new concept of dysphagia. To our knowledge, that was the first article that described the term "sarcopenic dysphagia," except those from Japan.

Dysphagia results in serious complications such as aspiration pneumonia, choking, dehydration, malnutrition, and lower quality of life, all of which are potentially lethal. A meta-analysis on aspiration pneumonia in frail older people revealed that dysphagia is a significant risk factor for aspiration pneumonia [13]. Furthermore, dysphagia negatively affects the nationwide cost of medication because of these complications, readmissions, higher drug intake, and prolonged hospitalization [14, 15]. Therefore, dysphagia is a serious problem that should be prevented and treated.

Many studies have been reported on dysphagia due to neurological diseases such as stroke, Parkinson's disease and other forms of dementia, amyotrophic lateral sclerosis, head and neck cancer, and esophageal cancer. However, articles on sarcopenic dysphagia are few because it is a new concept of dysphagia. We described the number of articles about dysphagia based on years of publication in **Table 1**. We used "aging" or "frail" or "sarcopenia" and "dysphagia"

	Total	2016	2015	2014
Stroke	1416	159	145	134
Head and neck cancer	1019	139	141	120
Parkinson's disease	472	50	53	46
Aging	305	31	31	30
Frail	75	8	6	8
Sarcopenia	38	13	11	6

We set the keywords related to sarcopenia (aging, frail, or sarcopenia) and major causes of dysphagia (stroke, head and neck cancer, or Parkinson's disease) for comparison of research interests. We described the number of articles overall and their years of publication in the last three years. Compared to stroke, Parkinson's disease, and head and neck cancer, articles related to sarcopenic dysphagia are less. The articles were accessed on January 7, 2017.

Table 1. Number of articles retrieved for the terms "dysphagia" or "swallowing" and each keyword on PubMed.

or "swallowing" as keywords for retrieving in PubMed. In addition, stroke or Parkinson's disease or head and neck cancer were used as keywords to compare these with the number of articles on dysphagia related to sarcopenia. Since sarcopenia is a geriatric syndrome [2], the number of older adults with sarcopenia would increase with a rapidly aging worldwide population. Similarly, the number of older adults with sarcopenic dysphagia would increase. Thus, it is important to investigate the clinical conditions and treatment strategies for sarcopenic dysphagia. In this chapter, we summarize dysphagia related to sarcopenia based on previous studies on mainly healthy or frail subjects or those with sarcopenia.

2. Epidemiology of sarcopenic dysphagia

2.1. Definition and prevalence

The current definition of sarcopenic dysphagia is "difficulty swallowing due to sarcopenia of general skeletal and swallowing muscles" [7, 12]. Although the diagnostic criteria for sarcopenia are defined by the cutoff value of muscle mass and physical function or muscle strength [2, 16], the diagnostic criteria for sarcopenic dysphagia have not been standardized. However, a few studies have attempted to investigate the prevalence of sarcopenic dysphagia; these included subjects without diseases directly affecting swallowing function, such as stroke, Parkinson's disease, and head and neck cancer. Maeda and Akagi [17, 18] reported its prevalence as 42.3 and 30%, respectively, in acute older inpatients at admission. In addition, in their prospective observational study [19], 26% of acute older inpatients developed sarcopenic dysphagia within 60 days of admission. Their studies mainly included older inpatients with acute internal diseases. For older inpatients, it is easy to develop sarcopenic dysphagia during hospitalization because of rest in bed and anorexia by illness. In our study subjects, from acute hospitals to a rehabilitation hospital [11], 32.2% of older inpatients had sarcopenic dysphagia on admission. Our study included many older inpatients with orthopedic disorders. These findings suggest that the prevalence of sarcopenic dysphagia is approximately 30–40% in older inpatients. In community-dwelling older adults, the review article reported that approximately 15% of them had dysphagia [20]. The risk factors of dysphagia included age, history of clinical disease, and physical frailty, including reduced activities of daily living. However, this review did not have sarcopenic dysphagia as an endpoint. Older inpatients are at a higher risk of sarcopenic dysphagia than community-dwelling older adults. The prevention, assessment, and intervention for sarcopenic dysphagia are important, especially in older inpatients.

2.2. Etiology

Several pathophysiological mechanisms are known for sarcopenia in general skeletal muscles. Sarcopenia is categorized as primary and/or secondary sarcopenia based on etiology [2]. The most prominent cause of primary sarcopenia is aging, while those of secondary sarcopenia are inactivity (bed rest, sedentary lifestyle, deconditioning, or zero-gravity conditions), malnutrition (inadequate dietary intake), and disease (advanced organ failure such as heart, lung, liver, kidney, brain, inflammatory disease, malignancy, or endocrine disease).

Several studies have shown associations of aging, inactivity, malnutrition, and disease with dysphagia [21–23]. The characteristic change in the swallowing mechanism in healthy older adults, because of aging, is referred to as "presbyphagia" [24]. Anatomical and functional changes due to aging render older adults at risk of dysphagia [25, 26]. Though aging causes reduced swallowing function, it does not cause dysphagia. In relation to inactivity, physical inactivity can cause sarcopenic dysphagia [19]. In our study in a rehabilitation hospital [11], physical activity level was independently associated with the functional level of oral intake of food and liquid. In addition, the duration of tentative nil per os (NPO) without dysphagia assessment in patients with aspiration pneumonia resulted in reduced swallowing ability during treatment [27]. Inactivity of swallowing muscles itself can cause disuse of themselves and appendicular skeletal muscles. Aspiration pneumonia in older adults usually results in bedrest and NPO for treatment. Although aspiration pneumonia is known to be caused by dysphagia, it can also cause sacropenic dysphagia because of inactivity and malnutrition with its treatment. In relation to nutritional status, mid-upper arm circumference was associated with swallowing function [10]. In addition, nutritional status was a factor of the prognosis of swallowing ability in older inpatients [19]. In other studies, malnutrition has been suggested to cause dysphagia [8, 28]. Veldee and Peth [8] postulated that swallowing muscles have moderate-to-high percentage of type II fibers because normal swallowing is characterized by rapid contraction of muscles. Furthermore, malnutrition can affect those swallowing muscles because type II fibers are reportedly affected by malnutrition more easily than type I fibers [29–32]. Malnutrition can be one of the main causes of sarcopenic dysphagia.

In relation to the disease, the prevalence of sarcopenia is high among chronically ill patients, ranging from 15 to 50% in patients with cancer and 30 to 45% in patients with liver failure [33]. In addition, cachexia is a metabolic syndrome characterized by loss of muscle mass with or without loss of fat mass, which can cause sarcopenia, and is prevalent in 50 to 80% of cases in several types of cancer [34]. Wakabayashi et al. [23] showed that loss of skeletal muscle mass was related to severe dysphagia in patients with cancer. Patients with chronic progressive diseases such as cancer can develop dysphagia more easily than those with other diseases, owing to sarcopenia. In older adults with Alzheimer's disease, decreased skeletal muscle mass resulted in poor swallowing functions [35]. Dysphagia in neurodegenerative disease can be caused by sarcopenia. Decreased general skeletal muscle mass was considered a risk factor for sarcopenic dysphagia in acute older inpatients [19]. Although the detailed pathophysiological mechanism of sarcopenic dysphagia from decreased general skeletal muscle mass is largely unclear, sarcopenic dysphagia can develop during general sarcopenia.

A high prevalence of sarcopenic dysphagia in older inpatients may be because hospitalization causes further inactivity and/or decrease in nutritional status and leads to severe sarcopenia. Almost all these studies revealed the associations between dysphagia and sarcopenia; however, these are not causal relationships because of the cross-sectional design of these studies. Further studies are required to explore causal relationships. We described the possible pathophysiological mechanism of sarcopenic dysphagia in **Figure 1**.

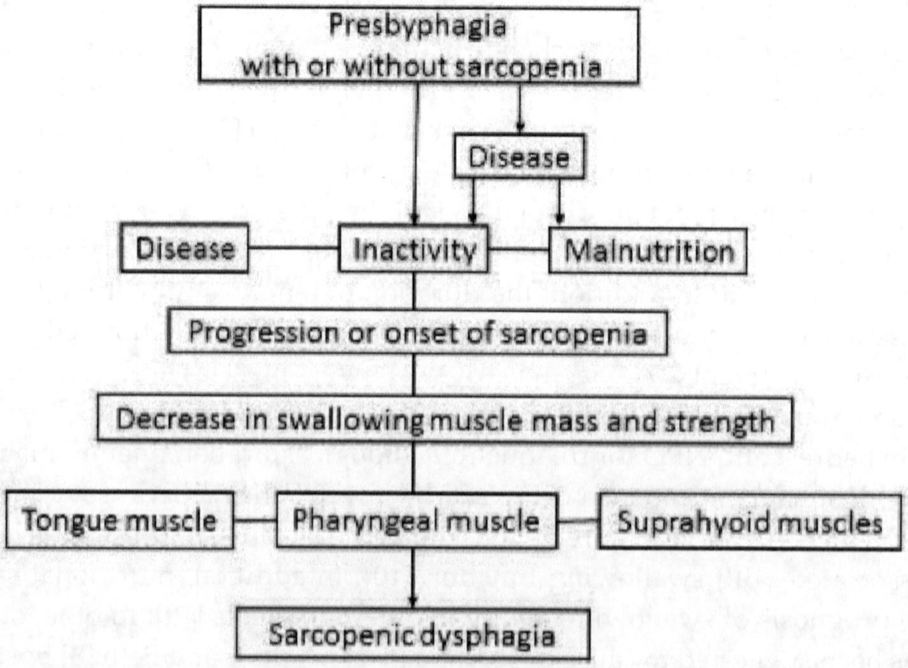

Figure 1. Possible mechanism of sarcopenic dysphagia. Older adults with presbyphagia can develop generalized sarcopenia due to disease, inactivity, or malnutrition. In the progress of generalized sarcopenia, sarcopenic dysphagia can develop due to decreased tongue, pharyngeal, and/or suprahyoid muscle function involved in swallowing.

3. Pathophysiology of sarcopenic dysphagia

3.1. Swallowing process

Swallowing is a complex process involving up to 30 striated muscles [12, 36], although swallowing is a continuous process generally conceptualized as occurring in several discrete phases. The first phase is the "preoral phase" wherein visual and olfactory qualities of food are recognized and they cause salivation, which is needed for bolus preparation [37]. The second phase is the "oral preparatory phase" wherein food is chewed and mixed with saliva to form a bolus that is easily transported to pharynx. The third phase is the "oral transit phase" wherein the tongue begins anterior-to-posterior propulsion of the bolus into pharynx. The fourth phase is the "pharyngeal phase" wherein numerous muscles function in a rapid sequence. The last phase is the "esophageal phase" wherein the bolus enters the esophagus and is transported toward the stomach by peristaltic contractions of the esophagus. Through swallowing, appropriate temporal coordination of feeding and breathing is needed to provide proper nutrition and to prevent aspiration because the pathways for food and air communicate in the pharynx [38].

3.2. Preoral phase to oral transit phase

In the preoral phase, cognitive function is related to dysphagia. In patients with congestive heart failure, cognitive dysfunction is a predictor of dysphagia [39]. In addition, sarcopenia has been independently associated with cognitive impairment in meta-analysis [40]. Thus, cognitive impairment can contribute to development of sarcopenic dysphagia. On transiting from the oral preparatory phase to the pharyngeal phase, several muscles are involved in swallowing, of which the tongue is a major muscle. The previous studies [9, 41] have found that individuals who aspirate have lower tongue strength than those who do not. Thus, tongue strength is a very important factor for swallowing. To our knowledge, Robbins et al. [42] are the first to indicate that tongue strength is affected by sarcopenia. In their study on healthy men, maximal isometric pressures were significantly greater at the tongue blade site in younger subjects, whereas peak swallow pressures remained similar across both young and older subjects. Nicosia et al. [43] also showed the same results in both healthy men and women. However, Robbins and colleagues [44] showed that both maximal isometric pressures and swallow pressures reduced with aging, and differences between maximal isometric pressures and swallow pressures were greater in younger adults than in older ones. Their studies have suggested diminished reserve of tongue strength in older adults. Buehring et al. [45] showed that both anterior and posterior maximum tongue pressure negatively correlated with age among community-dwelling individuals aged ≥ 70 years. Furthermore, Utanohara et al. [46] showed that men aged 20–40 years had higher anterior tongue pressure than the women, and anterior tongue pressure started to decrease from the age of 60 years in men and 70 years in women among healthy older adults. Their study indicated that tongue strength in men reduced with age at a faster rate than it did in women. Collectively, anterior and posterior tongue strength can decrease differently owing to age-related sarcopenia among men and women. Although a standard value of tongue strength in healthy older adults has not been established yet, Robbins et al. [41] considered tongue strength of <40 kPa as low, and Utanohara et al. [46] showed average tongue strength at 60 years of age was 37.6 ± 8.8 and 31.9 ± 8.9 kPa at 70 years of age. These values can be useful references in the clinical settings and in research. However, in our subjects aged ≥ 65 years [11], malnutrition was independently associated with low anterior tongue strength but not with age. Thus, decreased tongue strength in older adults can occur easily owing to malnutrition than because of aging.

The association between tongue strength and grip strength that represents whole body strength has been reported in several studies. Mendes et al. [47] showed that tongue and grip strength were reduced with increasing age. This study indicated that tongue strength was decreased owing to reduction in general muscle strength. Anterior tongue strength was significantly correlated with grip strength [11, 45, 47, 48]. However, Butler et al. [49] reported that posterior tongue strength, not anterior, was correlated with grip strength. The association between general muscle strength and tongue strength, whether anterior or posterior tongue, is under discussion. In addition to the difference of magnitude of tongue strength, Nicosia et al. [43] showed the difference of timing of tongue pressure generation between older and younger healthy adults. Time taken to reach maximal isometric pressure and swallowing pressure for liquids was longer in the older group than in the younger one. The timing of tongue strength generation may be also important in sarcopenic dysphagia.

Regarding tongue composition, a few studies have reported the distribution of tongue adipose tissue. Miller et al. [50] reported greater muscle tissue and correspondingly less adipose tissue in the posterior tongue than in the anterior tongue, whereas Nashi et al. [51] reported greater adipose tissue in the posterior tongue than in the anterior tongue on autopsy. As tongue muscle composition changed, amyloid deposits were found to be higher in older adults [52]. Owing to few studies on the tongue composition change by sarcopenia, further studies are required.

Regarding the association with appendicular skeletal muscle mass and tongue strength, Buehring et al. [45] showed that tongue strength was not significantly different in individuals who did or did not meet skeletal muscle mass criteria for sarcopenia. However, studies in older inpatients [11, 17] found a significant association between appendicular skeletal muscle mass and tongue strength in correlation analyses. In any case, the association between tongue strength and grip strength as one of sarcopenia indices is evident, and decreased tongue strength can be a symptom of sarcopenia and lead to sarcopenic dysphagia. Not only tongue strength but also tongue thickness was related to general muscle mass. Tamura et al. [53] showed that tongue thickness was significantly associated with mid-arm muscle area. Not only appendicular skeletal muscle mass but also tongue muscle mass can be affected by sarcopenia.

3.3. Pharyngeal phase

In the pharyngeal phase of swallowing, decreased pharyngeal strength has been shown to be related to aspiration status [54]. The suprahyoid muscles are important muscles responsible for pharyngeal strength required for swallowing. Feng and colleagues [55] examined the geniohyoid muscle—one of the suprahyoid muscles—using 80 computed tomography scans of the head and neck from healthy older and younger adults and revealed that the geniohyoid muscle atrophies with age in both the midsagittal and anterior coronal planes in men as well as women. In addition, atrophy of the geniohyoid muscle in the midsagittal plane was related to aspiration in men.

The movement of the hyoid bone, which is pulled upward and forward by the suprahyoid muscles, is assessed as an indicator of suprahyoid muscle function in videofluoroscopic swallowing studies (VFSS). VFSS is considered the gold standard examination for assessment of swallowing function because it is the only objective examination that evaluates the oral, palatal, pharyngeal, and pharyngoesophageal components of deglutition, comprehensively. Decreased range of motion and velocity of movement of the hyoid bone is observed more frequently in healthy older men than in younger men [56, 57]. In another study, the elevation of the hyoid was found to be greater in older adults both with and without dysphagia than in younger adults; however, in contrast to older adults without dysphagia, those with dysphagia were unable to use this strategy during deglutition of larger boluses [58]. In another study, the range of motion of the hyoid bone during swallowing was not significantly different between older and younger adults among both men and women. In contrast, the hyoid-larynx distance at rest was greater in both older men and women than in younger ones, and the change between the hyoid-larynx distance at rest and at the maximum approximation during swallowing was greater in older adults than in younger adults (men: mean 1.25 cm in younger men and 1.54 cm in older men; women: 1.07 cm in younger women and 1.19 cm in older women) [59]. The duration of supraglottic closure in VFSS was longer in older healthy adults than in younger healthy adults [60]. In addition, frail older adults showed slower laryngeal closure and upper esophageal sphincter opening and delayed maximal vertical hyoid motion (healthy, 0.310 ± 0.048 s; frail, 0.480 ± 0.055 s) than healthy adults. Tongue bolus propulsion strength measured by means of Newton's second law of motion in the pharyngeal phase in VFSS was 22.16 ± 2.54 mN in healthy older adults; frail older adults exhibited weaker tongue propulsion strength (8.99 ± 1.09 mN), leading to low bolus velocity and less kinetic energy [60]. There have been few studies on kinematic change related to sarcopenic dysphagia based on imaging findings; therefore, further research is warranted to investigate this issue.

In the assessment of dysphagia, jaw-opening strength was proposed as an indicator of suprahyoid muscle strength [61]. Based on measurement of jaw-opening strength in healthy adults, Iida et al. [62] suggested that suprahyoid muscle strength decreases with aging in both men and women. Machida et al. [63] demonstrated that low jaw-opening strength was associated with sarcopenia in older men. Suprahyoid muscle strength may decrease with aging and is further decreased in older men with sarcopenia. Hiramatsu et al. [64] demonstrated that the initiation of saliva swallowing was delayed and the number of saliva swallowings per 30 s decreased after meals in older adults but not in young adults (premeal, mean 7.61 and postmeal 7.30 in younger adults [no significant difference]; premeal, mean 5.35 and postmeal, mean 4.65 in older adults [significant difference, $p < 0.05$]). Their study indicated low endurance of swallowing muscles, including the suprahyoid muscles, in older adults. Low swallowing endurance can be an important component of sarcopenic dysphagia. Compared to studies on tongue muscles related to sarcopenia, fewer studies have been conducted on the suprahyoid muscles in relation to sarcopenia.

Kendall and Leonard [65] demonstrated that elderly patients with dysphagia of unknown etiology had delayed and incomplete pharyngeal constriction compared with both younger and age-matched controls without dysphagia. Leonard et al. [59] investigated spatial displacement variables in adults with no history of dysphagia and swallowing complaints. In their study, older adults with dysphagia exhibited poorer maximal pharyngeal constriction during swallowing as compared to healthy young controls. Dysfunction of pharyngeal constriction can be an important symptom of sarcopenic dysphagia. Based on the MRI scans of the neck in 60 women, Molfenter et al. [66] demonstrated that pharyngeal muscle thickness decreases and the size of the pharyngeal lumen increases with age. Such a structural change in the pharynx can result in incomplete pharyngeal constriction.

As for the sensory impairment associated with dysphagia, silent aspiration is a serious problem. Silent aspiration refers to aspiration before, during, or after swallowing in the absence of cough or visible signs of choking and distress. In a previous study, 32.5% of frail older adults with impaired safety swallow exhibited silent aspiration [60]. In a study on 76 healthy older adults [67], 83% (63/76) and 28% (21/76) exhibited penetration and silent aspiration, respectively. In addition, 85 and 61% of the subjects who exhibited penetration and aspiration, respectively, did not elicit a sensorimotor response. In another study with 56 healthy subjects [68], older adults showed a progressive decline in pharyngeal and supraglottic sensitivity measured using air pulse stimulation; sensory discrimination was 2.07 ± 0.20 mmHg in subjects aged 20–40 years and 2.68 ± 0.63 mmHg in subjects aged 61–90 years. Sarcopenia can lead to sensory decline in the pharynx and larynx and cause silent aspiration.

With regard to the changes in muscle tissue, sarcopenia or fatty degeneration after atrophy of striated muscles was observed to be accompanied by accumulation of macrophages [69, 70]. The numbers of macrophages per striated muscle fiber were 5–6 times greater in the larynx and pharynx than in other parts of the body (e.g. tongue, shoulder, and anus) in old men [71]. This kind of change in muscle tissue can lead to dysfunction of swallowing muscles with age.

3.4. Esophageal phase

Dysphagia caused by problems associated with the esophageal phase of swallowing is termed "esophageal dysphagia". Esophageal dysphagia can occur due to achalasia, diffuse esophageal spasm, nonspecific motor disorders, obstructive lesions such as stenosis or neoplasm, or gastroesophageal reflux disease [72]. Esophageal motility disorder with aging is termed "presbyesophagus" [73]. Neuromuscular dysfunction, decreased resting upper esophageal sphincter (UES) pressure, and delayed relaxation of the UES after swallowing are some age-related changes in swallowing [74, 75]. Sarcopenia can also alter esophageal functions. Sarcopenic esophageal dysphagia may be also important in addition to sarcopenic oropharyngeal dysphagia.

3.5. The coordination of swallowing with respiration

Disturbed respiration can cause aspiration in older adults [76]. The expiration-swallow-expiration (EX/EX) pattern is essential to prevent aspiration [77]. However, the probability of the non-EX/EX respiratory phase pattern has been found to be higher in the middle- and old-age groups than in the young-age group [78]. In addition, older adults had a longer swallowing apnea duration than younger adults for preventing aspiration [78]. Though the coordination of respiration and swallowing is regulated by the central pattern generator center in the brainstem, it can be altered in case of advanced age or disease [79]. This mechanism seems to be related to respiratory function change with age or disease. A few studies showed that respiratory muscle strength was related to sarcopenia [80, 81]. Sarcopenia can affect the safety swallowing respiratory pattern. The relationship between sarcopenic dysphagia and respiratory function should be investigated.

4. Treatment for sarcopenic dysphagia

A systematic review suggested that interventions such as resistance training, compound exercises (a mix of aerobic, flexibility, and/or balance training), and nutritional interventions (protein supplementation, essential amino acid [EAA, mainly leucine] supplementation, β-hydroxy β-methylbutyric acid [HMB; a bioactive metabolite of leucine] supplementation with arginine or alone or fatty acid supplementation) were effective for improvement of generalized muscle mass and strength or functions [82]. Among these interventions, supervised resistance exercise or composite exercise programs for at least 3 months and preferably longer, EAA (with leucine), and HMB were indicated to be more beneficial for improving muscle-related parameters in sarcopenia. In another review, Morley [83] suggested that resistance exercise is the most promising candidate for attenuating sarcopenia. In addition, supplementation with essential amino acids, creatine, vitamin D, or testosterone was also indicated to be effective.

With respect to treatment of dysphagia in relation to sarcopenia, the effectiveness of resistance training intervention to improve tongue muscle function has been demonstrated. Robbins et al. [9] used the Iowa Oral Performance Instrument to examine the effect of an 8-week progressive tongue resistance exercise program consisting of compressing an air-filled bulb between the tongue and hard palate in 10 healthy older adults aged 70–89 years. The frequency of exercise was 30 times in a single session, three times a day, and 3 days a week. The exercise intensity level in that study was 60% of the maximum pressure in the first week and 80% of the maximum pressure in the remaining 7 weeks. In this study, isometric tongue strength (baseline: mean 41 kPa; week 2: 44 kPa [nonsignificant difference]; week 4: 47 kPa [$p = 0.02$ compared to baseline]; week 6: 49 kPa [$p = 0.01$ compared to baseline]), tongue volume (change rate ranges from 2.16 to 10.68% upward), and peak swallowing pressure increased after the intervention. Tongue strength and thickness are decreased in sarcopenia but can have possible reversibility. The method used for measurement of tongue strength is described in **Figure 2**.

The effectiveness of the Shaker Exercise for strengthening the suprahyoid muscles is well-known in the field of dysphagia rehabilitation. The Shaker Exercise consists of an isometric component comprising three head lifts for 60 s each with a 60-s rest period between two consecutive head lifts and an isokinetic component comprising 30 consecutive head lifts at constant velocity (**Figure 3**). Shaker et al. [84] and Easterling [85] examined the effect of this

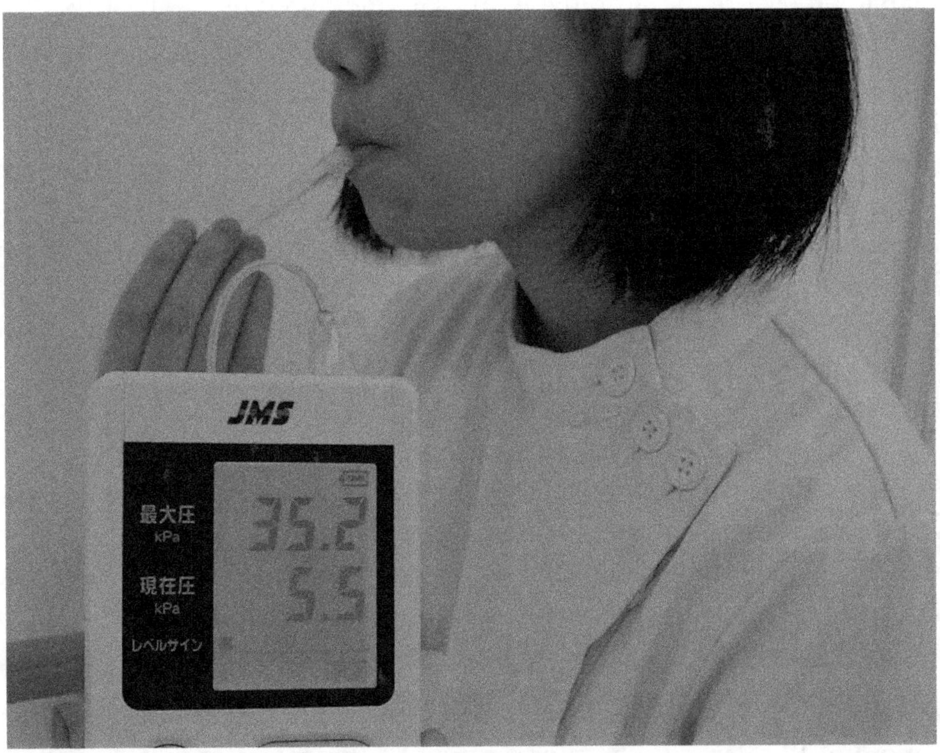

Figure 2. Tongue strength measurement. Compressing an air-filled bulb between the tongue and the hard palate and displaying the maximum tongue strength at the upper row (JMS, Hiroshima, Japan).

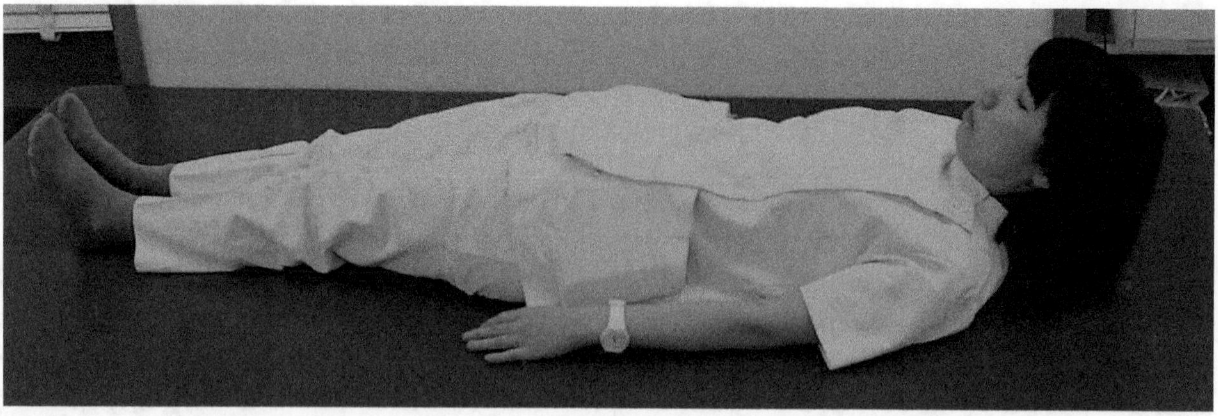

Figure 3. Shaker exercise. Lying on a bed and raising the head without lifting the shoulder, while looking at the toes.

exercise in healthy older adults. They showed that the anterior hyoid and larynx as well as the deglutitive anteroposterior UES opening diameter increased after this exercise was performed three times daily for 6 weeks. Wakabayashi et al. [86] demonstrated that dysphagia with aspiration was independently associated with both malnutrition and low head lifting strength. They suggested head lifting strength as an indicator of the severity of dysphagia in frail older adults. Strengthening the head lifting muscles can be an effective treatment for sarcopenic dysphagia. In recent years, a new method to strengthen the suprahyoid muscles—the Chin Tuck against Resistance (CTAR) exercise—has been developed [87]. This exercise involves squeezing a rubber ball placed between the chin and the manubrium sterni (**Figure 4**). The maximum activation level of the suprahyoid muscles measured using sEMG was significantly greater after this exercise than after both the isometric and isokinetic tasks in the Shaker Exercise; in addition, the CTAR exercise was less strenuous. CTAR was suggested to also be more specific in targeting the suprahyoid muscles than the Shaker exercise [88]. Instead of the rubber ball, a training device named ISO Swallowing Exercise Device (Alternative Speech and Swallowing Solutions, Inc.) was developed in America recently. The CTAR may be more feasible and efficient to improve swallowing function in older adults with sarcopenic dysphagia. The jaw-opening Exercise was developed as another training regimen for improving suprahyoid muscle strength [89]. This exercise is performed by opening the jaw to the maximum extent and maintaining this position for 10 s while feeling a sensation of stretching. This exercise is repeated 5 times with 10 s of rest as 1 set. Two sets of this exercise are needed to be performed daily. After this exercise, the upward movement of the hyoid bone and the opening of the UES significantly increased in all subjects. In addition, the time for pharynx passage also significantly decreased. In this study, among eight subjects with chronic dysphagia, four had dysphagia due to cerebrovascular disease and the remaining four had dysphagia due to possible sarcopenia. Further studies on interventions for people with sarcopenic dysphagia are warranted in the future.

For the treatment of dysphagia and prevention of aspiration pneumonia, compensatory strategies are important [7]. Particularly, modification of the consistency of ingested liquids is commonly used as a compensatory strategy. Rofes et al. [60] demonstrated that the prevalence of penetration and aspiration decreased by increasing the viscosity of ingested liquids

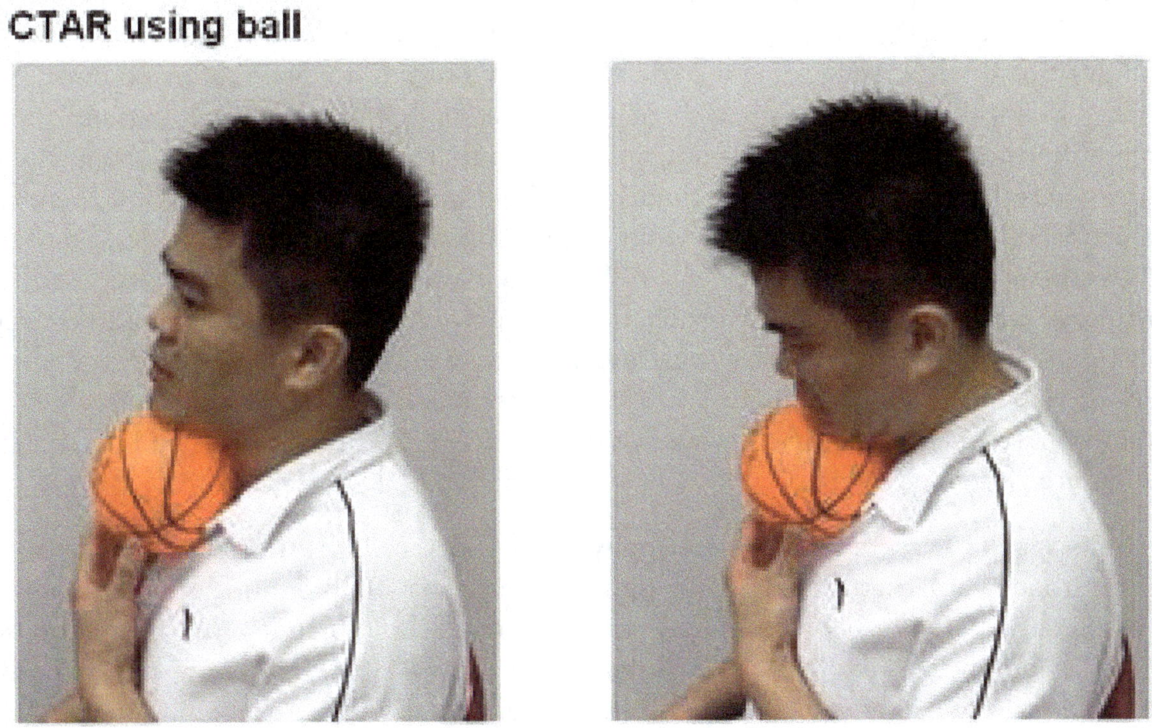

Figure 4. Chin tuck against resistance exercise. Squeezing a rubber ball placed between the chin and the manubrium sterni. Source: http://www.speechtherapyworks.com.sg/blog/new-dysphagia-exercise-chin-tuck-against-resistance-alternative-to-shaker-exercise/.

(liquid, nectar, and pudding viscosity) in frail older patients. In contrast, they also found that the prevalence of oral and pharyngeal residue increased with increase in viscosity. Thus, altering the consistency of ingested liquids can be effective for increasing the safety but not the efficiency of swallowing. The appropriate viscosity level should be determined by objective examination in older adults with sarcopenic dysphagia.

As treatments for sarcopenic dysphagia, nutritional and physical interventions have been indicated to be effective. Maeda and Akagi [90] describes the case of an 80-year-old woman who recovered from sarcopenic dysphagia with aggressive nutritional management and physical therapy in addition to dysphagia therapy. In their nutritional management, the total energy intake increased from 1200 to 1830 kcal/day, and the amount of protein intake increased from 0.84 ideal body weight (IBW)/day to 1.42 g/kg IBW/day. As a result, the oral intake level [91] improved from "nothing by mouth" level to "total oral diet with multiple consistencies, but requiring special preparation or compensations" level. Wakabayashi and Uwano [92] also described the case of a 71-year-old man who recovered from sarcopenic dysphagia with aggressive nutritional management and physical therapy in addition to dysphagia therapy. His energy intake was 986 kcal/day at the time of referral to the department of rehabilitation medicine and was increased to 2200 kcal/day. The oral intake level in this case improved from "nothing by mouth" level to "total oral diet with no restriction" level. In both the cases, physical function and nutritional status also improved with improvement in oral intake level. These cases indicate that nutritional management and physical rehabilitation in addition to dysphagia rehabilitation can be effective in the treatment of sarcopenic dysphagia. Our study [11] investigated the association between tongue strength, grip strength, and nutritional status, suggesting the effectiveness of physical rehabilitation and nutritional therapy in improving tongue strength. Yoshimura et al. [93] demonstrated that nutritional intervention added to resistance training improved muscle mass and activities of daily living more than resistance training alone in older inpatients in a rehabilitation hospital. Therefore, the combination of nutritional intervention and resistance training can also be effective in the treatment of sarcopenic dysphagia. Wakabayashi and Sakuma [94] have proposed that nutritional rehabilitation is useful for the treatment of sarcopenic dysphagia. In this concept, nutrition management, to increase muscle mass and strength, is proposed to be indispensable for rehabilitation. On the other hand, the effectiveness of nutritional intervention in sarcopenic dysphagia is unclear because of the lack of intervention studies and hence, such studies are warranted in future.

In adults aged 60 years or older, with atrophy of the vocal cords or sulcus vocalis with aging, self-controlled vocal exercise in the sitting position that consists of counting out loud from 1 to 10 while pulling up firmly on both sides of the seat reduced the frequency of hospitalization for aspiration pneumonia (2/199 in the intervention group and 18/216 in the control group) [95]. Subjects in the intervention group exercised for a total of two sets, both in the morning and in the evening for 6 months. The intrinsic laryngeal muscles commonly cause glottal closure insufficiency with aging [96–98]; therefore, sarcopenia can cause atrophy of the vocal cords. Because insufficient glottal closure increases the risk of aspiration [99], atrophy of the vocal cords can lead to aspiration pneumonia in older adults. The vocal exercise mentioned above can be an effective treatment for sarcopenic dysphagia.

As decrease in pharyngeal and supraglottic sensitivity was indicated in older adults with sarcopenic dysphagia, sensory stimulation may be an effective treatment. Ortega et al. [100] demonstrated the effectiveness of two sensory stimulation techniques. One was the chemical sensory stimulation with a natural TRPV1 agonist solution (natural capsaicinoids 1×10^{-5} M). In this study, capsaicin solution was obtained from an alimentary sauce containing 185.5 μg/g of capsaicinoid. Subjects consumed 10 mL of tomato juice mixed with the capsaicinoid sauce three times per day before each meal, 5 days per week for 2 weeks. The other technique was electrical stimulation in the thyrohyoid position using the Intelect VitalStim device (Chattanooga Group, Hixson, TN, USA), consisting of the application, at rest, of 80 Hz of transcutaneous electrical stimulus (biphasic, 700μs). Subjects received this therapy for 1 h per day, 5 days a week for 2 weeks. Aspiration was significantly reduced in the group that received a natural TRPV1 agonist solution (TRPV1 group; 38.46% vs. TSES group; 0%) and the prevalence of penetration decreased significantly in the group receiving electrical stimulation (TSES group; 87.5 vs. TRPV1 group; 25%). In addition, the time for laryngeal vestibule closure was significantly shortened in responder patients in the group receiving electrical stimulation (TSES group; 480 ± 167 ms vs. TRPV1 group; 295 ± 189.9 ms). Because the cause of dysphagia in the subjects in this study was aging (39.5%), or a combination of aging with previous stroke or neurodegenerative diseases, the effectiveness of these techniques for older adults with sarcopenic dysphagia should be examined.

In rehabilitation for sarcopenic dysphagia, risk management for aspiration pneumonia is also important. Frail older patients with oropharyngeal dysphagia have poorer oral health, higher oral bacterial load, and a higher prevalence of oral colonization by respiratory pathogens than healthy older adults [101]. Since these can be potential risk factors of aspiration pneumonia, oral care is important as a risk management strategy in the treatment of sarcopenic dysphagia.

The Dysphagia Working Group from the European Society for Swallowing Disorders and the European Union Geriatric Medicine Society has proposed that oropharyngeal dysphagia is a multifactorial geriatric syndrome [7] and is treatable only with a multidimensional approach. Further research is required to identify the components of this multidimensional approach.

5. Conclusions

Sarcopenic dysphagia is a swallowing disorder caused by sarcopenia of the swallowing muscles, including the general skeletal muscle. Its prevalence seems to be high, particularly in older adults after acute disease. Because sarcopenic dysphagia is caused mainly by inactivity and malnutrition, it is preventable and treatable in most cases. Among published articles on dysphagia, there have been few studies on sarcopenic dysphagia. With an increasing aging population, sarcopenic dysphagia has become an important public health issue. For adequate prevention, diagnosis, and treatment, further studies on the pathophysiology of and intervention for sarcopenic dysphagia are warranted in future.

Author details

Kotomi Sakai[1,2]* and Kunihiro Sakuma[3]

*Address all correspondence to: sakai.kotomi@hmw.gr.jp

1 Department of Rehabilitation, Setagaya Memorial Hospital, Tokyo, Japan

2 Department of Dysphagia Rehabilitation, Nihon University School of Dentistry, Tokyo, Japan

3 Institute for Liberal Arts, Environment and Society, Tokyo Institute of Technology, Tokyo, Japan

References

[1] Rosenberg IH. Sarcopenia: Origins and clinical relevance. The Journal of Nutrition. 1997;**127**:990-991

[2] Cruz-Jentoft AJ, Baeyens JP, Bauer JM, Boirie Y, Cederholm T, Landi F, Martin FC, Michel JP, Rolland Y, Schneider SM, Topinkova E, Vandewoude M, Zamboni M. Sarcopenia:

European consensus on definition and diagnosis: Report of the European Working Group on Sarcopenia in Older People. Age and Ageing. 2010;**39**:412-423

[3] Fielding RA, Vellas B, Evans WJ, Bhasin S, Morley JE, Newman AB, Abellan van Kan G, Andrieu S, Bauer J, Breuille D, Cederholm T, Chandler J, De Meynard C, Donini L, Harris T, Kannt A, Keime Guibert F, Onder G, Papanicolaou D, Rolland Y, Rooks D, Sieber C, Souhami E, Verlaan S, Zamboni M. Sarcopenia: An undiagnosed condition in older adults. Current consensus definition: Prevalence, etiology, and consequences. International Working Group on Sarcopenia. Journal of the American Medical Directors Association. 2011;**12**:249-256

[4] Chen LK, Liu LK, Woo J, Assantachai P, Auyeung TW, Bahyah KS, Chou MY, Chen LY, Hsu PS, Krairit O, Lee JS, Lee WJ, Lee Y, Liang CK, Limpawattana P, Lin CS, Peng LN, Satake S, Suzuki T, Won CW, Wu CH, Wu SN, Zhang T, Zeng P, Akishita M, Arai H. Sarcopenia in Asia: Consensus report of the Asian Working Group for Sarcopenia. Journal of the American Medical Directors Association. 2014;**15**:95-101

[5] Anker SD, Morley JE, Haehling SV. Welcome to the ICD-10 code for sarcopenia. Journal of Cachexia, Sarcopenia and Muscle. 2016;**7**:512-514

[6] WHO. International classification of functioning, disability and health [online]. 2016; **20**:22-27 http://www.who.int/classifications/icf/en/

[7] Baijens LWJ, Clavé P, Cras P, Ekberg O, Forster A, Kolb G, Leners JC, Masiero S, Mateos del Nozal J, Ortega O, Smithard DG, Speyer R, Walshe M. European Society for swallowing disorders—European Union geriatric medicine society white paper: Oropharyngeal dysphagia as a geriatric syndrome. Clinical Interventions in Aging. 2016;**11**:1403-1428

[8] Veldee MS, Peth LD. Can protein-calorie malnutrition cause dysphagia? Dysphagia. 1992;**7**:86-101

[9] Robbins J, Gangnon RE, Theis SM, Kays SA, Hewitt AL, Hind JA. The effects of lingual exercise on swallowing in older adults. Journal of the American Geriatrics Society. 2005;**53**:1483-1489

[10] Kuroda Y, Kuroda R. Relationship between thinness and swallowing function in Japanese older adults: Implications for sarcopenic dysphagia. Journal of the American Geriatrics Society. 2012;**60**:1785-1786

[11] Sakai K, Nakayama E, Tohara H, Maeda T, Sugimoto M, Takehisa T, Takehisa Y, Ueda K. Tongue strength is associated with grip strength and nutritional status in older adult inpatients of a rehabilitation hospital. Dysphagia. 2016. [Epub ahead of print]

[12] Clave P, Shaker R. Dysphagia: Current reality and scope of the problem. Nature Reviews of Gastroenterology and Hepatology. 2015;**12**:259-270

[13] van der Maarel-Wierink CD, Vanobbergen JN, Bronkhorst EM, Schols JM, de Baat C. Meta-analysis of dysphagia and aspiration pneumonia in frail elders. Journal of Dental Research. 2011;**90**:1398-1404

[14] Bonilha HS, Simpson AN, Ellis C, Mauldin P, Martin-Harris B, Simpson K. The one-year attributable cost of post-stroke dysphagia. Dysphagia. 2014;**29**:545-552

[15] Altman KW, Yu GP, Schaefer SD. Consequence of dysphagia in the hospitalized patient: Impact on prognosis and hospital resources. Archives of Otolaryngology—-Head & Neck Surgery. 2010;**136**:784-789

[16] Chen LK, Lee WJ, Peng LN, Liu LK, Arai H, Akishita M. Recent advances in sarcopenia research in Asia: 2016 update from the Asian Working Group for Sarcopenia. Journal of the American Medical Directors Association. 2016;**17**:767.e1-767.e7

[17] Maeda K, Akagi J. Decreased tongue pressure is associated with sarcopenia and sarcopenic dysphagia in the elderly. Dysphagia. 2015;**30**:80-87

[18] Maeda K, Akagi J. Sarcopenia is an independent risk factor of dysphagia in hospitalized older people. Geriatrics & Gerontology International. 2015;**4**:515-21

[19] Maeda K, Takaki M, Akagi J. Decreased skeletal muscle mass and risk factors of sarcopenic dysphagia: A prospective observational cohort study. The Journals of Gerontology Series A, Biological Sciences and Medical Sciences. 2016. [Epub ahead of print]

[20] Madhavan A, LaGorio LA, Crary MA, Dahl WJ, Carnaby GD. Prevalence of and risk factors for dysphagia in the community dwelling elderly: A systematic review. The Journal of Nutrition, Health & Aging. 2016;**20**:806-815

[21] Wakabayashi H, Matsushima M. Dysphagia assessed by the 10-item eating assessment tool is associated with nutritional status and activities of daily living in elderly individuals requiring long-term care. The Journal of Nutrition, Health & Aging. 2016; 20:22-27

[22] Aslam M, Vaezi MF. Dysphagia in the elderly. Gastroenterology & Hepatology. 2013; **9**:784-795

[23] Wakabayashi H, Matsushima M, Uwano R, Watanabe N, Oritsu H, Shimizu Y. Skeletal muscle mass is associated with severe dysphagia in cancer patients. Journal of Cachexia, Sarcopenia and Muscle. 2015;**6**:351-357

[24] Robbins J, Hamilton JW, Lof GL, Kempster GB. Oropharyngeal swallowing in normal adults of different ages. Gastroenterology. 1992;**103**:823-829

[25] Humbert IA, Robbins J. Dysphagia in the elderly. Physical Medicine and Rehabilitation Clinics of North America. 2008;**19**:853-866

[26] Ney DM, Weiss JM, Kind AJ, Robbins J. Senescent swallowing: Impact, strategies, and interventions. Nutrition in Clinical Practice: Official Publication of the American Society for Parenteral and Enteral Nutrition. 2009;**24**:395-413

[27] Maeda K, Koga T, Akagi J. Tentative nil per os leads to poor outcomes in older adults with aspiration pneumonia. Clinical Nutrition (Edinburgh, Scotland). 2016;**35**:1147-1152

[28] Hudson HM, Daubert CR, Mills RH. The interdependency of protein-energy malnutrition, aging, and dysphagia. Dysphagia. 2000;**15**:31-38

[29] Lewis MI, Sieck GC. Effect of acute nutritional deprivation on diaphragm structure and function. Journal of Applied Physiology. 1990;**68**:1938-1944

[30] Sieck GC, Lewis MI, Blanco CE. Effects of undernutrition on diaphragm fiber size, SDH activity, and fatigue resistance. Journal of Applied Physiology. 1989;**66**:2196-2205

[31] Drew JS, Farkas GA, Pearson RD, Rochester DF. Effects of a chronic wasting infection on skeletal muscle size and contractile properties. Journal of Applied Physiology. 1988;**64**:460-465

[32] Lewis MI, Li H, Huang Z-S, Biring MS, Cercek B, Fournier M. Influence of varying degrees of malnutrition on IGF-I expression in the rat diaphragm. Journal of Applied Physiology. 2003;**95**:555-562

[33] Peterson SJ, Braunschweig CA. Prevalence of sarcopenia and associated outcomes in the clinical setting. Nutrition in Clinical Practice: Official Publication of the American Society for Parenteral and Enteral Nutrition. 2016;**31**:40-48

[34] von Haehling S, Anker SD. Prevalence, incidence and clinical impact of cachexia: Facts and numbers-update 2014. Journal of Cachexia, Sarcopenia and Muscle. 2014;**5**:261-263

[35] Takagi D, Hirano H, Watanabe Y, Edahiro A, Ohara Y, Yoshida H, Kim H, Murakami K, Hironaka S. Relationship between skeletal muscle mass and swallowing function in patients with Alzheimer's disease. Geriatrics & Gerontology International. 2016. [Epub ahead of print]

[36] Matsuo K, Palmer JB. Anatomy and physiology of feeding and swallowing: Normal and abnormal. Physical medicine and Rehabilitation Clinics of North America. 2008; **19**:691-707

[37] Leopold NA, Kagel MC. Dysphagia – ingestion or deglutition? A proposed paradigm. Dysphagia. 1997;**12**:202-206

[38] Matsuo K, Palmer JB. Coordination of mastication, swallowing and breathing. The Japanese Dental Science Review. 2009;**45**:31-40

[39] Yokota J, Ogawa Y, Yamanaka S, Takahashi Y, Fujita H, Yamaguchi N, Onoue N, Ishizuka T, Shinozaki T, Kohzuki M. Cognitive dysfunction and malnutrition are independent predictors of dysphagia in patients with acute exacerbation of congestive heart failure. PloS One. 2016;**11**:e0167326

[40] Chang K-V, Hsu T-H, Wu W-T, Huang K-C, Han D-S. Association between sarcopenia and cognitive impairment: A systematic review and meta-analysis. Journal of the American Medical Directors Association. 2016;**12**:1164.e7-1164.e15

[41] Robbins J, Kays SA, Gangnon RE, Hind JA, Hewitt AL, Gentry LR, Taylor AJ. The effects of lingual exercise in stroke patients with dysphagia. Archives of Physical Medicine and Rehabilitation. 2007;**88**:150-158

[42] Robbins J, Levine R, Wood J, Roecker EB, Luschei E. Age effects on lingual pressure generation as a risk factor for dysphagia. The Journals of Gerontology Series A, Biological Sciences and Medical Sciences. 1995;**50**:M257-M262

[43] Nicosia MA, Hind JA, Roecker EB, Carnes M, Doyle J, Dengel GA, Robbins J. Age effects on the temporal evolution of isometric and swallowing pressure. The Journals of Gerontology Series A, Biological Sciences and Medical Sciences. 2000;**55**:M634-M640

[44] Robbins J, Humpal NS, Banaszynski K, Hind J, Rogus-Pulia N. Age-related differences in pressures generated during isometric presses and swallows by healthy adults. Dysphagia. 2016;**31**:90-96

[45] Buehring B, Hind J, Fidler E, Krueger D, Binkley N, Robbins J. Tongue strength is associated with jumping mechanography performance and handgrip strength but not with classic functional tests in older adults. Journal of the American Geriatrics Society. 2013;**61**:418-422

[46] Utanohara Y, Hayashi R, Yoshikawa M, Yoshida M, Tsuga K, Akagawa Y. Standard values of maximum tongue pressure taken using newly developed disposable tongue pressure measurement device. Dysphagia. 2008;**23**:286-290

[47] Mendes AE, Nascimento L, Mansur LL, Callegaro D, Jacob Filho W. Tongue forces and handgrip strength in normal individuals: Association with swallowing. Clinics (Sao Paulo, Brazil). 2015;**70**:41-45

[48] Crow HC, Ship JA. Tongue strength and endurance in different aged individuals. The Journals of Gerontology Series A, Biological Sciences and Medical Sciences. 1996; **51**:M247-M250

[49] Butler SG, Stuart A, Leng X, Wilhelm E, Rees C, Williamson J, Kritchevsky SB. The relationship of aspiration status with tongue and handgrip strength in healthy older adults. The Journals of Gerontology Series A, Biological Sciences and Medical sciences. 2011;**66**:452-458

[50] Miller JL, Watkin KL, Chen MF. Muscle, adipose, and connective tissue variations in intrinsic musculature of the adult human tongue. Journal of Speech, Language, and Hearing Research. 2002;**45**:51-65

[51] Nashi N, Kang S, Barkdull GC, Lucas J, Davidson TM. Lingual fat at autopsy. The Laryngoscope. 2007;**117**:1467-1473

[52] Yamaguchi A, Nasu M, Esaki Y, Shimada H, Yoshiki S. Amyloid deposits in the aged tongue: A postmortem study of 107 individuals over 60 years of age. Journal of Oral Pathology. 1982;**11**:237-244

[53] Tamura F, Kikutani T, Tohara T, Yoshida M, Yaegaki K. Tongue thickness relates to nutritional status in the elderly. Dysphagia. 2012;**27**:556-561

[54] Butler SG, Stuart A, Wilhelm E, Rees C, Williamson J, Kritchevsky S. The effects of aspiration status, liquid type, and bolus volume on pharyngeal peak pressure in healthy older adults. Dysphagia. 2011;**26**:225-231

[55] Feng X, Todd T, Lintzenich CR, Ding J, Carr JJ, Ge Y, Browne JD, Kritchevsky SB, Butler SG. Aging-related geniohyoid muscle atrophy is related to aspiration status in healthy

older adults. The Journals of Gerontology Series A, Biological Sciences and Medical Sciences. 2013;**68**:853-860

[56] Logemann JA, Pauloski BR, Rademaker AW, Colangelo LA, Kahrilas PJ, Smith CH. Temporal and biomechanical characteristics of oropharyngeal swallow in younger and older men. Journal of Speech, Language, and Hearing Research. 2000;**43**:1264-1274

[57] Kang BS, Oh BM, Kim IS, Chung SG, Kim SJ, Han TR. Influence of aging on movement of the hyoid bone and epiglottis during normal swallowing: A motion analysis. Gerontology. 2010;**56**:474-482

[58] Kendall KA, Leonard RJ. Hyoid movement during swallowing in older patients with dysphagia. Archives of Otolaryngology—Head & Neck Surgery. 2001;**127**:1224-1229

[59] Leonard R, Kendall KA, McKenzie S. Structural displacements affecting pharyngeal constriction in nondysphagic elderly and nonelderly adults. Dysphagia. 2004;**19**:133-141

[60] Rofes L, Arreola V, Romea M, Palomera E, Almirall J, Cabre M, Serra-Prat M, Clave P. Pathophysiology of oropharyngeal dysphagia in the frail elderly. Neurogastroenterology and Motility: The Official Journal of the European Gastrointestinal Motility Society. 2010;**22**:851-858, e230

[61] Hara K, Tohara H, Wada S, Iida T, Ueda K, Ansai T. Jaw-opening force test to screen for dysphagia: Preliminary results. Archives of Physical Medicine and Rehabilitation. 2014;**95**:867-874

[62] Iida T, Tohara H, Wada S, Nakane A, Sanpei R, Ueda K. Aging decreases the strength of suprahyoid muscles involved in swallowing movements. The Tohoku Journal of Experimental Medicine. 2013;**231**:223-228

[63] Machida N, Tohara H, Hara K, Kumakura A, Wakasugi Y, Nakane A, Minakuchi S. Effects of aging and sarcopenia on tongue pressure and jaw-opening force. Geriatrics & Gerontology International. 2017;**17**:295-301

[64] Hiramatsu T, Kataoka H, Osaki M, Hagino H. Effect of aging on oral and swallowing function after meal consumption. Clinical Interventions in Aging. 2015;**10**:229-235

[65] Kendall KA, Leonard RJ. Pharyngeal constriction in elderly dysphagic patients compared with young and elderly nondysphagic controls. Dysphagia. 2001;**16**:272-278

[66] Molfenter SM, Amin MR, Branski RC, Brumm JD, Hagiwara M, Roof SA, Lazarus CL. Age-related changes in pharyngeal lumen size: A retrospective MRI analysis. Dysphagia. 2015;**30**:321-327

[67] Butler SG, Stuart A, Leng X, Rees C, Williamson J, Kritchevsky SB. Factors influencing aspiration during swallowing in healthy older adults. The Laryngoscope. 2010;**120**:2147-2152

[68] Aviv JE, Martin JH, Jones ME, Wee TA, Diamond B, Keen MS, Blitzer A. Age-related changes in pharyngeal and supraglottic sensation. The Annals of Otology, Rhinology, and Laryngology. 1994;**103**:749-752

[69] Gumucio J, Flood M, Harning J, Phan A, Roche S, Lynch E, Bedi A, Mendias C. T lymphocytes are not required for the development of fatty degeneration after rotator cuff tear. Bone & Joint Research. 2014;**3**:262-272

[70] Siriett V, Salerno MS, Berry C, Nicholas G, Bower R, Kambadur R, Sharma M. Antagonism of myostatin enhances muscle regeneration during sarcopenia. Molecular Therapy: The Journal of the American Society of Gene Therapy. 2007;**15**:1463-1470

[71] Rhee S, Yamamoto M, Kitamura K, Masaaki K, Katori Y, Murakami G, Abe SI. Macrophage density in pharyngeal and laryngeal muscles greatly exceeds that in other striated muscles: An immunohistochemical study using elderly human cadavers. Anatomy & Cell Biology. 2016;**49**:177-183

[72] Greenslade J, Wyman A. Investigation of dysphagia. Surgery (Oxford). 2006;**24**:89-92

[73] DeVault KR. Presbyesophagus: A reappraisal. Current Gastroenterology Reports. 2002; **4**:193-199

[74] Fulp SR, Dalton CB, Castell JA, Castell DO. Aging-related alterations in human upper esophageal sphincter function. The American Journal of Gastroenterology. 1990;**85**: 1569-1572

[75] van Herwaarden MA, Katz PO, Matthew Gideon R, Barrett J, Castell JA, Achem S, Castell DO. Are manometric parameters of the upper esophageal sphincter and pharynx affected by age and gender? Dysphagia. 2003;**18**:211-217

[76] Nilsson H, Ekberg O, Bulow M, Hindfelt B. Assessment of respiration during video fluoroscopy of dysphagic patients. Academic Radiology. 1997;**4**:503-507

[77] Preiksaitis HG, Mills CA. Coordination of breathing and swallowing: Effects of bolus consistency and presentation in normal adults. Journal of Applied Physiology. 1996; **81**:1707-1714

[78] Wang CM, Chen JY, Chuang CC, Tseng WC, Wong AM, Pei YC. Aging-related changes in swallowing, and in the coordination of swallowing and respiration determined by novel non-invasive measurement techniques. Geriatrics & Gerontology International. 2015;**6**:736-744

[79] Shaker R, Li Q, Ren J, Townsend WF, Dodds WJ, Martin BJ, Kern MK, Rynders A. Coordination of deglutition and phases of respiration: Effect of aging, tachypnea, bolus volume, and chronic obstructive pulmonary disease. The American Journal of Physiology. 1992;**263**:G750-G755

[80] Izawa KP, Watanabe S, Oka K, Kasahara Y, Morio Y, Hiraki K, Hirano Y, Omori Y, Suzuki N, Kida K, Suzuki K, Akashi YJ. Respiratory muscle strength in relation to sarcopenia in elderly cardiac patients. Aging Clinical and Experimental Research. 2016; 28:1143-1148

[81] Elliott JE, Greising SM, Mantilla CB, Sieck GC. Functional impact of sarcopenia in respiratory muscles. Respiratory Physiology & Neurobiology. 2016;**226**:137-146

[82] Cruz-Jentoft AJ, Landi F, Schneider SM, Zuniga C, Arai H, Boirie Y, Chen LK, Fielding RA, Martin FC, Michel JP, Sieber C, Stout JR, Studenski SA, Vellas B, Woo J, Zamboni M, Cederholm T. Prevalence of and interventions for sarcopenia in ageing adults: A systematic review. Report of the International Sarcopenia Initiative (EWGSOP and IWGS). Age and Ageing. 2014;**6**:748-759

[83] Morley JE. Pharmacologic options for the treatment of sarcopenia. Calcified Tissue International. 2016;**98**:319-333

[84] Shaker R, Kern M, Bardan E, Taylor A, Stewart ET, Hoffmann RG, Arndorfer RC, Hofmann C, Bonnevier J. Augmentation of deglutitive upper esophageal sphincter opening in the elderly by exercise. The American Journal of Physiology. 1997;**272**:G1518-G1522

[85] Easterling C. Does an exercise aimed at improving swallow function have an effect on vocal function in the healthy elderly? Dysphagia. 2008;**23**:317-326

[86] Wakabayashi H, Sashika H, Matsushima M. Head lifting strength is associated with dysphagia and malnutrition in frail older adults. Geriatrics & Gerontology International. 2015;**4**:410-416

[87] Yoon WL, Khoo JKP, Rickard Liow SJ. Chin Tuck Against Resistance (CTAR): New Method for enhancing suprahyoid muscle activity using a Shaker-type exercise. Dysphagia. 2014;**29**:243-248

[88] Sze WP, Yoon WL, Escoffier N, Rickard Liow SJ. Evaluating the training effects of two swallowing rehabilitation therapies using surface electromyography – Chin Tuck Against Resistance (CTAR) Exercise and the Shaker exercise. Dysphagia. 2016;**31**:195-205

[89] Wada S, Tohara H, Iida T, Inoue M, Sato M, Ueda K. Jaw-opening exercise for insufficient opening of upper esophageal sphincter. Archives of Physical Medicine and Rehabilitation. 2012;**93**:1995-1999

[90] Maeda K, Akagi J. Treatment of sarcopenic dysphagia with rehabilitation and nutritional support: A comprehensive approach. Journal of the Academy of Nutrition and Diebetics. 2016;**116**:573-577

[91] Crary MA, Mann GD, Groher ME. Initial psychometric assessment of a functional oral intake scale for dysphagia in stroke patients. Archives of Physical Medicine and Rehabilitation. 2005;**86**:1516-1520

[92] Wakabayashi H, Uwano R. Rehabilitation nutrition for possible sarcopenic dysphagia after lung cancer surgery: A case report. American Journal of Physical Medicine & Rehabilitation/Association of Academic Physiatrists. 2016;**95**:e84-e89

[93] Yoshimura Y, Uchida K, Jeong S, Yamaga M. Effects of nutritional supplements on muscle mass and activities of daily living in elderly rehabilitation patients with decreased muscle mass: A randomized controlled trial. The Journal of Nutrition, Health & Aging. 2016; 20:185-191

[94] Wakabayashi H, Sakuma K. Rehabilitation nutrition for sarcopenia with disability: A combination of both rehabilitation and nutrition care management. Journal of Cachexia, Sarcopenia and Muscle. 2014;**5**:269-277

[95] Fujimaki Y, Tsunoda K, Kobayashi R, Tonghyo C, Tanaka F, Kuroda H, Numata T, Ishii T, Kuroda R, Masuda S, Hashimoto S, Misawa H, Shindo N, Mori T, Mori H, Uchiyama N, Kamei Y, Tanaka M, Hamaya H, Funatsuki S, Usui S, Ito I, Hamada K, Shindo A, Tokumaru Y, Morita Y, Ueha R, Nito T, Kikuta S, Sekimoto S, Kondo K, Sakamoto T, Itoh K, Yamasoba T, Matsumoto S. Independent exercise for glottal incompetence to improve vocal problems and prevent aspiration pneumonia in the elderly: A randomized controlled trial. Clinical Rehabilitation. 2016. [Epub ahead of print]

[96] Malmgren LT, Fisher PJ, Bookman LM, Uno T. Age-related changes in muscle fiber types in the human thyroarytenoid muscle: An immunohistochemical and stereological study using confocal laser scanning microscopy. Otolaryngology – head and neck surgery. Official Journal of American Academy of Otolaryngology-Head and Neck Surgery. 1999;**121**:441-451

[97] Malmgren LT, Jones CE, Bookman LM. Muscle fiber and satellite cell apoptosis in the aging human thyroarytenoid muscle: A stereological study with confocal laser scanning microscopy. Otolaryngology – head and neck surgery. Official Journal of American Academy of Otolaryngology-Head and Neck Surgery. 2001;**125**:34-39

[98] Martins RH, Benito Pessin AB, Nassib DJ, Branco A, Rodrigues SA, Matheus SM. Aging voice and the laryngeal muscle atrophy. The Laryngoscope. 2015;**125**:2518-2521

[99] Giraldez-Rodriguez LA, Johns M, 3rd. Glottal insufficiency with aspiration risk in dysphagia. Otolaryngologic Clinics of North America. 2013;**46**:1113-1121

[100] Ortega O, Rofes L, Martin A, Arreola V, Lopez I, Clave P. A Comparative study between two sensory stimulation strategies after two weeks treatment on older patients with oropharyngeal dysphagia. Dysphagia. 2016;**31**:706-716

[101] Ortega O, Sakwinska O, Combremont S, Berger B, Sauser J, Parra C, Zarcero S, Nart J, Carrion S, Clave P. High prevalence of colonization of oral cavity by respiratory pathogens in frail older patients with oropharyngeal dysphagia. Neurogastroenterology and Motility: The Official Journal of the European Gastrointestinal Motility Society. 2015;**27**:1804-1816

6

Rehabilitation in Sarcopenic Elderly

Raoul Saggini, Simona Maria Carmignano,
Lucia Cosenza, Tommaso Palermo and
Rosa Grazia Bellomo

Abstract

Sarcopenia is a complex problem and an important emerging field in rehabilitation of the elderly. In 2010, the European working group on sarcopenia in older people (EWGSOP) described sarcopenia as a syndrome characterised by progressive and generalised loss of skeletal muscle mass and strength, associated with a risk of adverse outcomes such as physical disability, poor quality of life and death. This field of rehabilitation has been defined as 'evaluative, diagnostic and therapeutic interventions whose purpose is to restore functional ability or enhance residual functional capability in elderly people with disabling impairments'. With growing numbers of frail older people, there is an increasing need for appropriate geriatric rehabilitation services. Definitely, sarcopenia needs a specific rehabilitation program to improve muscular mass and strength that must be integrated with a global approach with the aim to recover postural assessment, amplify sensory-motor systems, in order to gain the necessary information for proper motor planning, to reduce risk of falls. Several physical agents in medicine permit to treat sarcopenia, like vibrations or electrical stimulation. The aim of this chapter is to give an overview about rehabilitative medicine for sarcopenia, highlighting the state of the art, presenting the most significative clinical researches and giving some inputs to set a rehabilitation protocol.

Keywords: sarcopenia, physical energies, complex sensory-motor rehabilitation program, vibrations, electrical stimulation

1. Introduction

Sarcopenia (from the Greek sarx 'flesh' and penia 'loss') is a term used for the first time by Rosenberg to describe the age-related decrease in muscle mass. In fact, aging is associated with a progressive decline in muscle mass that can lead to a decrease in muscle quality and strength.

In 2010, the European working group on sarcopenia in older people (EWGSOP) described sarcopenia as a syndrome characterised by progressive and generalised loss of skeletal muscle mass and strength, associated with a risk of adverse outcomes such as physical disability, poor quality of life and death [1]. The reduction in muscle mass is associated with longer hospitalisation, increased need for rehabilitation care after hospital discharge, infective complications, prolonged duration of mechanical ventilation and higher mortality. There are several approaches to treat sarcopenia and it was demonstrated that, regardless of the type of intervention, treatment improves the quality of life preventing falls, disability and loss of independence among elderly patients [2]. Among interventions, resistance training has been shown to be the most effective to reduce the effects of sarcopenia, this because it induces skeletal muscle hypertrophy and enhances muscle strength; unfortunately, resistance training is not always feasible in sarcopenic elderly people [2]. Therefore, in these cases, physical therapies come to the rescue, i.e. vibrations or electrical stimulations. Particularly, it is possible to use focal vibrations, which excite the afferents coming from the neuromuscular spindle, leading to the activation of the proprioceptive sensory system. Electrical stimulation too is an alternative, even more effective than exercise alone, in strengthening muscles in sarcopenic patients [3]. These alternative approaches to exercise offered a safe addition to a traditional, high-intensity volitional strengthening program with the aim to implement muscular mass and strength. It is also a necessary adequate sensory-motor and functional recovery program to reach an acceptable walking ability. The ability to walk is the key to any human movement, despite the fact the human movements are not limited to bipedal locomotion; bipedal locomotion is a fundamental part of daily life and is a prominent target of public health physical activity guidelines [4]. In order to get a better walking performance and a postural global improvement, two integrate procedures may be used: normalisation of the foot-ground reaction to control vertical and shear forces on the foot during the stance phase; second one is the microgravitary environment that determines the sensory-motor and functional recovery of the posture during walking activity in combination to the development of proprioceptive information from periphery to the cortical central system [4]. Definitely, sarcopenia needs a specific rehabilitation program to improve muscular mass and strength that must be integrated with a global approach with the aim to recovery postural assessment, amplify sensory-motor systems, in order to gain the necessary information for proper motor planning, to reduce risk of falls.

2. Background

Aging, as mentioned, is characterised by a progressive loss of skeletal muscle mass and strength, thus leading to the loss of functional capacity. In sarcopenia, the loss of skeletal muscle mass must be due to a chronic disruption in the balance between muscle protein synthesis and degradation.

In active and healthy elderly patients, the mechanism underlying the loss of muscle mass does not seem to be bound to a disorder of protein metabolism in the basal state (fasting). Rather, it was proposed that muscle in the elderly presents a deficiency in the ability to regulate protein synthesis in response to an anabolic stimulus, such as physical activity or food intake [1].

According to epidemiological data in literature, the prevalence of sarcopenia in people ranging in ages from 60 to 70 turns out to be 5–13%, while in patients over 80, it varies between 11 and 50% [2]. In 2000, the number of people worldwide over the age of 60 years was estimated at 600 million, a value that is forecast to rise to 1.2 billion in 2025 and 2 billion in 2050 [5]. Making an approximate estimate about the prevalence, people with sarcopenia nowadays are more than 50 million that should increase to over 200 million in the next 40 years.

The impact of sarcopenia in elderly affects multiple aspects; in fact, its influence can be seen in terms of morbidity [6], disability [7], increasing in costs related to health care [8] and mortality [9].

The underlying causes of sarcopenia and frailty are multifactorial. Although the progressive loss of muscle mass that occurs with aging is well-known for many years, but it is only with the latest techniques and prospective-longitudinal studies that changes related to aging in muscle composition have begun to be described [10].

Several reviews have highlighted cellular and molecular mechanisms underlying the weakness and muscle atrophy related to aging [11]. It has been seen that the loss of muscle strength and mass are the consequence of a progressive atrophy due to a loss of individual muscle fibres associated to a reduction of some motor units; this implies fat and other non-contractile tissue (i.e. fibrous tissue) infiltrations which involves a reduction of 'muscle quality' [1].

Therefore, changes in musculoskeletal age are initially neuromuscular and subsequently others several factors intervene (**Figure 1**) such as neural transmission, protein synthesis and

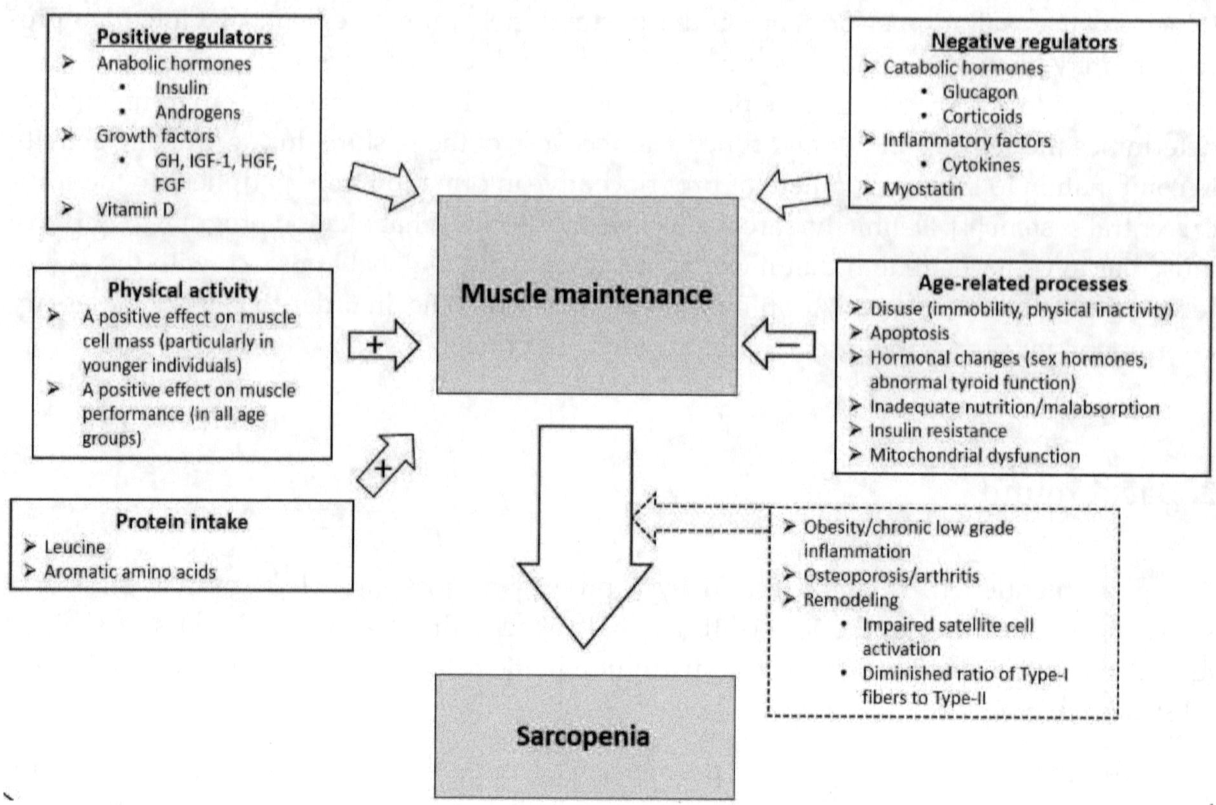

Figure 1. Factors that affect the muscle maintenance and/or the onset of sarcopenia. + positive influence, − negative influence. GH growth hormone, IGF-1 insulin-like growth factor 1, HGF: hepatocyte growth factor, FGF: fibroblast growth factor.

degradation, muscle architecture, composition of muscle fibres, increasing in production of reactive oxygen species, apoptosis of muscle cells, alteration in excitation-contraction coupling and metabolism [11].

In generic terms, sarcopenia is the age-associated loss of skeletal muscle mass and function; this decline is progressive and generalised with the possible risk of adverse outcomes such as physical disability, poor quality of life and even death [12, 13]. The causes are multifactorial and can include disuse, changing endocrine function, chronic diseases, inflammation, insulin resistance and nutritional deficiencies. The pathogenic mechanisms underlying sarcopenia are different from acute muscular atrophy resulting from disuse, cachexia, denervation or other conditions.

In order to make the diagnosis of sarcopenia, the European working group on sarcopenia in older people (EWGSOP) recommends verifying the simultaneous presence of both low muscle mass and reduction in muscle function (understood as strength or performance). Thus, the diagnosis requires the satisfaction of the criterion 1 in combination of criterion 2 or criterion 3 (**Table 1**).

The reason why are necessary at least two criteria for the diagnosis is that the force does not depend only on the muscle mass and also the relationship between strength and mass is not linear [14]. In fact, alterations in muscle quality have a central role in the loss of strength in elderly. Hughes et al. [15] showed that only a variation of 5% in strength depends on muscle mass. Muscle weakness may lead to reduced function, decreased physical activity and immobility, thus leading to secondary muscular 'ex non usu' atrophy. Consequently, diminished muscle mass is the result, but also the cause of age-related loss of strength. This is due to increased levels of pro-inflammatory cytokines and to a damage of type 2 muscle fibres. Furthermore, the growth in muscle mass is not directly related to an increment in strength, which may be increased even in the absence of a visible variation of muscle mass [16]. Neurological changes, hormonal and metabolic milieu, pro-inflammatory cytokines, fat infiltration (lipotoxicity) may conduce to a progressive muscle weakness in elderly [13]. Therefore, defining sarcopenia only in terms of loss of muscle mass is too simplistic and may be of limited clinical value. Precisely for this reason, some authors argue that the term dynapenia would be preferable to describe the loss of strength and function associated with aging [17]. However, 'sarcopenia' is a term so widely spread that replacing it could generate more confusion.

Sarcopenia staging, which reflects the severity degree of the disease, is a concept that can be of assistance in clinical management of the condition; specifically, the EWGSOP suggests a division into 'pre-sarcopenia', 'sarcopenia' and 'severe sarcopenia' (**Table 2**). 'Pre-sarcopenia' stage is characterised by low muscle mass without influencing on muscle strength or physical

Diagnosis is based on documentation of criterion 1 plus criterion 2 or 3
1. Low muscle mass
2. Low muscle strength
3. Low physical performance

Table 1. EWGSOP diagnostic criteria.

Stage	Muscle mass	Muscle strength	Performance
Pre-sarcopenia	↓		
Sarcopenia	↓	↓	Or ↓
Severe sarcopenia	↓	↓	↓

Table 2. EWGSOP stages of sarcopenia.

performance; this phase can only be identified by techniques that measure muscle mass accurately (see later). Concerning to standard populations, 'sarcopenia' stage is characterised by low muscle mass with low muscle strength or low physical performance. The last stage, when the three criteria (low muscle mass, low muscle strength and low physical performance) are present concomitantly, is defined as 'severe sarcopenia'. Recognising different stages of sarcopenia is essential to choose the most appropriate treatment and setting, thus enabling the achievement of therapeutic goals. Staging also allows to program scientific research focused on a particular stage or to evaluate any changes over time [18].

Generally, all the syndromes associated with prominent muscle loss are described as sarcopenia. Only research on the etiopathological mechanisms of age-related sarcopenia can lead to distinction from secondary forms, so the most appropriate therapy for each of them can be chosen such as cachexia, frailty and sarcopenic obesity.

The parameters of sarcopenia are muscle mass and function. The measurable variables are mass, strength and physical performance; for diagnostic and research purposes, it is important to identify the best diagnostic test that is able to measure them accurately. It is also important to recognise changes by repeating the same measures over time in the same individuals [18].

Only a few clinical trials are underway to evaluate the potential for sarcopenia treatments compared to the great impact that reduced mobility and functionality have on the quality of life of older people. The absence of standardised primary outcomes is a major challenge for the design of such studies. For intervention trials, EWGSOP presently recommends three primary outcome variables: muscle mass, muscle strength and physical performance (**Table 3**). Further studies could lead to the finding of outcomes currently considered secondary, but which may play a central role in the diagnostic and prognostic phase of this clinical condition.

Among methods of evaluation computed tomography (CT) and magnetic resonance imaging (MRI) can distinguish fat from other soft tissues of the body, thus representing validate methods for estimating muscle mass for research scope. The high costs and risks related to exposure to radiation (TC), limit their use in clinical practice. Dual energy X-ray absorptiometry (DEXA) distinguishes adipose tissue, bone mineral mass and lean body mass. It can be used both in research and in clinical practice and exposes patients to a smaller quantity of radiations. However, the access to this method is limited for severely obese individuals; furthermore, the equipment is not portable, which limits its use in epidemiological studies on a large scale.

Bioimpedance analysis (BIA) is a test that is not expensive, easy to use, easily reproducible and suitable for both ambulatory patients and bedridden. The bioelectrical impedance measurement

Variable	Exams	Clinical practice
Muscle mass	Computed tomography (CT) Magnetic resonance imaging (MRI) Dual energy X-ray absorptiometry (DXA) Bioimpedance analysis (BIA) Total or partial body potassium per fat-free tissue	BIA DXA Anthropometry
Muscle strength	Handgrip strength Knee flexion/extension Peak expiratory flow	Handgrip strength
Physical performance	Short Physical Performance Battery (SPPB) Usual gait speed Timed up and go test Stair climb power test	SPP Usual gait speed Timed up and go test

Table 3. Measurements of muscle mass, strength and performance in research and clinical practice.

techniques have been studied for many years and the BIA results in standard conditions correlate with the predictions of the MRI [19].

Among measurements to assess muscle strength, it is necessary to emphasise the importance of handgrip test; even if lower limbs are more relevant than the upper limbs in physical function and walking, the evaluation of strength by isometric handgrip has been widely used. Measured under standard conditions, with a well-studied model of dynamometer hand, it is closely correlated with lower limb muscles power and with the area of calf section.

The short physical performance battery (SPPB) is one of the most valid techniques to measure physical performance. It consists of a brief set of tests evaluating the functionality of the lower limbs. This battery is composed of three different sections. The first one is the assessment of balance in three tests: (a) maintenance of balance in stand position with feet together side-by-side for 10 seconds; (b) maintenance of balance in semi-tandem position (heel of one foot against side of big toe of the other) for 10″; (c) maintenance of balance in tandem position (feet aligned heel to toe) for 10″. The second section evaluates gait speed measuring the time required to walk 4 m linear at a normal pace. Finally, the third one measures the time required to perform five rises from a chair to an upright position as fast as possible without the use of the arms.

Other tests can be used in clinical practice, as they require a very simple execution setting. One of these is the sit to stand test, which evaluates the ability to move from sit to stand position without using arms. The timed up-and-go test (TUG), which evaluates the dynamic balance by measuring the time required to complete a series of tasks (getting up from a chair, walking a short distance, turning around an obstacle, walking back and sitting down again) [20, 21].

Specific mode and intensity of physical activity can act synergistically to maintain and even increase muscle mass, strength and power, both in healthy individual and in elderly patients with limited functionality. These interventions also have been found effective for all ages and there is evidence for similar responses in both female and male [22].

During aging, a sedentary lifestyle is associated with a decrease in lean body mass and with an increase in fat mass, which ultimately leads to an increase in mortality and functional limitations. This is demonstrated in studies showing the reduction of cardiovascular-related risk and all causes of mortality in individuals highly physically active than those moderately active or worse sedentary.

Physical activity, in particular resistance exercises, is a powerful stimulus to promote muscle protein anabolism, resulting in specific metabolic and morphological adaptations of the skeletal muscle tissue. Resistance type exercise training can effectively increase muscle strength and muscle mass, thus improving physical performance and functional capacity. To stimulate muscle hypertrophy and to increase strength in elderly patients, it is known [23] that the traditional exercise of resistance at low speed (i.e. performing concentric and eccentric to each muscle in 2–3″) is found to be a type of intervention that is safe, feasible and effective. The physiological response to resistance exercises may consist in an increase in protein synthesis, in an activation and proliferation of satellite cells, in a production of anabolic hormones and in a decreased activity of catabolic cytokines. Resistance exercises in elderly subjects appear to lead to an increased number of mitochondria and a reduction in oxidative stress. Recent scientific evidences suggest that muscle performance is a determining factor regarding the functional capabilities. A new and effective approach to increase power in elderly subjects is found to be the fast-contraction-velocity exercise. In addition, the aerobic exercise can generate benefits on elderly muscles through an increment in mitochondrial energy production, increased insulin sensitivity and/or reduction of the oxidative stress [24].

In elderly patients, the clinical relevance of a nutritional and rehabilitative intervention based on exercise, resides with the long-term effects on not only strength and muscle mass but also on the implications concerning functional capacity and risk of developing chronic metabolic diseases. It is well known that the ability to respond to an anabolic stimulus, through the activation of muscle protein synthesis, is kept up even in elderly (though to a lesser extent) [24]. Definitely, it is possible to affirm that resistance-type exercise interventions have been shown effective in increasing skeletal muscle mass, training muscle strength and/or improving functional capacity in elderly [24].

3. Rehabilitation

3.1. Scientific researches

Over the years, we have therefore investigated the effects of exercise and mechanical stimulation in primary prevention and treatment of sarcopenia.

In 2006, the first study [25] evaluated the selective development of muscle strength in 20 female subjects with severe atrophy of the femoral quadriceps muscle, with a mean age of 31 years. Subjects were randomly divided in two groups, named A and B. Group A performed 10 rehabilitation sessions, 5 times per week, lasting 10 minutes each, with mechano-sound vibration (without performing voluntary contraction) with a defined frequency of 300 Hz. Group B performed 10 sessions of strengthening every other day through isokinetic Cybex equipment at 90°/second in concentric-eccentric mode. The evaluation was performed at first visit (T0), after the treatment period (T1) and at a 6 months follow-up (T2) by isokinetic testing (Cybex) with flexion-extension movement of right and left knee at 180 and 60°/second, in both study groups. At T1 evaluation, it was found in both groups a significant increase in muscle strength and working ability as well as an improvement in muscular coordination. The increase in contractile strength in group A was comparable to that obtained with a conventional rehabilitation protocol (group B). Differences between the two groups were the longest duration of treatment effectiveness (about 6 months) and the faster achievement of these results, already during the protocol, in Group A. High speed contractile improvements induced by the local vibrational method appeared more effective; in fact, in group A, contralateral muscle strength improved too, unlike the group B.

In a 2008 study, we compared the efficacy of three methods of training in elderly subjects with postural instability and sarcopenia [26]. Nineteen subjects (11F and 8M, aged between 64 and 80 years) took part in the study. Evaluations at T0 and T1 have been carried out through clinical examination, needle biopsy of the vastus lateralis muscle (measuring specific development of the individual fibres), expression of myosin heavy chains, transcriptional and regenerative capacity profile of satellite cells. Subjects were divided randomly into three groups of six subjects each; group A performed aerobic training (endurance), group B anaerobic training (power), group C mechano-sound vibration at a frequency of 300 Hz. The protocol frequency was three sessions per week for all study groups. The results obtained showed that the development of single fibre strength did not change in any of the training protocols; gene expression profiles showed, for each type of intervention, the stimulation of a specific metabolic pathway, as both resistance and vibration training increased aerobic metabolism, while resistance training stimulated creatine metabolism. All trainings protocols stimulated in a different way the expression of sarcomeric and cytoskeletal proteins; in particular, mechano-sound vibration training has stimulated proteins associated with the Z-line. It was also found that satellite cells contribute to regeneration and trophism of muscle fibre. The results therefore suggested that all training protocols are effective in contrasting the progression of sarcopenia and each one is able to stimulate specific molecular signals. The effects are specific because there is a relationship between the type of exercise and the metabolism stimulated.

In another study, we further evaluated the effect of focused vibration on elderly skeletal muscle [27]. Eleven subjects (5F and 4M, aged between 65 and 82 years), diagnosed with sarcopenia in accordance with the guidelines of the Centers for Disease Control and Prevention (CDC) were evaluated and treated. Inclusion criteria for the study were patients older than 18 years, diagnosis of sarcopenia in absence of joint pathology. Exclusion criteria were cardiovascular and/or metabolic diseases, hereditary or acquired muscular disorders, respiratory and psychiatric disorders, treatment with testosterone or other drugs affecting muscle mass. Mechanical vibrations were applied at local level at a frequency of 300 Hz on thigh muscles for a period of 12 weeks, starting from a 15-minute per session once a week to progressively reach 3 sessions per week. The evaluation consisted of clinical examination, resting ECG and isometric tests. These were carried out the week before the beginning of the study (T0, pre-session), at the end of the therapeutic protocol (T1, post-session) and

16 weeks after the end of treatment (T2, follow-up). Moreover, it was evaluated the body mass index (BMI), the measurement of the circumference of proximal and distal thigh and it was performed the vastus lateralis muscle biopsy. Maximal isometric strength evaluation of lower limb extensor muscles showed an increase in strength since 4 weeks of treatment in women and after 8 weeks in men; increasing strength reached a plateau phase at week 12. As it regards the circumferences, it was found a significant increase of the distal circumference of 0.5–3 cm and a non-significant increase of the thigh circumference at the proximal zone. Vastus lateralis biopsy results showed the increase of muscle fibre section width (T0: 3667 ± 310.7, T1: 4238 ± 357.4 μm^2); changing in myosin chains, which switched from the isoform slow (MyHC-1) to the isoform fast (MyHC-2X). Other interesting observations were the stimulation of genes involved in energetic metabolism (PIK3R3; GSK-3), in protein synthesis and degradation, in calcium homeostasis (ACTA2; MLCB; ARL5A; LCCP; TTID; POP3; RyR3; CHERP) and in oxidative stress processes (P12; PRDX3; MSRA). It was also found a down-regulation of the gene coding for nitric oxide synthase (NOS-1). The results showed that sarcopenic skeletal muscle reduced metabolic power because of several factors, such as a reduction in blood supply, fibrosis processes and atrophy development. Muscle tissue undergoes continuous oxidative phenomena; this leads to imbalance between oxidant and antioxidant capacity; in fact, in elderly, several genes coding for antioxidant factors are down-regulated. The reduced expression of NOS leads to a reduction of the amount of nitric oxide circulating, compromising vasodilatation. Therefore, focused mechano-sound vibration, increasing the expression of genes coding for antioxidant factors, while enhancing the maximal isometric force, can be considered effective in combating sarcopenia.

In a more recent study of 2013, we compared the effectiveness of three types of training on strength and balance ability on a population of elderly male subjects suffering from sarcopenia [4]. In this study, 40 male subjects (mean age 71 years) diagnosed with sarcopenia, in accordance with the guidelines of the CDC, were evaluated and treated. Inclusion criteria of the study were patients over 18 years, sarcopenia diagnosis in absence of joint disorders. Exclusion criteria were cardiovascular or metabolic diseases, hereditary or acquired muscular disorders, respiratory and psychiatric disorders, treatment with testosterone or other substances affecting muscle mass. Forty participants were included randomly into one of the four study groups. Each group performs a specific protocol. Group A carried out a comprehensive sensorimotor training on I-Moove® with 'Reebost' program (for balance and flexibility) for 20 minutes, after warming-up with cycle-ergometer (5 minutes) and stretching of the lower limbs; frequency of sessions was 2 times per week for 12 weeks. Group B performed aerobic endurance training with leg-press and leg-extension: 2 times a week for 12 weeks. Group C underwent training vibration with a frequency of 300 Hz (average size of the transducer of 23.7 cm^2) lasting 15 minutes per session, 1 session a week for the first 8 weeks and 3 sessions per week in the last four weeks; group D (control group) did not perform any kind of rehabilitation program. The assessment was carried out using clinical examination, maximal isometric tests performed on leg-extension equipped with load cell, BMI measurement, gait analysis, stabilometry. At the end of treatment was highlighted statistically significant increase in bilateral isometric force equal to 45% in group B (which performed resistance training) and 43%

in group C, which was treated with mechano-sound vibrations. In the group, which carried out the sensorimotor training on I-Moove (group A), the improvement was only 15%, while no change was observed in the control group. About balance and stability, it was found a significative improvement of the sway area and path length, measured by stabilometry, in groups A and C; no improvements were found in groups B and D. Another observation was the increase in half-step length in all three trained groups (108% in group A, 65% in group B, 92% in group C); step width increased only in the I-Moove group. Significant reduction of 24% in time of contact to the ground was observed only in the vibration training group. The study showed that an overall sensorimotor stimulation produced by focused acoustic vibration and proprioceptive training, carried out with I-Moove, is an effective approach to increase strength and balance in sarcopenic elderly, which could result in a better quality of life.

As a part of primary prevention, we also evaluated the influence of exercise and focused acoustic vibration on blood concentration of some hormones [28]. Aim of the study was to evaluate the effects of focused acoustic vibrations, set to a frequency of 300 Hz, on muscle performance and blood hormone concentrations in healthy young adult males in acute and long-term observations. In this study, 36 male patients (average age 21.5 years) were evaluated and treated; they usually performed moderate intensity level of physical activity (1–2 times per week). The participants were divided into 2 groups: group A performed focused mechano-acoustic vibrations every 3 days for 4 weeks (10 sessions overall); instead, group B performed resistance training every 3 days for 4 weeks (10 sessions). The assessment was carried out every 3 days, during therapeutic session, through haematochemical parameters (to quantify hormone levels), counter-movement jump (CMJ) and maximal voluntary isometric contraction (MVC); assessments were performed before each session, immediately after it and 1 hour after the end of treatment. All subjects also performed isokinetic and MVC tests after 4 weeks of training and at 2 months follow-up. Group A showed a significant increase in growth hormone (GH) and creatine-phosphokinase levels and a reduction of cortisol levels ($P < 0.05$); no change was highlighted in group B. In both groups, it was observed a significant improvement in MVC test ($P < 0.05$). After 4 weeks, the results showed evidence of an increase in isokinetic tests and in maximal strength test in both groups; the improvement persisted in the next 2 months. These results indicate that focused mechano-acoustic vibrations can influence the concentration of particular hormones and can improve neuromuscular performance. The benefit gained is maintained over the medium to long term and it was comparable to what happens after a resistance training treatment.

Other authors have also studied the effectiveness of vibration therapy in improving strength and muscle tone in patients suffering from sarcopenia. Wei et al. [29] try to determine the optimal combination of frequency and exposure time of a whole-body vibration (WBV) training program to improve muscle performance in elderly with age-related muscle loss. A total of 80 community-dwelling older adults with sarcopenia were randomly divided into four groups, 20 patients each: first group treated with WBV set to low-frequency and long duration (20 Hz × 720 seconds), second group treated at medium-frequency and medium duration (40 Hz × 360 seconds), third group set to high-frequency and short duration (60 Hz × 240 seconds) and control group did not perform any training. The treatment period lasted 12 weeks and a follow-up was scheduled at additional 12 weeks. There was a significant time per group interaction effect in isokinetic knee extension at 180°/second. The study found significant time effects in all muscle strength outcome variables. Comparing second group (WBV set at 40 Hz for 360 seconds) with control group, the authors found that the percentage of change from baseline values were significant on isokinetic knee extension tests (at 180 and 60°/second). Therefore, they concluded that the best combination for WBV exercise is to set medium frequency and medium duration (40 Hz × 360 seconds), because of it shows the best outcome among all other combinations tested; moreover, the improvements in knee extension performance can be maintained for 12 weeks after cessation of WBV training.

The effectiveness of electrostimulation in rehabilitation has been long known, especially in muscle strengthening. Kern et al [30] analysed (at functional, structural and molecular level) the effects of electrical stimulation training on healthy seniors with normal lifestyle, without routine sport activity. The study found that electrical stimulation was able to improve muscle torque and functional performances and it increased muscle fibres and most importantly fast fibres, which are related to the power of skeletal muscle. At molecular level, electrical stimulation induced up-regulation of insulin-like growth factor 1 (IGF-1) and modulation of MuRF-1, a muscle-specific atrophy-related gene. Furthermore, it induced up-regulation of relevant markers of differentiating satellite cells and of extracellular matrix remodelling, which might guarantee shape and mechanical forces of trained skeletal muscle as well as maintenance of satellite cell function, reducing fibrosis. This study provide evidence that electrostimulation is a safe method to counteract muscle decline associated with aging.

In 2015, Barberi et al. [31] analysed some downstream pathways activated by IGF-1. They demonstrated that electrical stimulation increases not only anabolic pathways, but it also reduces muscle catabolism. Extracellular matrix during physical exercise shows remodelling processes. The authors demonstrated that this occur also with electrostimulation, due to enhance of collagen expression; in fact, they observed an up-regulation of three different forms of collagen (I, III and VI) in electrical stimulated muscle. The question was if this increase in collagen was due to stimulated fibrosis by electrical stimulation. However, biopsy did not demonstrate any accumulation of fibrotic tissue. Further supporting the morphological evidences, Barberi et al. analysed miR29, one of the most important controllers of fibrosis. Actually, the electrical stimulation regulates miR29, which might down-regulate fibrosis. Then authors verified electrical stimulation in increasing activity of satellite cells, such as physical exercise. In fact, electrostimulation increased the number of these cells, and this is also demonstrated by the increase of their molecular markers (myogenin, miR-206 and miR-1). In conclusion, the electrical stimulation can be applied to elderly sarcopenic patients, which might not carry out normal physical activity, modulating similar factors associated with exercise. In particular, IGF-1 once stimulated through electrostimulation, activates anabolic pathway, increasing protein synthesis and satellite cells. All these modifications lead to an increase in muscle performance.

As part of a bio-progressive rehabilitative approach, treatment of sarcopenic patients may not be limited to muscle strengthening or pain resolution. It appears clear; therefore, the need for a global approach to the patient, which also guarantees postural and gait rehabilitation. To do this, we usually consider the use of SPAD® (dynamic anti-gravitary postural system), the function of which is to provide postural stability and to increase exteroceptive and proprioceptive sensitivity. SPAD® [32] is composed by a conveyor belt, surmounted by a lifting structure, which forces the patient to walk in a straight line on a treadmill, while six proprioceptive blocks (four anterior and two on the back) act on the rotation components.

In a 2008 study [33], the aim was to define the possibility of using SPAD system in elderly rehabilitation. Group A was treated with SPAD system, while group B performed a proprioceptive rehabilitative protocol on Galileo platform (WBV at 28 Hz). Patients were evaluated at the beginning of the treatment (T0), at the end (T1) and at 6 months follow-up (T2) through gait analysis, stabilometry and isokinetic test (Cybex® system). After treatment period, both groups showed a significative improvement in gait alignment, a reduction of sway area and ellipse surface in stabilometry and a significative improvement in isokinetic tests. At follow-up evaluation, better results were found in group A (maintenance of previous results) than in group B, especially in gait and balance. These results show the effectiveness of both treatments suggested, with a better outcome at follow-up in the group that performed a rehabilitative protocol with SPAD system. In conclusion, it can be stated that SPAD treatment allows to comprehensively address the problem of postural disability evident in aging, as it acts on deep spine muscles, improving lower limb muscles tone and associating a motor-vestibular rehabilitation. This means a greater capacity of mobility with a better quality of life for elderly people.

3.2. Rehabilitative protocols

Scientific data illustrated above and those collected by our personal experience allowed us to summarise that each type of physical agents in medicine has a proper applicability in terms of cost/benefit ratio. To modulate muscle activity, enhancing muscle tone, the approach applied is:

Step 1. Focused mechano-acoustic vibrations

Step 2. Focused mechano-acoustic vibrations + SPAD

Step 3. Electrical stimulation + whole-body vibrations + SPAD

With regard to the focused mechano-acoustic vibration, the frequencies related to effects on muscles can be schematically summarised as follows:

- 120 Hz, muscle relaxation
- 200 Hz, strengthening of slow muscle fibres
- 300 Hz, strengthening of fast muscle fibres

Therefore, the treatment protocol we recommend, using Vibration Sound System®, in elderly patients suffering from sarcopenia, consists of 200 Hz for 10 minutes, 300 Hz for 10 minutes and 120 Hz for 5 minutes, applied with segmental strips in standing and/or supine position (**Figure 2**). The aim of this treatment is muscle strengthening and corticalisation.

Integrated protocols involve the use of focal vibrations in combination with active exercises and systems that increase proprioceptive stimulation to determine the synergy between stimuli.

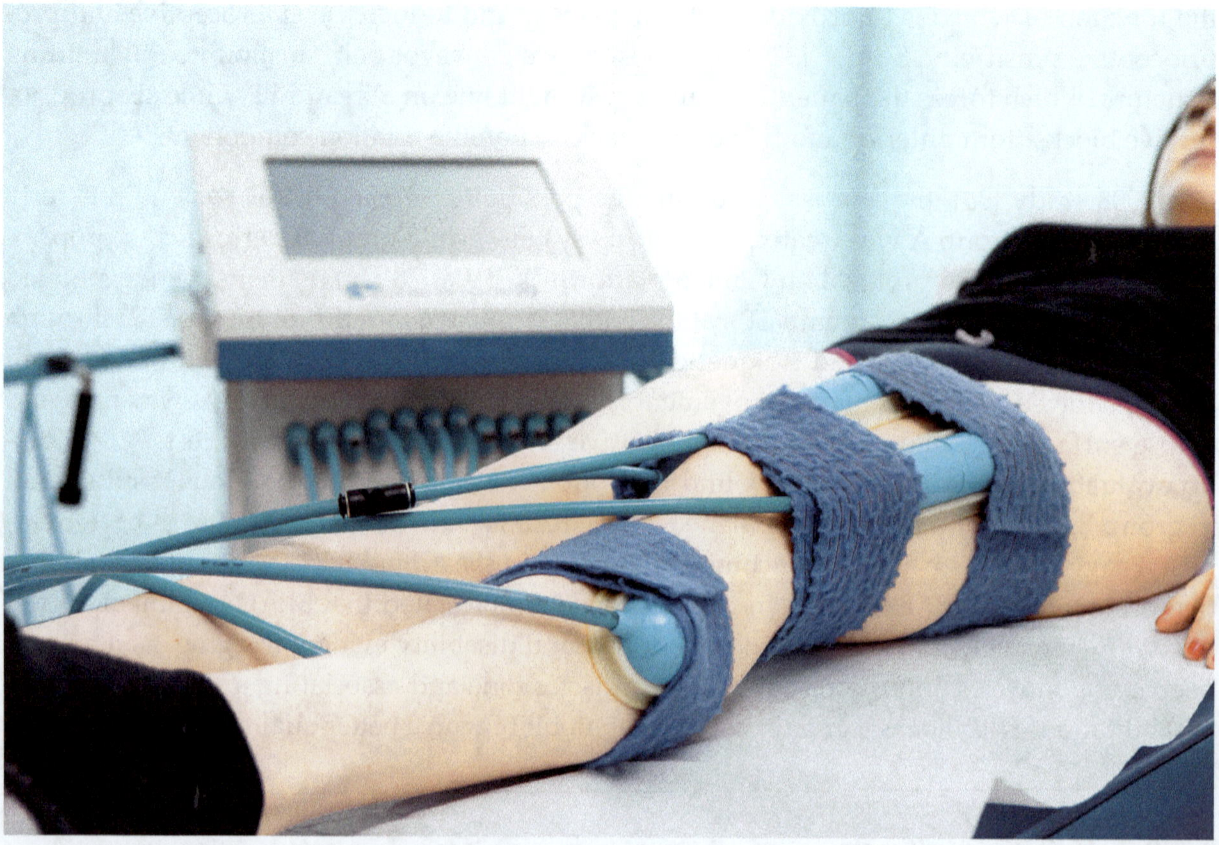

Figure 2. Focused mechano-acoustic vibrations, in supine position.

For example, if the clinical conditions of the patient permit it, we work with Vibration Sound System® to carry out eccentric exercises in upright position.

Treatment goals include increased strength through muscle hypertrophy and improved flexibility. This is also achieved through stretching exercises that improve the absorption of energy and the muscular movement range, and thus the power. Therefore, the reduction of the risk of falling, as well as the improvement of coordination, is achieved.

Another type of integrated protocol, to recover kinetic and kinematic characteristics of gait, includes the use of Vibration Sound System® with a proprioceptive system called Synergy Mat (Human Tecar® Unibell srl, Calco, Italy). It is composed by mats and pillows and it allows training, rehabilitation and natural and harmonious re-education of the body. Different surfaces give the possibility to work barefoot on different levels of instability, responding to the needs of personalised training and rehabilitation (**Figure 3**). Different densities correspond to different level of movement absorption, providing protection of the joints and increasing energy expenditure time. The variety of interchangeable elements that composed the Synergy Mat set (mats and pillows) provides many combinations of routes adapted to the user-specific needs.

To better understand the potential of vibrations and even the feasibility to integrate them with other rehabilitative systems (such as synergy mat), **Table 4** provides a list of protocols related to specific objectives and a brief description of exercises.

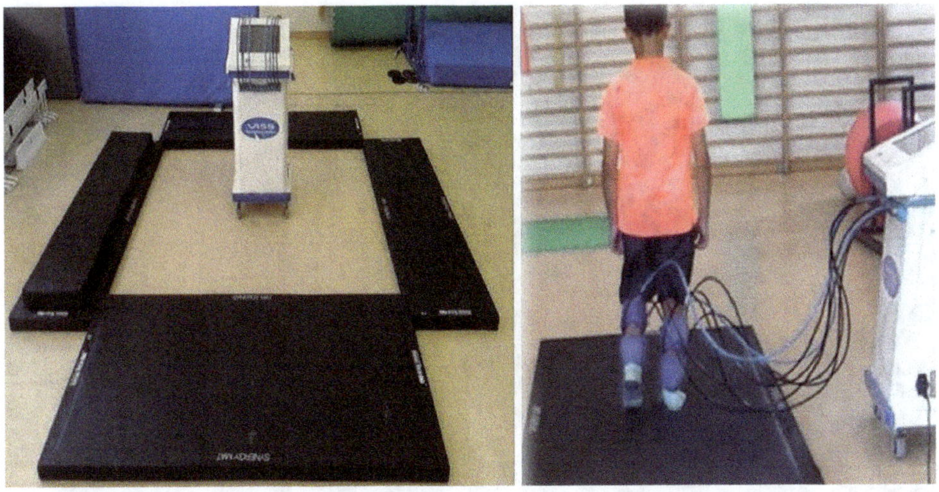

Figure 3. Another possible way to use focused mechano-acoustic vibrations in association with synergy mat.

Aim	Frequencies	Description
Muscle relaxation	50–120 Hz for 10 minutes (applied with an hand piece)	Treatment of tender points and fatigue
	120–200 Hz for 10 minutes (applied with an hand piece)	Treatment of trigger points and taut bands
Muscle strengthening, upright position	200 Hz for 10 minutes 300 Hz for 10 minutes 120 Hz for 5 minutes (applied with segmental strips)	Strengthening of slow muscle fibres Strengthening of fast muscle fibres Deconditioning
Muscle strengthening and corticalisation	200 Hz for 10 minutes 300 Hz for 10 minutes 120 Hz for 5 minutes (applied with segmental strips)	Working with squats through active work or isometric muscle contraction
Proprioceptive exercise in combination with *Synergy Mat* (Human Tecar® Unibell srl, Calco, Italy)	60–80–100–120–140–160–180–200–220–240–260–280–300 Hz, to increase every 2 minutes (applied with segmental strips)	Mono- and bipedal walking on unstable proprioceptive platforms

Table 4. Treatment protocols proposed using mechano-acoustic vibrations.

As mentioned, the second-line treatment we suggest for sarcopenia is the association of focused mechano-acoustic vibrations with SPAD® (**Figure 4**). This system has two alternative and complementary support systems: pneumatic and mechanical, which allow using consistently rates of body weight support even higher than 50%. The aim of this therapy is the recruitment of specific muscle chains, postural reprogramming and optimisation of motor coordination with restoration of the proprioceptive stimuli and physiological recovery of gait motor patterns. Therefore, the goals are both mechanical (partial decompression of lumbar spinal structures during the walk due to the microgravitary environment created) and proprioceptive (automatic-induced adaptations related to walking, once the mechanical action of relieves has achieved the percentage of body weight support established).

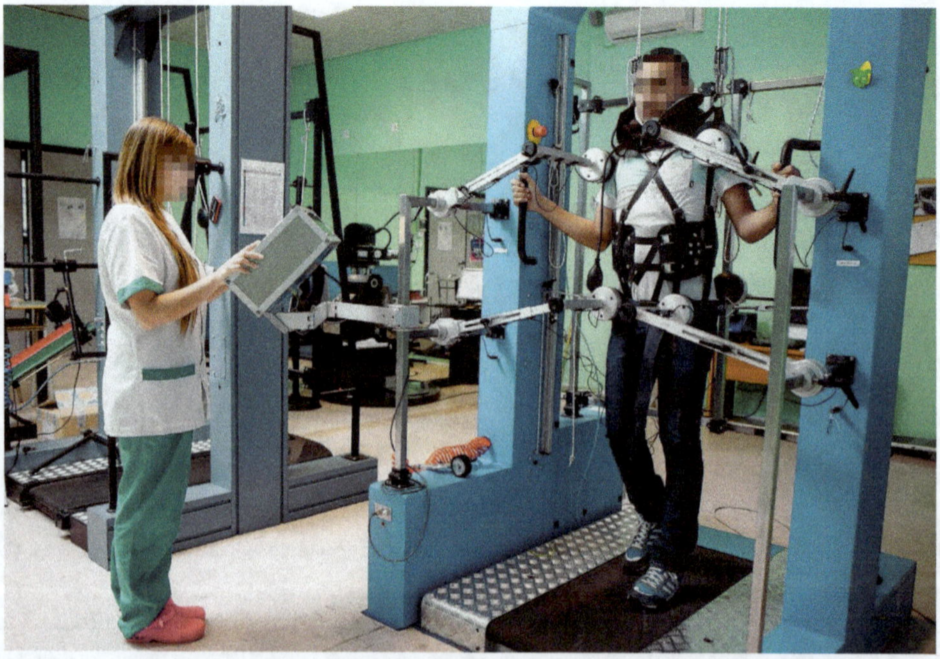

Figure 4. SPAD® system.

Third-line treatment consists of whole-body vibrations, electrical stimulation and SPAD.

Currently available WBV devices (**Figure 5**) deliver vibrations at a range of frequencies from 15 to 60 Hz and displacements from <1 to 10 mm. Considering several combinations of amplitudes and frequencies with current technology, it is clear that there are a wide variety of WBV protocols that could be used in elderly patients suffering from sarcopenia. The duration of treatment varies between individuals as well as frequencies (range 15–45 Hz); moreover, sessions of short duration (2–20 minutes), interspersed in variable-duration periods of rest, are recommended. The exercise on WBV platform would have to be performed in standing with hips and knees in slight flexion, to ensure better transmissibility of the forces to hips and spine. **Table 5** shows our WBV protocols to treat sarcopenia.

Neuromuscular electrical stimulation is defined as the use of electrical stimulation to activate muscles through intact peripheral nerve. Conventional exercise programs to increase strength are based on the overload principle of eliciting a small number of contractions of high-intensity (at least 70% of a maximal contraction 3–10 repetitions or fewer) in a treatment session performed 3–5 times per week. The same frequency of sessions can be applied when using electrical stimulation to increase strength in healthy and healthy-but-injured patients.

Our therapeutical approach involves the use of alternating currents of medium frequency produced by Horizontal Therapy (Hakomed®, **Figure 6**). The rationale is that each induced frequency generates a specific effect; for strengthening, in example, the frequencies at which muscles have to work are 20 or 100 Hz. In particular, our protocol for sarcopenia consists of a stimulation at 20 Hz for 30 minutes per session; this program includes a stimulation phase and a rest phase of 30 seconds each.

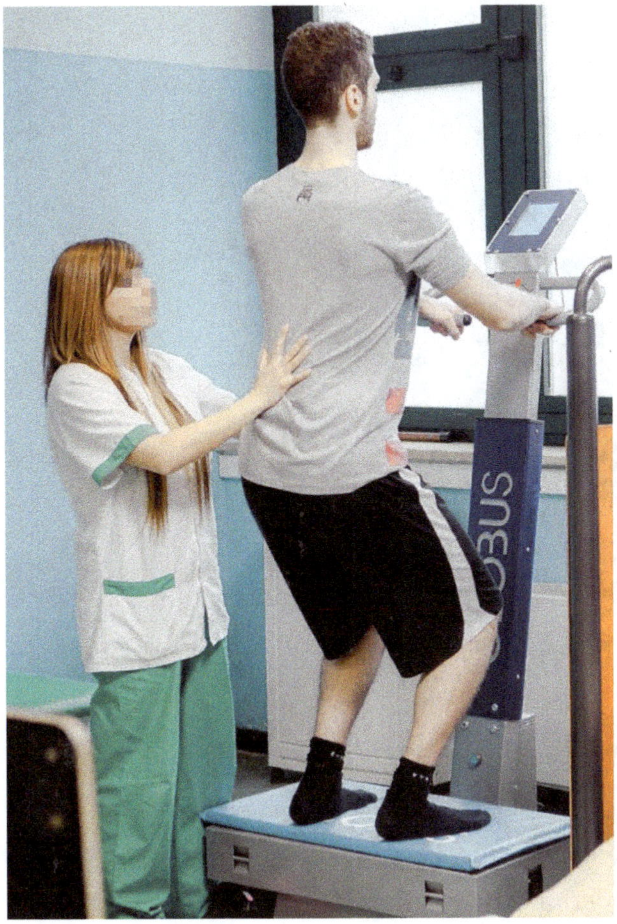

Figure 5. Whole-body vibrations (WBV).

Aim	Parameters	Protocol
Strength training	*Frequency*: 15–12 Hz. *Duration*: 3–5 minutes. *Amplitude*: medium to high, depending on comfort.	Starting position: exercises out of force and power series alternately. Sets of 10, three sets per exercise. 10-to-20-second rest between sets. 1–3-minute rest between the sets. Additional weights 70% of individual's maximal strength.
Stretching/balance exercises	*Frequency*: 15–30 Hz. *Duration*: 3–5 minutes for each exercise. *Amplitude*: low to medium.	Starting position: in standing, carry out exercises from balance and stretching series. The number of repetitions is individually tailored. Importantly, the whole body is gradually brought to an end-of-range stretching position. Balance: placing one foot alternately on the lowest position, slightly lift the other foot and hold at 5 Hz without support for 5–30 seconds.
Power training	*Frequency*: 18–30 Hz. *Duration*: 5–6 minutes. *Amplitude*: medium to high.	Carry out exercises without weights, concentrating on speed and changes in direction.

Table 5. Treatment sequence for the use of whole-body vibration in sarcopenia.

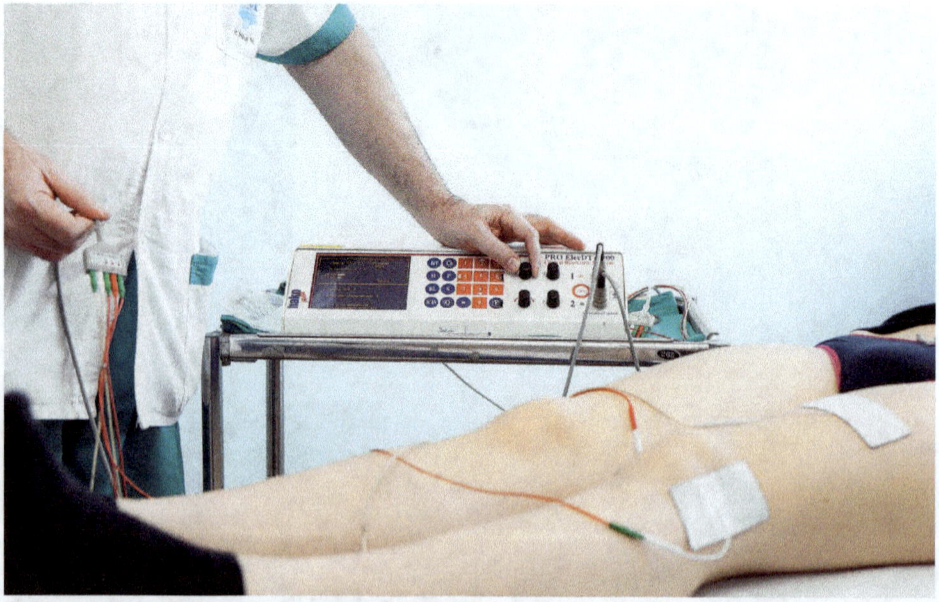

Figure 6. Horizontal therapy.

4. Conclusions

Sarcopenia is a complex problem and an important emerging field in rehabilitation of elderly. The progressive and generalised loss of skeletal muscle mass and strength is associated with the risk of physical disability, poor quality of life and death.

For these reasons, adopting the correct therapeutic solutions results of fundamental importance; to do this is necessary to know, not only the possible pharmacological interventions, but also the therapeutic possibilities that can be used thanks to the increased knowledge in the field of physical therapy. The role of rehabilitation specialist must be to integrate various therapeutic options in order to set a more suitable rehabilitative approach with the purpose of recovery postural assessment and amplify sensory-motor systems.

Author details

Raoul Saggini[1*], Simona Maria Carmignano[2], Lucia Cosenza[2], Tommaso Palermo[2] and Rosa Grazia Bellomo[3]

*Address all correspondence to: saggini@unich.it

1 Department of Medical Sciences, Oral and Biotechnology, "G. d'Annunzio" University, Chieti, Italy

2 School of Specialties in Physical and Rehabilitation Medicine, "G. d'Annunzio" University, Chieti, Italy

3 Department of Medical Sciences, Oral and Biotechnology, "G. d'Annunzio" University, Chieti, Italy

References

[1] Lynch GS, editor. Sarcopenia – Age-Related Muscle Wasting and Weakness. New York: Springer; 2011

[2] Morley JE. Sarcopenia: Diagnosis and treatment. The Journal of Nutrition Health and Aging. 2008;**12**:452-456

[3] Canning A, Grenier S. Does neuromuscular electrical stimulation improve muscular strength gains of the vastus medialis muscle. International Journal of Physical Medicine and Rehabilitation. 2014;**2**:4

[4] Bellomo RG, Iodice P, Maffulli N, Maghradze T, Coco V, Saggini R. Muscle strength and balance training in sarcopenic elderly: A pilot study with randomized controlled trial. European Journal of Inflammation. 2013;**11(1)**:193-201

[5] World Health Organization. Ageing and Life Course [Internet]. 2009. Available from: http://www.who.int/ageing/en/

[6] Sayer AA, Dennison EM, Syddall HE, et al. Type 2 diabetes, muscle strength, and impaired physical function: The tip of the iceberg? Diabetes Care. 2005;**28**:2541-2542

[7] Janssen I, Heymsfield SB, Ross R. Low relative skeletal muscle mass (sarcopenia) in older persons is associated with functional impairment and physical disability. Journal of the American Geriatrics Society. 2002;**50**:889-896

[8] Janssen I, Shepard DS, Katzmarzyk PT, et al. The healthcare costs of sarcopenia in the United States. Journal of the American Geriatrics Society. 2004;**52**:80-85

[9] Gale CR, Martyn CN, Cooper C, et al. Grip strength, body composition, and mortality. International Journal of Epidemiology. 2007;**36**:228-235

[10] Rizzoli R, Reginster JY, Arnal JF, Bautmans I, Beaudart C, Bischoff-Ferrari H, et al. Quality of life in sarcopenia and frailty. Calcified Tissue International. 2013 Aug;**93**(2):101-120

[11] Ryall JG, Schertzer JD, Lynch GS. Cellular and molecular mechanisms underlying age-related skeletal muscle wasting and weakness. Biogerontology. 2008;**9**:213-228

[12] Delmonico MJ, Harris TB, Lee JS, et al. Alternative definitions of sarcopenia, lower extremity performance, and functional impairment with aging in older men and women. Journal of the American Geriatrics Society. 2007;**55**:769-774

[13] Goodpaster BH, Park SW, Harris TB, et al. The loss of skeletal muscle strength, mass, and quality in older adults: The health, aging and body composition study. The Journals of Gerontology Series A Biological Sciences and Medical Sciences. 2006;**61**:1059-1064

[14] Janssen I, Baumgartner R, Ross R, et al. Skeletal muscle cutpoints associated with elevated physical disability risk in older men and women. American Journal of Epidemiology. 2004:**159**:413-421

[15] Hughes VA, Frontera WR, Roubenoff R, Evans WJ, Singh MA. Longitudinal changes in body composition in older men and women: Role of body weight change and physical activity. The American Journal of Clinical Nutrition. 2002;**76**:473-481

[16] Trappe S, Godard M, Gallagher P, Carroll C, Rowden G, Porter D. Resistance training improves single muscle fiber contractile function in older women. American Journal of Physiology Cell Physiology. 2001;**281**:C398-C406

[17] Clark BC, Manini TM. Sarcopenia ≠ dynapenia. The Journals of Gerontology Series A Biological Sciences and Medical Sciences. 2008;**63**:829-834

[18] Cruz-Jentoft AJ, Baeyens JP, Bauer JM, et al. Sarcopenia: European consensus on definition and diagnosis: Report of the European Working Group on Sarcopenia in Older People. Age and Ageing. 2010;**39**(4):412-423

[19] Janssen I, Heymsfield SB, Wang ZM, Ross R. Estimation of skeletal muscle mass by bioelectrical impedance analysis. Journal of Applied Physiology. 2000;**89**:465-471

[20] Guralnik JM, Simonsick EM, Ferrucci L, Robert J, Glynn LF, et al. A short physical performance battery assessing lower extremity function: Association with self-reported disability and prediction of mortality and nursing home admission. The Journals of Gerontology. 1994:**49**:M85-94

[21] Mathias S, Nayak US, Isaacs B. Balance in elderly patients: The "get-up and go" test. Archives of Physical Medicine and Rehabilitation. 1986;**67**:387-389

[22] Chodzko-Zajko WJ, Proctor DN, Fiatarone Singh MA, Minson CT, Nigg CR, Salem GJ, Skinner JS. American College of Sports Medicine position stand. Exercise and physical activity for older adults. Medicine and Science in Sports and Exercise. 2009;**41**:1510-1530

[23] Forbes SC, Little JP, Candow DG. Exercise and nutritional interventions for improving aging muscle health. Endocrine. 2012 Aug;**42**(1):29-38

[24] Snijders T, Verdijk LB, van Loon LJ. The impact of sarcopenia and exercise training on skeletal muscle satellite cells. Ageing Research Reviews. 2009 Oct;**8**(4):328-338

[25] Saggini R, Iodice P, Cancelli F, Di Baldassarre V, Bellomo RG. Lo sviluppo selettivo di forza muscolare nel contesto riabilitativo: metodologie a confronto. Europa Medicophysica. Giugno. 2006;**42**(Suppl. 1):357-358

[26] Saggini R, Bellomo RG, Coco V, Savoia V, Iodice P, Fanò G. Instabilità posturale, sarcopenia e cadute. Geriatric Medicine. Gennaio/Aprile. 2008;**1**(Suppl.):21-25

[27] Pietrangelo T, Mancinelli R, Toniolo L, Cancellara L, Paoli A, Puglielli C, et al. Effects of local vibrations on skeletal muscle trophism in elderly people: Mechanical, cellular, and molecular events. International Journal of Molecular Medicine. 2009 Oct;**24**(4):503-512

[28] Iodice P, Bellomo RG, Gialluca G, Fanò G, Saggini R. Acute and cumulative effects of focused high-frequency vibrations on the endocrine system and muscle strength. European Journal of Applied Physiology. 2011;**111**:897-904

[29] Wei N, Pang MY, Ng SS, Ng GY. Optimal frequency/time combination of whole-body vibration training for improving muscle size and strength of people with age-related muscle loss (sarcopenia): A randomized controlled trial. Geriatrics & Gerontology International; 2016 [Epub ahead of print]. DOI: 10.1111/ggi.12878

[30] Kern H, Barberi L, Löfler S, et al. Electrical stimulation counteracts muscle decline in seniors. Frontiers in Aging Neuroscience. 2014;**6**:189

[31] Barberi L, Scicchitano BM, Musaro A. Molecular and cellular mechanisms of muscle aging and sarcopenia and effects of electrical stimulation in seniors. European Journal of Translational Myology. 2015;**25**(4):5227

[32] Di Pancrazio L, Bellomo RG, Franciotti R, Iodice P, Galati V, et al. Combined rehabilitation program for postural instability in progressive supranuclear palsy. NeuroRehabilitation. 2013;**32**:855-860

[33] Saggini R, Bellomo RG, Savoia V, Iodice P, Di Pancrazio L, et al. Instabilità posturale, sarcopenia e cadute. European Journal of Medical Physics. 2008;**44**(Suppl. 1):21-25

7

Understanding Cachexia, Sarcopenia and Physical Exercise in Patients with Cancer

Shinichiro Morishita, Atsuhiro Tsubaki and Jack B. Fu

Abstract

Many patients with cancer experience muscle wasting and weakness. Muscle wasting in patients with cancer can be caused by cachexia and sarcopenia. Both cachexia and sarcopenia involve inflammation and oxidative stress. However, they differ in the underlying mechanisms that lead to muscle wasting. Cachexia involves the release of inflammatory cytokines due to cancer, while sarcopenia involves inflammation due to aging. Physical exercise has shown effectiveness for improving physical function, ability, and quality of life (QOL) in patients with cancer cachexia. On the other hand, no studies have investigated the relationship between physical exercise and sarcopenia in elderly patients with cancer. Previous studies showed effectiveness for improving physical function in elderly patients with cancer. In the future, more studies are required on physical exercise in sarcopenic elderly patients with cancer.

Keywords: cachexia, sarcopenia, physical exercise, quality of life, patients with cancer

1. Introduction

Muscle wasting and weakness are common in many disease states and conditions including aging and cancer [1]. Muscle wasting in advanced cancer is related to age, sex, tumor type, and inflammation [2]. It can be caused by inflammation and malnutrition in patients with cancer [3]. Patients with cancer have problems including anorexia, weight loss, negative nitrogen balance, and skeletal muscle wasting [4]. The loss of muscle and fat tissue due to chronic illness is referred to as cachexia, and the general loss of muscle mass with advancing age is referred to as sarcopenia [5]. Sarcopenia diagnosis requires documentation of low muscle mass along with either low muscle strength or low physical performance [6]. Cachexia and sarcopenia share some pathological muscle wasting mechanisms characterized by inflammation and oxidative stress [7, 8]. In both cachexia and sarcopenia, muscle loss can lead to frailty and adversely affect various clinical outcomes [9]. Many oncologists and rehabilitation staffs confuse cancer cachexia with simple starvation or physiological processes such as sarcopenia. Since cancer cachexia and sarcopenia can both involve muscle wasting, we speculate that the two conditions can be confused in patients with cancer. However, sarcopenia and cachexia should not be confused in patients with cancer (**Figure 1**). Instead, it should be understood that the loss of skeletal muscle mass occurs in patients with cancer (cachexia) as well as during aging (sarcopenia). Cachexia involves muscle wasting and weakness as a result of cancer-related inflammation, while sarcopenia involves muscle wasting and weakness as a result of age-related inflammation. Thus, the underlying pathological processes leading to muscle wasting and weakness differ between the two conditions.

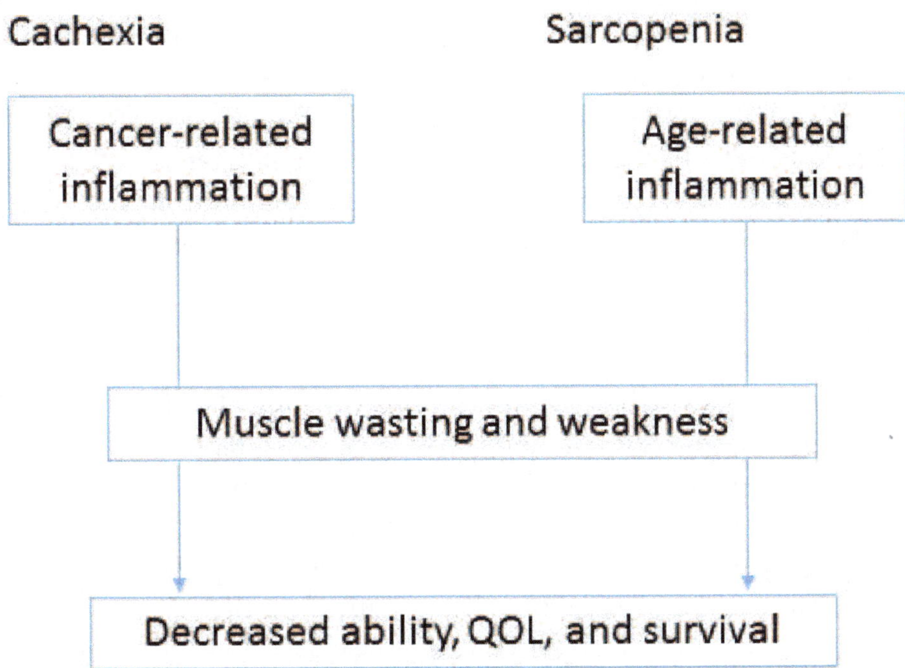

Figure 1. Muscle wasting due to cancer cachexia and sarcopenia.

2. Cachexia

Cachexia is associated with cancer and other chronic diseases, and cachexia patients lose weight and experience a decline in their overall health. The mechanism of cancer cachexia is known to involve inflammatory cytokines such as tumor necrosis factor-alpha and interleukin-6 [10]. Cancer cachexia is a complex syndrome that describes the progressive muscle wasting and weakness observed in many patients with cancer and accounts for at least 20% of cancer deaths [11, 12]. It is caused by numerous complex interactions of tumor and host factors [13, 14], and results in anorexia, wasting syndrome, and subsequent related issues [15].

It is a multifactorial syndrome defined by an ongoing loss of skeletal muscle mass (with or without loss of fat mass) that cannot be fully reversed by conventional nutritional support [16]. A panel of experts has also defined consensus criteria for diagnosing cachexia in patients with cancer [16]: (1) weight loss > 5% over the past 6 months (in the absence of simple starvation); (2) BMI < 20 kg/m^2 and any degree of weight loss > 2%; or (3) appendicular skeletal muscle index consistent with sarcopenia (males < 7.26 kg/m^2; females < 5.45 kg/m^2), and any degree of weight loss > 2%. A defining feature of cancer cachexia is the loss of muscle, but fat may also be lost [17]. Weight loss is involuntary, meaning that there is no desire or attempt to lose weight. Cancer cachexia usually worsens over time, and as weight loss increases, cancer cachexia patients also experience difficulties in daily activities.

Cancer cachexia has three clinical stages: precachexia, cachexia, and refractory cachexia [16]. The condition may occur in stages that are defined by differences in food intake, weight loss, and ability to function. In addition to muscle wasting and appetite loss, patients who have cancer anorexia–cachexia have a poor overall quality of life (QOL) and experience fatigue. They find it difficult to perform regular daily activities [18], and experience a significant symptom burden [19, 20]. Patients with cancer cachexia have significant decrease in physical function [21, 22], with low grip strength, and shorter walking distance even when controlling for muscle wasting [23, 24]. Also, cancer cachexia patients demonstrate lower physical activity [25–27]. In the early or mild stage, patients with cancer may only notice a slight loss of appetite. At the moderate stage, patients will notice more weight loss and often eat less than at the early and mild stages. In the severe stage, muscle wasting becomes markedly increased compared to the moderate stage, and the condition may be resistant to normal treatments such as dietary supplementation and nutritional support. Patients with cancer do not experience weight gain. Furthermore, patients may also have great difficulties in performing routine activities [16, 28]. Cachexia can reduce the physical activities of daily living (ADL) in patients with cancer [29]. Many patients with cancer cachexia experience decrease in physical function and ADL after muscle wasting. Thus, in addition to nutritional support, physical exercise may also contribute to improve the physical function in patients with cancer cachexia.

3. Sarcopenia

Sarcopenia, derived from a Greek word meaning "poverty of flesh," is characterized by the triad of progressive loss of skeletal muscle mass, muscle strength, and physical performance [30]. It is defined as age-related muscle wasting; thus, sarcopenia frequently occurs in elderly people. European Working Group on Sarcopenia in Older People (EWGSOP) recommends that the diagnosis of sarcopenia in elderly patients should be based on the presence of both low muscle mass and low muscle function (strength or performance) [6]. EWGSOP uses these characteristics to further classify the condition into the stages of presarcopenia, sarcopenia, and severe sarcopenia [6]. Sarcopenia has emerged as an important prognostic factor in elderly advanced patients with cancer [6]. Modalities used to assess sarcopenia include magnetic resonance imaging, computed tomography, dual-energy X-ray absorptiometry, and bioelectrical impedance analysis [31]. Sarcopenia is associated with poor performance status, toxicity from chemotherapy, and short time of tumor control [32, 33].

Sarcopenia is now recognized as a multifactorial geriatric syndrome [34, 35], and is a common clinical symptom of elderly patients with cancer [36]. It has been reported to serve as an independent risk factor for poor prognosis indicative of disease and death [37]. It typically co-occurs with cachexia in patients with cancer [38]. However, changes in muscle mass and physical performance may occur before clinically overt cachexia in patients with cancer [35]. In recent years, clinical research on the application of exercise, nutritional support, and drugs, as well as other comprehensive interventions in sarcopenia patients have demonstrated good results [39]. A significant proportion of elderly patients with cancer are at risk of sarcopenia development. However, despite its potential impact on their quality of life [2, 40], limited data are available regarding the factors associated with sarcopenia in elderly patients with cancer, who might have more problems such as malnutrition than non sarcopenic patients.

4. Physical exercise

Physical exercise has the potential to help maintain or slow the loss of physical function [41] as well as sustain and build muscle mass [42]. Aerobic and resistance exercise have been found to better improve upper and lower body strength than usual care in patients with cancer [42]. Aerobic exercise training for skeletal muscles improves wasting in cardiac and cancer cachexia patients [43]. Resistance exercise attenuates muscle wasting associated with a variety of catabolic conditions [44]. Physical exercise has been shown to be effective in improving physical activity levels in cancer survivors [45]. Physical activity intervention significantly improved quality of life for cancer cachexia patients [46, 47]. A systematic review found that physical activity has benefits including improvement in physical activity levels, aerobic fitness, muscle strength, functional quality of life, anxiety, and self-esteem [48] (**Figure 2**).

Physical activity correlated with maximum exercise capacity, weight loss, blood hemoglobin concentration, C-reactive protein, and QOL-related factors of physical functioning and bodily pain in patients with cancer with progressive cachexia [49]. Physical exercise may promote a disruption in the cycle of events leading to cachexia advancement (i.e. muscle tissue loss via anorexigenic proinflammatory cytokines) and, in turn, enhanced functionality and thus, improved QOL in patients with cancer [50]. It has been suggested to counteract sustained disease-related inflammation and the effect of exercise training in cancer cachexia [51]. Furthermore, it has been shown an association with the reduced levels of C-reactive protein in patients with cancer [52].

In patients with cancer, physical exercise represents a function-preserving, anti-inflammatory, and metabolism-modulating strategy with a low cost [53]. It may reverse protein degradation while increasing protein synthesis and lean body mass, thus counteracting the wasting seen in cachexia [54]. It is necessary to develop a better understanding of how to support patients with cancer in starting and maintaining physical activity and exercise programs. It is uncertain whether physical activity during and following cancer treatment has the same benefits

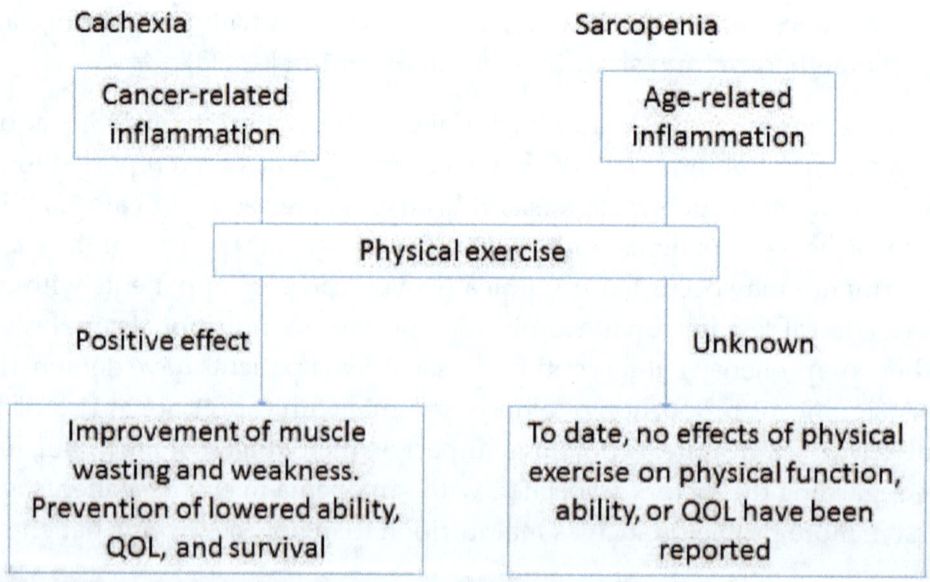

Figure 2. The effectiveness of physical exercise for patients with cancer with cachexia and sarcopenia.

in the weight-stable and weight-losing patients. The question also remains as to whether physical exercise has any health benefit in people with cancer cachexia or those at risk of cancer cachexia. Research investigating physical exercise in patients with cancer undergoing treatment has demonstrated improvements in physical performance, fatigue, and functional quality of life. It is unclear whether these benefits are experienced by patients with cancer cachexia. There is insufficient evidence to establish the safety and effectiveness of physical exercise in cancer cachexia patients, and future trials on exercise and supportive care interventions are required in this population. Aerobic and resistance exercise regimens may have positive effects on decreasing cancer-related fatigue and muscle wasting in patients with cancer cachexia.

To date, no studies have shown a relationship between physical exercise and cancer sarcopenia. In elderly patients with cancer, physical exercise has several benefits including improving immune function [55], hemoglobin and red blood cell count [56], and physical activity [57], not but VO2peak, 1 repetition maximum, functional capacity, anxiety level, or emotional well-being [58]. Physical exercise seems to improve physical function and immune function in elderly patients with cancer [59]. However, it has not shown effectiveness for sarcopenic patients with cancer.

5. Summary and conclusion

Muscle wasting is often encountered in patients with cancer. Both cachexia and sarcopenia lead to muscle wasting in patients with cancer. However, the different mechanisms of muscle wasting in patients with cancer should be recognized. Physical exercise might be effective for improving physical function, physical activity, ADL, and QOL in patients with cancer cachexia. In the future, more studies are required on physical exercise in sarcopenic elderly patients with cancer. Studies investigating the combined effect of physical exercise and nutritional therapies such as branched chain amino acids in cancer rehabilitation are required to improve patient outcomes in the future.

Author details

Shinichiro Morishita[1]*, Atsuhiro Tsubaki[1] and Jack B. Fu[2]

*Address all correspondence to: ptmorishin@yahoo.co.jp

1 Institute for Human Movement and Medical Sciences, Niigata University of Health and Welfare, Niigata, Japan

2 Department of Palliative, Rehabilitation & Integrative Medicine, University of Texas MD Anderson Cancer Center, Houston, TX, USA

References

[1] Lynch GS, Schertzer JD, Ryall JG: Therapeutic approaches for muscle wasting disorders. Pharmacol Ther 2007, **113**(3):461-487.

[2] Wallengren O, Iresjö BM, Lundholm K, Bosaeus I: Loss of muscle mass in the end of life in patients with advanced cancer. Support Care Cancer 2015, **23**(1):79-86.

[3] Argilés JM, López-Soriano FJ, Busquets S: Muscle wasting in cancer: The role of mitochondria. Curr Opin Clin Nutr Metab Care 2015, **18**(3):221-225.

[4] Fearon KC, Baracos VE: Cachexia in pancreatic cancer: New treatment options and measures of success. HPB (Oxford) 2010, **12**(5):323-324.

[5] Muscaritoli M, Anker SD, Argilés J, Aversa Z, Bauer JM, Biolo G, Boirie Y, Bosaeus I, Cederholm T, Costelli P et al: Consensus definition of sarcopenia, cachexia and pre-cachexia: Joint document elaborated by Special Interest Groups (SIG) "cachexia-anorexia in chronic wasting diseases" and "nutrition in geriatrics". Clin Nutr 2010, **29**(2):154-159.

[6] Cruz-Jentoft AJ, Baeyens JP, Bauer JM, Boirie Y, Cederholm T, Landi F, Martin FC, Michel JP, Rolland Y, Schneider SM et al: Sarcopenia: European consensus on definition and diagnosis: Report of the European Working Group on Sarcopenia in Older People. Age Ageing 2010, **39**(4):412-423.

[7] Bowen TS, Schuler G, Adams V: Skeletal muscle wasting in cachexia and sarcopenia: Molecular pathophysiology and impact of exercise training. J Cachexia Sarcopenia Muscle 2015, **6**(3):197-207.

[8] Argilés JM, Busquets S, Stemmler B, López-Soriano FJ: Cachexia and sarcopenia: Mechanisms and potential targets for intervention. Curr Opin Pharmacol 2015, **22**:100-106.

[9] Rolland Y, Abellan van Kan G, Gillette-Guyonnet S, Vellas B: Cachexia versus sarcopenia. Curr Opin Clin Nutr Metab Care 2011, **14**(1):15-21.

[10] Argilés JM, Busquets S, López-Soriano FJ: Cytokines as mediators and targets for cancer cachexia. Cancer Treat Res 2006, **130**:199-217.

[11] Shum AM, Polly P: Cancer cachexia: Molecular targets and pathways for diagnosis and drug intervention. Endocr Metab Immune Disord Drug Targets 2012, **12**(3):247-259.

[12] Murphy KT, Lynch GS: Update on emerging drugs for cancer cachexia. Expert Opin Emerg Drugs 2009, **14**(4):619-632.

[13] Tisdale M: Cancer cachexia. Curr Opin Gastroenterol 2010, **26**(2):146-151.

[14] Tisdale M: Mechanisms of cancer cachexia. Physiol Rev 2009, **89**(2):381-410.

[15] Fearon K, Arends J, Baracos V: Understanding the mechanisms and treatment options in cancer cachexia. Nat Rev Clin Oncol 2013, **10**(2):90-99.

[16] Fearon K, Strasser F, Anker SD, Bosaeus I, Bruera E, Fainsinger RL, Jatoi A, Loprinzi C, MacDonald N, Mantovani G et al: Definition and classification of cancer cachexia: An international consensus. Lancet Oncol 2011, **12**(5):489-495.

[17] Evans WJ, Morley JE, Argilés J, Bales C, Baracos V, Guttridge D, Jatoi A, Kalantar-Zadeh K, Lochs H, Mantovani G et al: Cachexia: A new definition. Clin Nutr 2008, **27**(6):793-799.

[18] Vaughan VC, Martin P, Lewandowski PA: Cancer cachexia: Impact, mechanisms and emerging treatments. J Cachexia Sarcopenia Muscle 2013, **4**(2):95-109.

[19] LeBlanc TW, Nipp RD, Rushing CN, Samsa GP, Locke SC, Kamal AH, Cella DF, Abernethy AP: Correlation between the international consensus definition of the Cancer Anorexia-Cachexia Syndrome (CACS) and patient-centered outcomes in advanced non-small cell lung cancer. J Pain Symptom Manage 2015, **49**(4):680-689.

[20] Tarricone R, Ricca G, Nyanzi-Wakholi B, Medina-Lara A: Impact of cancer anorexia-cachexia syndrome on health-related quality of life and resource utilisation: A systematic review. Crit Rev Oncol Hematol 2016, **99**:49-62.

[21] Dalton JT, Barnette KG, Bohl CE, Hancock ML, Rodriguez D, Dodson ST, Morton RA, Steiner MS: The selective androgen receptor modulator GTx-024 (enobosarm) improves lean body mass and physical function in healthy elderly men and postmenopausal women: Results of a double-blind, placebo-controlled phase II trial. J Cachexia Sarcopenia Muscle 2011, **2**(3):153-161.

[22] Dobs AS, Boccia RV, Croot CC, Gabrail NY, Dalton JT, Hancock ML, Johnston MA, Steiner MS: Effects of enobosarm on muscle wasting and physical function in patients with cancer: A double-blind, randomised controlled phase 2 trial. Lancet Oncol 2013, **14**(4):335-345.

[23] Wallengren O, Lundholm K, Bosaeus I: Diagnostic criteria of cancer cachexia: Relation to quality of life, exercise capacity and survival in unselected palliative care patients. Support Care Cancer 2013, **21**(6):1569-1577.

[24] Mantovani G: Randomised phase III clinical trial of 5 different arms of treatment on 332 patients with cancer cachexia. Eur Rev Med Pharmacol Sci 2010, **14**(4):292-301.

[25] Maddocks M, Byrne A, Johnson CD, Wilson RH, Fearon KC, Wilcock A: Physical activity level as an outcome measure for use in cancer cachexia trials: A feasibility study. Support Care Cancer 2010, **18**(12):1539-1544.

[26] Johns N, Greig C, Fearon KC: Is tissue cross-talk important in cancer cachexia? Crit Rev Oncog 2012, **17**(3):263-276.

[27] Fearon KC: The 2011 ESPEN Arvid Wretlind lecture: Cancer cachexia: The potential impact of translational research on patient-focused outcomes. Clin Nutr 2012, **31**(5):577-582.

[28] Tan BH, Fearon KC: Cachexia: Prevalence and impact in medicine. Curr Opin Clin Nutr Metab Care 2008, **11**(4):400-407.

[29] Massa E, Madeddu C, Lusso MR, Gramignano G, Mantovani G: Evaluation of the effectiveness of treatment with erythropoietin on anemia, cognitive functioning and functions studied by comprehensive geriatric assessment in elderly cancer patients with anemia related to cancer chemotherapy. Crit Rev Oncol Hematol 2006, **57**(2):175-182.

[30] Iannuzzi-Sucich M, Prestwood KM, Kenny AM: Prevalence of sarcopenia and predictors of skeletal muscle mass in healthy, older men and women. J Gerontol A Biol Sci Med Sci 2002, **57**(12):M772–M777.

[31] Cruz-Jentoft AJ, Landi F, Schneider SM, Zúñiga C, Arai H, Boirie Y, Chen LK, Fielding RA, Martin FC, Michel JP et al: Prevalence of and interventions for sarcopenia in ageing adults: A systematic review. Report of the International Sarcopenia Initiative (EWGSOP and IWGS). Age Ageing 2014, **43**(6):748-759.

[32] Peng PD, van Vledder MG, Tsai S, de Jong MC, Makary M, Ng J, Edil BH, Wolfgang CL, Schulick RD, Choti MA et al: Sarcopenia negatively impacts short-term outcomes in patients undergoing hepatic resection for colorectal liver metastasis. HPB (Oxford) 2011, **13**(7):439-446.

[33] Miyamoto Y, Baba Y, Sakamoto Y, Ohuchi M, Tokunaga R, Kurashige J, Hiyoshi Y, Iwagami S, Yoshida N, Watanabe M et al: Negative impact of skeletal muscle loss after systemic chemotherapy in patients with unresectable colorectal cancer. PLoS One 2015, **10**(6):e0129742.

[34] Cruz-Jentoft AJ, Landi F, Topinková E, Michel JP: Understanding sarcopenia as a geriatric syndrome. Curr Opin Clin Nutr Metab Care 2010, **13**(1):1-7.

[35] Collins JT, Noble S, Chester J, Davies HE, Evans WD, Lester J, Parry D, Pettit RJ, Byrne A: Association of sarcopenia and observed physical performance with attainment of multidisciplinary team planned treatment in non-small cell lung cancer: An observational study protocol. BMC Cancer 2015, **15**:544.

[36] Gibson DJ, Burden ST, Strauss BJ, Todd C, Lal S: The role of computed tomography in evaluating body composition and the influence of reduced muscle mass on clinical

outcome in abdominal malignancy: A systematic review. Eur J Clin Nutr 2015, **69**(10):1079-1086.

[37] Zhuang CL, Huang DD, Pang WY, Zhou CJ, Wang SL, Lou N, Ma LL, Yu Z, Shen X: Sarcopenia is an independent predictor of severe postoperative complications and long-term survival after radical gastrectomy for gastric cancer: Analysis from a large-scale cohort. Medicine (Baltimore) 2016, **95**(13):e3164.

[38] Evans WJ: Skeletal muscle loss: Cachexia, sarcopenia, and inactivity. Am J Clin Nutr 2010, **91**(4):1123S–1127S.

[39] Burton LA, Sumukadas D: Optimal management of sarcopenia. Clin Interv Aging 2010, **5**:217-228.

[40] Ugolini G, Pasini F, Ghignone F, Zattoni D, Bacchi Reggiani ML, Parlanti D, Montroni I: How to select elderly colorectal cancer patients for surgery: A pilot study in an Italian academic medical center. Cancer Biol Med 2015, **12**(4):302-307.

[41] Maddocks M, Murton AJ, Wilcock A: Therapeutic exercise in cancer cachexia. Crit Rev Oncog 2012, **17**(3):285-292.

[42] Stene GB, Helbostad JL, Balstad TR, Riphagen II, Kaasa S, Oldervoll LM: Effect of physical exercise on muscle mass and strength in cancer patients during treatment–A systematic review. Crit Rev Oncol Hematol 2013, **88**(3):573-593.

[43] Alves CR, da Cunha TF, da Paixão NA, Brum PC: Aerobic exercise training as therapy for cardiac and cancer cachexia. Life Sci 2015, **125**:9-14.

[44] al-Majid S, McCarthy DO: Cancer-induced fatigue and skeletal muscle wasting: The role of exercise. Biol Res Nurs 2001, **2**(3):186-197.

[45] Bourke L, Homer KE, Thaha MA, Steed L, Rosario DJ, Robb KA, Saxton JM, Taylor SJ: Interventions for promoting habitual exercise in people living with and beyond cancer. Cochrane Database Syst Rev 2013, **9**:CD010192.

[46] Lowe SS: Physical activity and palliative cancer care. Recent Results Cancer Res 2011, **186**:349-365.

[47] Aapro M, Arends J, Bozzetti F, Fearon K, Grunberg SM, Herrstedt J, Hopkinson J, Jaquelin-Ravel N, Jatoi A, Kaasa S et al: Early recognition of malnutrition and cachexia in the cancer patient: A position paper of a European School of Oncology Task Force. Ann Oncol 2014, **25**(8):1492-9.

[48] Speck RM, Courneya KS, Mâsse LC, Duval S, Schmitz KH: An update of controlled physical activity trials in cancer survivors: A systematic review and meta-analysis. J Cancer Surviv 2010, **4**(2):87-100.

[49] Fouladiun M, Körner U, Gunnebo L, Sixt-Ammilon P, Bosaeus I, Lundholm K: Daily physical-rest activities in relation to nutritional state, metabolism, and quality of life in cancer patients with progressive cachexia. Clin Cancer Res 2007, **13**(21):6379-6385.

[50] Battaglini CL, Hackney AC, Goodwin ML: Cancer cachexia: Muscle physiology and exercise training. Cancers (Basel) 2012, **4**(4):1247-1251.

[51] Lira FS, Neto JC, Seelaender M: Exercise training as treatment in cancer cachexia. Appl Physiol Nutr Metab 2014, **39**(6):679-686.

[52] Maddocks M, Jones LW, Wilcock A: Immunological and hormonal effects of exercise: Implications for cancer cachexia. Curr Opin Support Palliat Care 2013, **7**(4):376-382.

[53] Lira FS, Antunes BeM, Seelaender M, Rosa Neto JC: The therapeutic potential of exercise to treat cachexia. Curr Opin Support Palliat Care 2015, **9**(4):317-324.

[54] Gould DW, Lahart I, Carmichael AR, Koutedakis Y, Metsios GS: Cancer cachexia prevention via physical exercise: Molecular mechanisms. J Cachexia Sarcopenia Muscle 2013, **4**(2):111-124.

[55] Bigley AB, Spielmann G, LaVoy EC, Simpson RJ: Can exercise-related improvements in immunity influence cancer prevention and prognosis in the elderly? Maturitas 2013, **76**(1):51-56.

[56] Mohamady HM, Elsisi HF, Aneis YM: Impact of moderate intensity aerobic exercise on chemotherapy-induced anemia in elderly women with breast cancer: A randomized controlled clinical trial. J Adv Res 2017, **8**(1):7-12.

[57] Ying H, Wang Y, Ning X, Zhou J, Zhao L, Shao Y, Bai C, Chen S: Changes of exercise and the clinical effects among eldly non-small cell lung cancer survivors. Zhongguo Fei Ai Za Zhi 2010, **13**(1):64-68.

[58] Quist M, Adamsen L, Rørth M, Laursen JH, Christensen KB, Langer SW: The impact of a multidimensional exercise intervention on physical and functional capacity, anxiety, and depression in patients with advanced-stage lung cancer undergoing chemotherapy. Integr Cancer Ther 2015, **14**(4):341-349.

[59] Miki E, Kataoka T, Okamura H: Feasibility and efficacy of speed-feedback therapy with a bicycle ergometer on cognitive function in elderly cancer patients in Japan. Psychooncology 2014, **23**(8):906-913.

8

Pancreatic Cancer Cachexia: Current Concepts and Clinical Management

Michelle Guan, Arvind M. Shinde and
Andrew E. Hendifar

Abstract

There has been great progress over the last decade in understanding the pathophysiology of cachexia associated with pancreatic cancer. However, there is a large need to find better therapeutic options to successfully manage this complex and challenging condition. Patients with pancreatic cancer have some of the highest prevalence and often the most severe degrees of cachexia, which is described as a multifactorial metabolic syndrome that is associated with unintended weight loss of adipose tissue and skeletal muscle in the setting of anorexia. This chapter will review the current concepts surrounding pancreatic cancer cachexia, its clinical diagnosis, pathophysiology, and its known and proposed therapeutics. A multimodal approach utilizing nutritional support and pharmaceutical therapies is proposed to lead to the most successful management of pancreatic cancer cachexia.

Keywords: pancreatic cancer, cachexia, anorexia, metabolic syndrome, catabolism

1. Introduction

In western countries, pancreatic cancer represents the fourth leading cause of cancer-related death [1]. Among the many complications associated with this disease, cachexia marked by progressive weight loss represents one of the most distressing features related to pancreatic cancer. Cachexia is a multidimensional wasting syndrome that is characterized by unintended loss of both adipose tissue and lean body mass (LBM) that cannot be fully reversed through conventional nutritional support. It is a complex metabolic disorder frequently described in pancreatic cancer and represents a significant physical and psychological burden in approximately 80% of pancreatic cancer patients during the disease progression [2]. The complications associated with cachexia, which include immobility, impaired immunity, and severe respiratory muscle impairment leading to cardiopulmonary failure, result in death in up to one-third of pancreatic cancer patients [3]. Cachectic patients are observed to have lower physical function, decreased tolerance to chemotherapy and radiation treatment, and generally worse prognosis than those with stable weight. Poorer outcomes after pancreaticoduodenectomy have also been observed in patients with preoperative signs of cachexia [4].

While research over the past decade has provided new insights regarding the pathogenesis of pancreatic cancer cachexia, the mechanistic pathology of this condition is still not entirely understood. In this chapter, we will provide a review of the current concepts, potential therapeutic targets, and management of this significant clinical condition.

2. Classification and progression of cancer cachexia

Cachexia has been established to be a common adverse effect of cancer. An international consensus in 2011 defined cachexia as a multifactorial condition recognized by ongoing skeletal muscle loss irreversible by standard nutritional support and eventual functional impairment [5]. The diagnostic criterion established for cancer cachexia is weight loss greater than 5% within 6 months or weight loss greater than 2% in patients already showing depletion (body mass index (BMI) < 20 kg/m^2) or evidence of sarcopenia determined by a dual energy X-ray absorptiometry (DEXA). A skeletal muscle index less than 7.26 kg/m^2 in males and 5.45 kg/m^2 in females is classified as cachexia and the majority of pancreatic cancer patients show signs of cachexia at the time of diagnosis [2].

Cachexia typically develops progressively through a continuum by way of three clinically relevant stages: precachexia, cachexia, and refractory cachexia [5]. A combination of degree of ongoing weight loss as well as depletion of energy stores and body protein mass (using BMI) can be used to classify the severity of the condition. At the precachexia stage, patients show metabolic signs such as anorexia and impaired glucose tolerance prior to significant unintended weight loss. Patients who continue to lose weight and meet the diagnostic criterion described above then transition to full-on cachexia. The cachexia is considered clinically refractory when the cancer is characterized as preterminal or when the individual becomes unresponsive to anticancer therapy. With the presence of uncontrollable catabolism and a life expectancy of less than 3 months, therapeutic interventions usually focus on palliating the symptoms and further preventing the complications of cachexia.

3. Assessment of cancer cachexia

A patient should be assessed for the following features to be characterized with cachexia: anorexia or reduced food intake, catabolic drivers, muscle mass and strength, and functional and psychosocial ability [5]. A recent study indicated that patients who exhibit these components have significantly worse prognosis. Weight loss (>10% weight loss), reduced food intake

(<1500 kcal/day), and indication of systematic inflammation (C-reactive protein (CRP) > 10 mg/L) reduced subjective and objective functional ability in patients with at least two of these components [2].

Many underlying factors could contribute to anorexia or reduced food intake. Pancreatic cancer patients suffer from a reduced drive to eat, chemosensory disturbances (e.g., taste and smell), dysphagia, decreased gastrointestinal (GI) motility (e.g., early satiety and nausea), pain, and fatigue [5]. To detect the presence of these factors, food intake should be assessed routinely by the patient or a family member. At the minimum, the patient should estimate their overall food intake in comparison to their normal intake or have a family member perform a percentile calculation of food consumed during each meal [6]. The early detection of secondary causes of reduced food intake, such as stomatitis, constipation, dyspnoea, and poor dietary habits is important since some complications may be readily reversible [5].

A key component of pancreatic cancer cachexia is hypercatabolism due to tumor metabolism, systemic inflammation, or other tumor-mediated effects. Systemic inflammation is often indexed using serum C-reactive protein (CRP) levels [7]. Indirect indices such as responsiveness to chemotherapy and rate of disease progression should also be evaluated.

As cancer cachexia is characterized by ongoing muscle wasting, a routine assessment of muscle mass is performed with the various techniques currently available. The methods to measure muscle mass include cross-sectional imaging with computed tomography (CT) or magnetic resonance imaging (MRI); appendicular skeletal muscle index obtained from DEXA, anthropometry (mid-upper muscle area); and bioimpedance analysis to obtain a whole body fat-free mass index [5, 8–10]. An imaging-based method is typically selected to quantify changes in body composition by factors such as skeletal muscle wasting, altered body fat distribution, and pathological accumulation of lipids in various tissues. An MRI provides a measurement of quadriceps muscle volume with a coefficient of variation <1% while diagnostic CT scans estimate the cross-sectional area of the abdominal muscle at the L3 area, which can be extrapolated to the lean body mass of the entire body. Muscle strength is typically assessed with an upper-limb hand-grip dynamometry [5].

Among pancreatic cancer patients, those who are overweight were found to be more likely to develop a condition termed as sarcopenic obesity or cachexia hidden in the context of obesity. Sarcopenic obesity is the substantial muscle loss and dysfunction associated with pathological accumulation of adipose tissue. While sarcopenia alone is not associated with decreased survival, being both overweight and sarcopenic does have a significant effect on mortality. With approximately 40% of obese pancreatic patients with detectable sarcopenic obesity, this condition needs to be recognized early on as it was also found to be an important prognostic factor for decreased survival [11]. A comprehensive approach including history, physical examination, and various imaging tests to properly identify this phenomenon can potentially increase the survival of pancreatic cancer patients.

Cancer cachexia contributes substantially to a decreased quality of life by adversely effecting physical and psychosocial functioning. As it is associated with symptoms such as fatigue, weakness, and poor physical performance, it leads to altered body images and can significantly impact the patient's relationships and emotional well-being [12]. A recent study that used an advanced ambulatory pedometer technology found that physical activity was reduced by around 40% in cachectic cancer patients [13]. Since increased bed rest is known to reduce protein synthesis and contribute to the decrease in skeletal muscle mass in healthy patients, this decrease in physical function in cachectic patients adversely affects performance status, quality of social interactions, and ability to performance daily living tasks [14]. Currently, the most widely accepted method for assessing the effects of cancer cachexia is the routine use of patient-reported physical functioning, specifically using the European Organization for Research and Treatment of Cancer (EORTC) quality of life questionnaire (QLQ)-C30 or the Eastern Cooperative Oncology Group (ECOG) questionnaire [15–17]. Physical functioning can also be assessed with physician-reported physical activity (the Karnofsky performance score) and objective methodologies including electric activity meters or checklists of specific activities [17].

4. Mechanisms of cancer cachexia

The pathophysiology of cancer cachexia is characterized by a negative protein and energy balance created by a combination of reduced food intake and abnormal metabolism that is mainly driven by a large increase in the rate of skeletal muscle proteolysis [5, 18, 19]. Anorexia and hypercatabolism have been found in cachectic patients to be driven by mechanical factors such as cytokines, circulating hormones, neuropeptides, neurotransmitters, and tumor-derived factors. Recent studies have also identified other processes that potentially contributed to the pathophysiology of pancreatic cancer cachexia, including neural invasion and abnormalities in muscle microenvironment [20–25]. The following section will review these currently proposed mechanisms that interact and contribute to the development of this disease.

4.1. Mechanical factors

Cancer-associated weight loss can be promoted and maintained by reduced food intake, which can be a result of loss of appetite driven by abnormal mechanical digestion [26]. Tumorigenesis is the main cause of these digestive abnormalities and frequently results in the obstruction of the pancreatic duct and/or GI tract, especially the second portion of the duodenum. This can directly lead to symptoms of pain, fatigue, nausea, dysphagia, gastroparesis, duodenal stenosis, pancreatic insufficiency and malabsorption, and constipation [27]. A pancreaticoduodenectomy to resect a pancreatic head mass is often performed following an obstruction and unfortunately can exacerbate pancreatic insufficiency and reduce oral intake [28, 29].

4.2. Cytokines and systemic inflammation

The hypercatabolic component of cachexia is largely caused by the systemic inflammation response, which in turn promotes fat and protein degradation. Serum C-reactive protein is utilized to indirectly index systemic inflammation, and elevated CRP levels (CRP > 10 mg/L) have been related to cachexia and poor performance in pancreatic cancer patients [2]. Elevated levels of the cytokines IL-6 and IL-10 have also been associated with weight loss, poor prognosis, and decreased survival in patients [7, 30]. The cytokines that are generated by tumor cells or released by the host in response to cancer have been found to contribute to pathways that result in anorexia and hypercatabolism. These pathways can be separated into the hypothalamus-mediated central pathways and the peripheral pathways, which control lipolysis and proteolysis.

4.2.1. Centrally mediated pathways

The hypothalamus typically plays a role in energy intake by responding to peripheral signals regarding energy and adiposity status. A mechanical response is produced via these signaling pathways and abnormalities in these pathways can lead to anorexia. Current findings indicate that systemic inflammation plays a role in inducing cancer anorexia through the activation of a complex neurochemical cascade [24, 25, 31, 32]. Interference with the hypothalamus' normal response to peripheral signals is suggested to be a direct consequence of elevated tumor-mediated cytokine expression, which actively promotes anorexigenic pathways and inhibits orexigenic pathways [24, 25].

Derangements in the ability of the hypothalamus to transduce peripheral signals into neuronal responses may also be associated with cancer anorexia. There are two pathways that are responsible for energy expenditure and food intake within the hypothalamus: neuropeptide Y (NPY)/agouti-related peptide (AgRP) neurons that stimulate energy intake and proopiomelanocortin (POMC)/cocaine and amphetamine-regulated transcript (CART) neurons that inhibit intake. Research suggests that the hyperactivation of the POMC/CART pathways through the IL-1 and other pro-inflammatory cytokines could contribute to developing cancer cachexia [20–23].

Energy homeostasis is also regulated by a protein called leptin through feedback signaling via the central nervous system (CNS). By controlling the synthesis and activation of hypothalamic neuropeptides, such as NPY and corticotropin-releasing factor (CRF), leptin reduces appetite and increases energy expenditure. Since leptin is primarily released by adipose tissue, a lower body fat mass due to starvation leads to lower leptin levels, which allows for the production, release, and action of a potent orexigenic peptide called NPY. NPY then promotes the activation of the NPY/AgRP pathway that stimulates energy intake. Low levels of leptin also decrease the activity of anorexigenic neuropeptides that decrease appetite, which include CRF and melanocortin. Studies have found that cytokines, including tumor necrosis factor-alpha (TNF-α) and interleukin1 (IL-1), increase leptin mRNA expression in adipocytes and in plasma despite decreased adiposity [33–36]. Cancer anorexia might therefore be a consequence of increased leptin levels since compensatory mechanisms that typically occur with reduced food intake are inhibited. However, there is also evidence showing that cytokines can induce anorexia without leptin [37]. In some animal and clinical studies, leptin levels were found to not be elevated in tumor-bearing rats and patients with cancer cachexia [38–41]. Recent research demonstrated that in cancer cachexia, IL-1 and TNF-α mimic leptin signaling and result in the interference of the orexigenic pathway, which is normally a response to reduced leptin levels [24, 42]. This suggests that even during starvation, the inhibition of the orexigenic response and activation of the anorexigenic pathway can occur and lead to unopposed anorexia and elevated energy expenditure.

Serotonin may also contribute to the pathogenesis of cancer anorexia, specifically through the melanocortin system. Research has shown that IL-1 releases hypothalamic serotonin and indirectly alters food intake [43]. High levels of serotonin create a continuous activation of POMC/CART neurons, which causes decreased appetite and anorexia [44]. Additionally, higher levels of tryptophan, which is a precursor of serotonin, were also found in plasma and cerebrospinal fluids of cancer patients with cachexia compared to those without cachexia or healthy controls [45]. After tumor removal, tryptophan concentrations were normalized and subsequently improved appetite [46]. These facts concurrently suggest that serotonin plays a pivotal role in the development of cancer cachexia and is also a potential therapeutic target.

These hypothalamic pathways and neuropeptides were also found to have catabolic effects. The POMC/CART anorexigenic pathway activates the sympathetic nervous system and leads to the induction of mitochondrial uncoupling proteins, including UCP-1 and UCP-2 [47, 48]. By dissipating the proton gradient generated during respiration across the inner mitochondrial membrane and uncoupling respiration from ATP synthesis, UCP-1 and UCP-2 result in thermogenesis and energy expenditure in brown adipose tissue (BAT) [47, 48]. Increases in BAT thermogenesis have been associated with a cachectic state in both humans and experimental animals [49, 50].

4.2.2. Peripheral pathways

Not only have cytokines been proven to corroborate and sustain the neurochemical changes associated with cancer cachexia, but they have also been found to induce lipolysis, muscle catabolism, and the hepatic acute phase protein response (APPR) through multiple pathways [51–57]. The combined action of these cellular activities results in the development of progressive muscle and adipose tissue loss.

4.2.2.1. TNF-α

The cytokine TNF-α has been shown to result in profound metabolic changes, even when administered in low doses. Characterized as a potent anorexigenic agent, it promotes lipolysis, impairs lipogenesis, and increases mobilization of lean tissue reserves from skeletal muscle. TNF-α has been shown to induce lipolysis *in vitro* with increases in glycerol production in mouse and human adipocytes, likely through downregulation of perilipin [51]. Since perilipin typically coats intracellular lipid droplets, the decreased expression of perilipin thus enables the lipolysis regulator hormone-sensitive lipase (HSL) to access the surface of lipid droplets for breakdown [51, 52]. By acting as an inhibitory agent on adipocyte differentiation, TNF-α also results in impaired lipogenesis [53, 54].

Research has also indicated that TNF-α contributes to the muscle wasting that characterizes cancer cachexia. Mouse models demonstrated that TNF-α may promote muscle protein degradation by producing reactive oxygen species (ROS). Nuclear factor κB (NFκB) is activated as a result of this oxidative stress and then subsequently upregulates the ubiquitin-mediated proteasome pathway [55, 56]. Moreover, TNF-α has been shown to upregulate the expression of the 1/2- and 2.4-kb transcripts of ubiquitin and the ubiquitin ligase atrogin 1/MAFbx in skeletal muscle [55, 56]. *In vitro* experiments that involved NFκB-mediated downregulation of MyoD transcripts have also shown the ability of TNF-α to interfere with myogenesis [57].

While these studies indicate that TNF-α is involved in lipolysis and proteolysis, its relevance in cancer cachexia is still not well established. While some studies measuring TNF-α serum levels in pancreatic cancer patients with cachexia found the predicted inverse relationship between TNF-α levels and body weight as well as BMI; other studies involving advance-staged cancer patients demonstrate no such correlation between circulating TNF-α levels, weight loss, and anorexia. Because of the conflicted results produced from these studies, the significance of TNF-α in cancer cachexia still remains an active area of debate.

4.2.2.2. IL-6

Another important pro-inflammatory cytokine implicated in facilitating cachexia is IL-6, which has been associated with weight loss and reduced survival in pancreatic cancer patients [7, 30, 58]. The secretion of IL-6 is known to be induced by TNF-α and works synergistically with TNF-α in many of its cellular functions, including the triggering of other cytokines. Although the role of IL-6 in lipolysis is still unclear, a recent study using cachectic tumor-bearing mice demonstrated enhanced IL-6 signaling in brown adipose tissue, which suggests that IL-6 may be directly involved in activating thermogenesis [59]. More importantly, IL-6 is known to activate the hepatic APPR and stimulate tissue catabolism. The C-26 tumor-bearing mouse model of cancer cachexia established an IL-6 dependent loss of skeletal muscle during cancer cachexia and treatment with an IL-6 targeting antibody attenuated the development of weight loss [60]. Another study confirmed increased CRP levels and IL-6 production in pancreatic cancer patients with cachexia [7]. There is a strong correlation between heightened peripheral blood mononuclear cells (PBMCs) production of IL-6 and the presence of increased APPR [7, 58, 61]. The stimulation of APPR thus promotes the production of acute phase proteins like CRP and gives rise to hypercatabolism at the expense of skeletal muscle [62]. A twofold to threefold increase in fibrinogen production and elevated serum CRP is observed as a consequence of APPR activation [63]. The hepatic synthesis of acute phase proteins occurs due to the mobilization of peripheral amino acid reserves from lean muscle and contributes greatly to the observed weight loss. Both the overproduction of IL-6 and APPR thus have been shown to result in poor responses to chemotherapy in those surviving with pancreatic cancer cachexia [7].

4.3. Tumor-derived factors

In addition to cytokines and systemic inflammation, tumor-derived factors also contribute to the metabolic abnormalities leading to pancreatic cancer cachexia. Two of the most studied factors are lipid mobilizing factor (LMF) and proteolysis-inducing factor (PIF). Other factors that potentially lead to pancreatic cancer cachexia are still being established.

4.3.1. Lipid mobilizing factor

Another molecule associate with cancer is LMF, which was isolated from both a mouse model of cancer cachexia (MAC16 adenocarcinoma) and the urine of patients with unresectable pancreatic cancer and weight loss [64]. Given that LMF was found only in pancreatic patients with weight loss and not in those without weight loss or even normal individuals, LMF/ZAG was identified as a serum protein that is a potential marker of pancreatic cancer cachexia [64, 65]. Additional immunohistochemical findings identified LMF/ZAG expression in pancreatic cancer cells and in the peritumoral stroma, with cachectic pancreatic cancer patients demonstrating stronger immunostaining results than those without cachexia or normal subjects [65].

LMF/ZAG has also been demonstrated through *in vivo* findings to cause selective reduction of carcass fat without altering levels of body water and nonfat mass [66]. This lipolysis is activated by the stimulation of adenylate cyclase in a GTP-dependent fashion and is proposed to be mediated by β3 adrenergic receptors [66–68]. When mice are treated with LMF/ZAG, elevated serum levels of glycerol and 3-hydroxybutyrate are observed as well as an increase of oxygen usage by BAT is observed, demonstrating the role of LMF/ZAG in stimulating lipid utilization [66]. This increase in lipid oxidation and utilization has been shown to be mediated by the $^{14}CO_2$ from [14C-carboxy]triolein and also potentially by β3 adrenergic receptors [69]. This function occurs with the increased expression of mitochondrial UCPs, particularly UCP-1, UCP-2, and UCP-3 in BAT, and UCP-2 in the skeletal muscle and liver [70]. LMF/ZAG also enhances the response of adipose tissues to the lipolytic effects of other stimuli such as catecholamines [66]. The plasma membranes of adipocytes contain Gs α-subunits (Gαs) that stimulate adenylate cyclase and Gi α-subunits (Gαi) that inhibit adenylate cyclase. LMF/ZAG favors mobilization of lipid stores from adipocytes and promotes hypercatabolism by increasing Gαs and decreasing Gαi expression [71]. By promoting both the lipid and substrate utilization as well as mitochondrial oxidative pathways in BAT, LMF/ZAG results in lipolysis, elevated energy expenditure, and a hypercatabolic state.

4.4. Proteolysis-inducing factor

In 1996, PIF was isolated from a murine tumor (MAC16) originating in an adenocarcinoma murine model of cachexia and was discovered to induce skeletal muscle catabolism in MAC16 [72]. In humans, PIF was also discovered in cachectic cancer patients, but not from patients with weight loss due to trauma, cancer patients with little or no weight loss or normal individuals [73]. Moreover, this compound was detected in the urine of 80% of pancreatic cancer patients with significantly higher total weight loss and rate of weight loss than those whose urine did not contain PIF [74]. Immunochemistry analysis also revealed the presence of PIF in the cytoplasm of GI tumors such as pancreatic adenocarcinoma [75].

PIF has been found to induce cachectic symptoms when injected intravenously in normal mice; body composition analysis revealed that PIF extracted from the urine of cachectic cancer patients induced reductions in lean body mass without reduction in food and water intake in murine models [76]. This decrease in muscle mass involved two components: an increase in protein degradation by 50% and a reduction in protein synthesis by 50% observed in gastrocnemius muscle [77]. Additional studies regarding the PIF-mediated reduction in protein mass implicate the ubiquitin-proteasome proteolytic pathway. Upon the administration of PIF in normal mice, mRNA levels for ubiquitin, $E2_{14k}$, and the C9 proteasome subunit are increased. An increase in the expression of the ubiquitin-proteasome pathway in skeletal muscle may contribute to this protein degradation; some studies suggest that this process is found to be mediated by the activation of NFκB [78–80]. While a reduction in protein mass as well as the depletion of myosin is observed, actin levels continue to remain unchanged with the administration of PIF [80].

The role of NFκB in protein degradation following administration of PIF is still not entirely elucidated. However, it is known that arachidonic acid originating from membrane phospholipids is released and then rapidly metabolizes into eicosanoids such as hydroxyeicosatetraenoic acid (15 -HETE) with phospholipase A_2 (PLA_2), which has also been shown to increase in the presence of PIF [81]. 15-HETE was also shown to cause the nuclear accumulation of NFκB and thus protein degradation [82]. The muscle degradation due to the PIF-induced expression of the ubiquitin-proteasome pathway is also largely reliant on NADPH oxidase and production of ROS [81, 83]. Protein kinase C (PKC) is necessary for the activation of NADPH oxidase and may also be dependent on 15-HETE. The generation of ROS stimulates IκB kinase (IKK) and phosphorylates and degrades IκB; this process then releases NFκB from its inactive cytosolic complex [84].

PIF results in the reduction of protein mass not only by causing degradation, but also by inhibiting protein synthesis. PIF activates double-stranded RNA-dependent protein kinase (PKR) through phosphorylation, which leads to the phosphorylation of eIF2; this in turn inhibits translation and subsequently protein synthesis [85]. PKR is also able to elevate the expression and activity of the ubiquitin-proteasome pathway by activating IKK, which then generates excessive NFκB [86].

APPR that is associated with cachectic pancreatic cancer patients may also be driven by PIF, which was found to play a role in excessively generating hepatic cytokines. Human hepatocyte cultures that were treated with PIF had increased NFκB, signal transducers, and activators of transcription (STAT3), which resulted in an increased production of IL-6, IL-8, and CRP, as well as decreased production of transferrin [87]. The same treatment given to human Kupffer cells and monocytes similarly resulted in an increased production of TNF-α, IL-6, and IL-8 [88].

4.5. Other proposed mechanisms

4.5.1. Pax7 dysregulation

Other contributory factors to muscle loss within a cachectic setting have also been investigated in recent studies and further characterize the muscle microenvironment. In pancreatic cancer patients with cachexia, activation of NFκB in satellite muscle progenitor cells resulted in muscle wasting caused by the dysregulation of the self-renewing transcription factor Pax7, which suppressed expression of MyoD and myogenin [89, 90]. These processes subsequently prevented the muscle progenitor cells that typically commit to a myogenic program from completing differentiation and inhibited myoblast fusion, which ultimately impaired muscle regeneration [90]. Furthermore, Pax7 was shown to be induced by serum factors from both cachectic mice and patients in an NFκB-dependent manner [90]. However, the exact circulating factors contributing to NFκB activation and Pax7 dysregulation still require further research.

4.5.2. *Neural invasion*

Pancreatic cancer patients often develop signs of neural invasion that can result in nerve damage from intraneural tumors of pancreatic cancer. Recent studies suggest that this process involving nerve damage is associated with cachexia as well as astrocyte activation and microglia stimulation in the spinal cord. These activated astrocytes may then stimulate the sympathetic nervous system, which has previously been shown to induce lipolysis and muscle atrophy [47, 91]. However, the mechanisms that potentially lead to cachexia still require further investigation.

4.6. Management of cancer cachexia

Since cachexia is a multifactorial condition, treatments involving combinations of therapies are more likely to be successful. Current therapeutic strategies involve an integrated and multimodal approach including oncological therapy for control of the tumor, nutritional support, and pharmacological treatment. The best supportive care practices also involve the management of the secondary causes of anorexia, such as pain, nausea, pancreatic insufficiency, and constipation.

4.6.1. *Nutritional support*

Nutritional deficit is one of the highest concerns among pancreatic cancer patients [92]. Involving dieticians and nutrition assessment programs early on in the disease progression is essential for the successful management of pancreatic cancer cachexia. These programs can provide essential dietary suggestions as well as recommendations for oral nutritional supplementation, enteral nutrition, and parenteral nutrition [93–96].

When concerned with appetite and weight management, professional dietary guidance can significantly increase oral caloric and protein intake [97]. Pancreatic cancer patients who were enrolled in studies requiring them to take oral nutritional supplementation found improvements in weight and appetite [98, 99]. Specifically, including L-Carnitine and omega-3 fatty acids as an addition to patients' diets may provide benefits [100, 101]. In a multicenter, randomized, double-blind trial that enrolled patients with advanced pancreatic cancer, L-Carnitine supplementation was found to significantly improve weight and body mass composition, which ultimately resulted in an increased global quality of life [101].

For patients with swallowing difficulties or severe dysphagia, a nasogastric tube or gastrostomy tube can be utilized to administer nutritional support. However, enteral feeding can be linked to morbidity resulting from aspiration, pneumonia, and diarrhea. For patients with bowel dysfunction and progressive weight loss despite enteral support, parenteral nutrition may be used to limit nutritional deterioration and provide temporary benefits [102].

While nutritional interventions can provide temporary stabilization in nutritional status and certain metabolic indices for cachectic cancer patients, response is often limited in these patients and is frequently lower than responses observed in noncancer patients receiving equivalent nutritional support [103]. A unimodal approach is still not sufficient and patients with pancreatic cancer cachexia will therefore require a combination of therapies to successfully manage the cachexia.

4.6.2. Pharmacological approach

Since nutritional interventions produce only limited responses, many studies attempted to manipulate the process of cachexia using a variety of pharmacological agents. The mechanisms of these drugs are all based on modulation of cytokines, hormones, or other pathways involved in the pathophysiology of cancer cachexia.

4.6.2.1. Progestogens

Megestrol acetate (MEGACE) is a synthetic and orally active derivative of the naturally occurring hormone progesterone. It was first developed for the treatment of breast cancer and later for endometrial cancer, MEGACE is now used to stimulate appetite and increase weight in cancer-associated anorexia, as well as for other chronic conditions such as the human acquired immunodeficiency syndrome (AIDS) after being approved by the Food and Drug Administration (FDA) in 1993. Multiple trials have demonstrated that MEGACE (480–800 mg/day) resulted in significant improvements in appetite, food intake, nausea, and weight gain among pancreatic patients with cancer cachexia [27, 104–107]. This efficacy of MEGACE appears to be dose-dependent [106]. MEGACE is generally well-tolerated with low incidence of side effects, including rash, adrenal insufficiency, hyperglycemia, and thromboembolic events, which only have an incidence of less than 5% [105]. Since its approval, many studies have confirmed the effectiveness of MEGACE at increasing weight and thus quality of life when compared to other drugs potentially used for the management of cancer cachexia (cisapride, dronabinol, corticosteroids, and nandrolone) [108, 109]. Body composition analysis has also confirmed that the weight gain observed following MEGACE intake is predominately due to increases in adipose tissue and less from increases in body fluid [110]. However, there were no improvements in survival found in those who were treated with MEGACE [107, 109].

Some studies suggest that the mechanisms by which MEGACE stimulates appetite and weight gain is related to decreased production and release of pro-inflammatory cytokines (IL-1, IL-6, and TNF-α) as well as the stimulation of NPY in the hypothalamus [111–113]. Another progestogen, medroxyprogesterone acetate, was demonstrated through *in vitro* experiments to decrease the production of cytokines and serotonin by PBMC of cancer patients [112, 113].

4.6.2.2. Corticosteroids

Corticosteroids are one of the most widely used appetite stimulants and are effective in inducing food intake and weight gain [114–116]. However, these do not result in lasting changes (less than 4 weeks) and may cause long-term side effects, such as insulin resistance, fluid retention, steroid-induced myopathy, skin fragility, adrenal insufficiency, and sleep and cognitive disorder [116]. The exact mechanisms of action of corticosteroids in a cancer cachexia context still remains unclear, but is likely to be related to the inhibition of IL-1, TNF-α, and leptin as well as the stimulation of NPY [117]. Because of their short duration of effectiveness, corticosteroids may be useful for patient with short expected survival.

4.6.2.3. *Cannabinoids*

Cannabinoids, which are also called dronabinols, are a class of diverse chemical compounds that have a known effect on reducing nausea as well as weight gain and stabilization. A phase II trial found that dronabinol improved anorexia in 68% of patients, but also resulted in dangerous toxicity levels in 16% of patients who eventually suspended treatment [118]. In addition, dronabinol is associated with many adverse side effects, including euphoria, hallucination, psychosis, vertigo, and cardiovascular disorders. The mechanism of action appears to be mediated by interaction with endorphin receptors, interference with IL-1 production, activation of cannabinoid receptors associated with the neurochemical circuit of leptin, and inhibition of prostaglandin synthesis.

In a controlled clinical trial, dronabinol was compared to megestrol acetate in cachectic cancer patients [119]. A total of 469 patients were enrolled in the study and were instructed to take megestrol acetate 800 mg/day or dronabinol 2.5 mg/12 h or both. The findings indicate that megestrol is superior to dronabinol in terms of increasing appetite and weight: 75 vs. 49% ($P = 0.0001$) increase in appetite, respectively and 11 vs. 3% ($P = 0.02$) increase in weight gain of at least 10% from baseline, respectively [114]. There were no differences in appetite and weight between the combination treatment group compared to the megestrol acetate only group (66 vs. 75%, $P = 0.17$, for appetite and 8 vs. 11%, $P = 0.43$, for =10% weight gain, respectively). While megestrol acetate seems to be more effective than dronabinol, cannabinoid is still able to stimulate in appetite and reduce nausea. It is available as an alternative option as an appetite stimulant and antiemetic.

4.6.2.4. *Anti-inflammatory agents*

Systemic inflammation plays an important role in the pathophysiology of pancreatic cancer cachexia. Pro-inflammatory cytokines, including TNF-α, IL-1, and IL-6, have been implicated in the progression of cancer cachexia in a potentially synergistic way. These findings have prompted the development of treatments to curtail the inflammatory response by inhibiting the synthesis or action of cytokines.

Research has indicated that nonsteroidal anti-inflammatory drugs (NSAIDs), including cyclooxygenase-2 (COX-2) inhibitors, indomethacin, and ibuprofen, have the ability to reduce acute phase proteins and cytokines [120–122]. The inhibition of prostaglandin synthesis has been shown *in vivo* to attenuate tumor progression and decrease incidence of cancer cachexia [123, 124]. NSAIDs inhibition of prostaglandin synthesis blocks downstream effects of systemic inflammation; thereby interfering with the cytokines that depend on signal transduction mediated by eicosanoids. In cachectic patients with metastatic solid tumors, indomethacin use may prolong survival and offer palliative support to those with advanced cancer, including pancreatic cancer patients [125]. Other controlled clinical trials have shown that ibuprofen can reduce CRP levels, increase body weight and muscle mass, and improve global quality of life, especially when combined with progestogens [122, 126, 127]. McMillan et al. conducted a multicenter, randomized, control trial that involved 73 cachectic patients with advanced GI cancers, predominately pancreatic cancer (67% of patients) [126]. This study reported that taking a combination of ibuprofen (1200 mg/day) and megestrol acetate (480 mg/day) resulted in more significant improvements in weight and increased quality of life compared to those only consuming megestrol acetate [128]. Similar side effects were present in both groups, including venous thrombosis, upper GI bleeding, and ascites. However, due to disease progression, there was a high attrition rate with 63% failing to complete the 12-week assessment. These provide promising results that would benefit greatly from larger studies that can better evaluate the clinical role of NSAIDs in the management of pancreatic cancer cachexia.

Research has also shown that thalidomide has anti-inflammatory and complex immunomodulatory properties. Thalidomide results in the downregulation of the production of TNF-α as well as other pro-inflammatory cytokines in monocytes, inhibits NFκB, downregulates cyclooxygenase 2, and inhibits angiogenesis [129]. Many controlled trials showed that thalidomide is well-tolerated and successful in improving appetite, weight gain, and sensation of well-being [130, 131]. One specific double-blind, placebo-controlled, randomized clinical trial of thalidomide recruited 50 pancreatic cancer patients with cachexia to take either 200 mg/day of thalidomide or a placebo [131]. The study found that after 4 weeks, patients in the thalidomide group had significant increases in weight compared to the placebo group (0.37 vs. −2.21 kg, $P = 0.005$) and significant improvements in lean body mass (1.0 cm^3 in arm muscle mass vs. −4.46 cm^3, $P = 0.002$) [131]. There were some adverse reactions to thalidomide, including peripheral neuropathy, dizziness, somnolence, constipation, rash, and possible increased risk of venous thromboembolism in the setting of malignancy. These preliminary results are encouraging, but merits further investigation to confirm the efficacy of thalidomide in treating pancreatic cancer cachexia.

Some therapeutic approaches also involve pharmaconutrients with anti-inflammatory activity, such as the omega-3 fatty acids eicosapentaenoic acid (EPA) and docosahexaenoic acid (DHA). Both found abundantly in fish oil, EPA and DHA both have immunomodulatory properties that allow for the suppression of pro-inflammatory cytokines, including IL-1, TNF-α, and IL-6 by PBMC [132, 133]. Research on EPA has also suggested its ability to inhibit the downstream effects of LMF and PIF [134–136]. In past studies involving patients with unresectable pancreatic cancer, fish oil supplementation containing both EPA and DHA as well as high-purity EPA administration have both been associated with weight stabilization [137, 138]. A study conducted by Barber et al. further demonstrated the efficacy of EPA, which were taken through oral supplementation, at producing significant increases in weight, dietary intake, and performance status in cachectic patients with advanced pancreatic cancer [100]. However, recent data from a multicenter, double-blind, placebo-controlled, randomized clinical trial provided conflicting results suggested that single agent EPA administration is not effective in treating cancer cachexia [139]. Another multicenter clinical trial that compared EPA, megestrol acetate, and a combination treatment determined that megestrol acetate alone resulted in more weight gain than EPA administration or a combination therapy [140]. While the role of EPA in the management cancer cachexia still remains unclear, recent data demonstrates EPA's lack of effectiveness as a single agent or even in combination regimens for the management of pancreatic cancer cachexia.

As the mechanisms involved in the development and progression of cancer cachexia continues to be elucidated, the management of this multifactorial syndrome has made improvements towards developing a multimodal approach. Recent data from a large multicenter trial suggests that a combination therapy with megestrol acetate (320 mg/day), EPA supplementation, L-carnitine (4 g/day), and thalidomide (200 mg/day) provides more effective results in improving lean body mass and appetite than single agents [141]. Future progress in the field of cancer cachexia will be realized through the development of combined pharmacological therapies given along with nutritional supplementation in the context of supportive care.

5. Future directions

Despite a significant increase in research on cancer cachexia, there are currently no therapies available for pancreatic cancer cachexia that results in lasting effects on weight management and improvements in prognosis. Developing an effective and powerful treatment for this disease still remains an ongoing challenge.

Recent studies have focused on targeted therapies with anti-inflammatory activity. IL-6 has been identified as a promising target, but most of the studies investigating IL-6 antibodies have involved nonsmall cell lung cancer (NSCLC) patients with cachexia [142–145]. In a phase II randomized, double-blind, placebo-controlled trial with NSCLC patients, the humanized monoclonal IL-6 antibody called ALD518 (also known as BMS-945429) was evaluated for its safety and efficacy in treating cancer cachexia. This safe and well-tolerated antibody effectively increased hemoglobin levels and prevented loss of lean body mass [142, 143]. Rigas et al. also reported statistically significant improvements in fatigue score in the ALD518 group vs. placebo group that persisted over a 12-week period [142].

Another agent that was found to have anti-inflammatory properties is OHR/AVR118, which is an immune modulator that targets both TNF-α and IL-6. In a phase II study by Chasen et al. administering OHR/AVR118 in cachectic patients with advanced cancer resulted in improvements in anorexia, dyspepsia, strength, and depression [146]. A current phase IIb study is advancing the understanding of the role and efficacy of OHR/AVR118 in enhancing appetite as well as improving weight, lean body mass, strength, and quality of life [147]. Additional research is still needed to evaluate the safety and efficacy of these agents in pancreatic cancer patients with cachexia.

Studies have discovered the therapeutic potential of inhibiting myostatin and activin type IIB (ActRIIB) in treating cancer cachexia. ActRIIB is a high affinity activin receptor that mediates signaling through a subset of TGF-β ligands including myostatin and activin and both play a critical role in regulating muscle mass [148]. These ligands inhibit myogenesis and the Akt/mTOR pathway involved in muscle protein synthesis and upregulate the expression of ubiquitin ligases that degrade muscle. In several models of cancer cachexia, Zhou et al. reported the prevention of muscle wasting as well as prolonged survival through the pharmacological inhibition of the ActRIIB pathway [148]. One myostatin inhibitor BYM338 has been developed by Novartis (Hanover, NJ, USA) and is currently being investigated for the efficacy of myostatin inhibitors in attenuating loss of body mass. This compound is currently being evaluated in a multicenter, randomized, double-blind, placebo-controlled phase II trial that involves cachectic patients with either stage IV NSCLC or stage III/IV pancreatic cancer [149]. LY2495655 is another humanized antimyostatin antibody currently investigated in a multicenter, randomized, double-blind, placebo-controlled phase II trial that recruited patients with locally advanced or metastatic pancreatic cancer. Patients were administered with one of two different doses of LY2495655 in combination with gemcitabine to evaluate potential dose-dependent effects on survival, lean body mass, and physical performance [150].

6. Conclusion

Cancer cachexia is still regarded as noncurable and is diagnosed in approximately 80% of pancreatic cancer patients. Among these patients, 30% eventually die from cachexia-related complications [2, 151]. As a multifactorial condition, pancreatic cancer cachexia is complex disease that is associated with anorexia and excessive catabolism mediated by mechanical factors, pro-inflammatory cytokines, neuropeptides, hormones, and tumor-derived factors. The pathophysiology of cachexia in pancreatic cancer is characterized by compromised energy homeostasis driven by decreased food intake and abnormal metabolism. This negative protein and energy balance leads to unintentional skeletal muscle and adipose tissue mass, which greatly decreases the overall prognosis of pancreatic cancer patients.

While the management of cancer cachexia has improved dramatically in the past decade, more research is still needed to further understand the complex mechanisms involved in the pathogenesis and maintenance of pancreatic cancer cachexia. Current research identifies targeted immunotherapy as a promising treatment option for cachexia and successful intervention of this condition will most likely involve a multimodal approach to aid in developing potential therapeutics. Future progress in the management of cancer cachexia will likely be realized through a combined approach that includes nutritional support, multiple agents, and targeted therapies to improve the quality of life and general outlook of patients with pancreatic cancer.

Author details

Michelle Guan[1,2]*, Arvind M. Shinde[1] and Andrew E. Hendifar[1,2]

*Address all correspondence to: michelle8guan@gmail.com

1 Samuel Oschin Comprehensive Cancer Center, Cedars Sinai Medical Center, Los Angeles, CA, USA

2 Department of Medicine, David Geffen School of Medicine, Los Angeles, CA, USA

References

[1] Jemal A, Murray T, Ward E, Samuels A, Tiwari RC, Ghafoor A, et al. Cancer statistics, 2005. CA Cancer J Clin. 2005;**55**(1):10-30. DOI: 10.3322/canjclin.55.1.10.

[2] Fearon KC, Voss AC, Hustead DS, Group CC. Definition of cancer cachexia: effect of weight loss, reduced food intake, and systemic inflammation on functional status and prognosis. Am. J. Clin. Nutr. 2006b;**83**(6):1345-1350.

[3] Bachmann J, Heiligensetzer M, Krakowski-Roosen H, Büchler MW, Friess H, Martignoni ME. Cachexia worsens prognosis in patients with resectable pancreatic cancer. J. Gastrointest. Surg. 2008;**12**(7):1193-1201. DOI: 10.1007/s11605-008-0505-z.

[4] Pausch T, Hartwig W, Hinz U, Swolana T, Bundy BD, Hackert T, et al. Cachexia but not obesity worsens the postoperative outcome after pancreatoduodenectomy in pancreatic cancer. Surgery. 2012;**152**(3):S81–S88. DOI: 10.1016/j.surg.2012.05.028.

[5] Fearon K, Strasser F, Anker SD, Bosaeus I, Bruera E, Fainsinger RL, et al. Definition and classification of cancer cachexia: an international consensus. Lancet Oncol. 2011;**12**(5):489-495. DOI: 10.1016/S1470- 2045(10)70218-7.

[6] Bruera E, Sweeney C. Cachexia and asthenia in cancer patients. Lancet Oncol. 2000;**1**:138-147. DOI: 10.1016/S1470-2045(00)00033-4.

[7] Moses AG, Maingay J, Sangster K, Fearon KC, Ross JA. Pro-inflammatory cytokine release by peripheral blood mononuclear cells from patients with advanced pancreatic cancer: relationship to acute phase response and survival. Oncol. Rep. 2009;**21**(4):1091-1095. DOI: 10.3892/or_00000328.

[8] Simons JP, Schols AM, Westerterp KR, ten Velde GP, Wouters EF. The use of bioelectrical impedance analysis to predict total body water in patients with cancer cachexia. Am. J. Clin. Nutr. 1995;**61**(4):741-745.

[9] Prado CM, Birdsell LA, Baracos VE. The emerging role of computerized tomography in assessing cancer cachexia. Curr. Opin. Support. Palliat. Care. 2009;**3**(4):269-275. DOI: 10.1097/SPC.0b013e328331124a.

[10] Di Sebastiano KM, Mourtzakis M. A critical evaluation of body composition modalities used to assess adipose and skeletal muscle tissue in cancer. Appl. Physiol. Nutr. Metab. 2012;**37**(5):811-821. DOI: 10.1139/h2012-079.

[11] Tan BH, Birdsell LA, Martin L, Baracos VE, Fearon KC. Sarcopenia in an overweight or obese patient is an adverse prognostic factor in pancreatic cancer. Clin. Cancer Res. 2009;**15**(22):6973-6979. DOI: 10.1158/1078- 0432.CCR-09-1525.

[12] Donohoe CL, Ryan AM, Reynolds JV. Cancer cachexia: mechanisms and clinical implications. Gastroenterol. Res. Pract. 2011;**2011**;601434. DOI: 10.1155/2011/601434.

[13] Dahele M, Skipworth RJ, Wall L, Voss A, Preston T, Fearon KC. Objective physical activity and self-reported quality of life in patients receiving palliative chemotherapy. J. Pain Symptom Manage. 2007;**33**(6):676-685. DOI: 10.1016/j.jpainsymman.2006.09.024.

[14] Biolo G, Ciocchi B, Stulle M, Piccoli A, Lorenzon S, Dal MV, et al. Metabolic consequences of physical inactivity. J. Ren. Nutr. 2005;**15**(1):49-53.

[15] Aaronson NK, Ahmedzai S, Bergman B, Bullinger M, Cull A, Duez NJ, Filiberti A, Flechtner H, Fleishman SB, de Haes JC, et al. The European organization for research and treatment of cancer QLQ-C30: a quality-of-life instrument for use in international clinical trials in oncology. J. Natl. Cancer Inst. 1993;**85**(5):365-376.

[16] Luckett T, King MT, Butow PN, Oguchi M, Rankin N, Price MA, Hackl NA, Heading G. Choosing between the EORTC QLQ-C30 and FACT-G for measuring health-related quality of life in cancer clinical research: issues, evidence and recommendations. Ann. Oncol. 2011;**22**(10):2179-2190. DOI: 10.1093/annonc/mdq721.

[17] West H, Jin JO. Performance status in patients with cancer. JAMA Oncol. 2015;**1**(7):998. DOI:10.1001/jamaoncol.2015.3113.

[18] Fearon KC. Cancer cachexia: developing multimodal therapy for a multidimensional problem. Eur. J. Cancer. 2008;44(8):1124-1132. DOI: 10.1016/j.ejca.2008.02.033.

[19] Fearon KC. The 2011 ESPEN Arvid Wretlind lecture: cancer cachexia: the potential impact of translational research on patient-focused outcomes. Clin. Nutr. 2012;33:577– 582. DOI: 10.1016/j.clnu.2012.06.012.

[20] Wisse BE, Frayo RS, Schwartz MW, Cummings DE. Reversal of cancer anorexia by blockade of central melanocortin receptors in rats. Endocrinology. 2001;**142**(8):3292-3301. DOI: 10.1210/endo.142.8.8324.

[21] Marks D, Cone RD. The role of the melanocortin-3 receptor in cachexia. Ann. N.Y. Acad. Sci. 2003;**994**:258-266. DOI: 10.1111/j.1749- 6632.2003.tb03188.x.

[22] Marks DL, Butler AA, Turner R, Brookhart G, Cone RD. Differential role of melanocortin receptor subtypes in cachexia. Endocrinology. 2003;**144**(4):1513-1523. DOI: 10.1210/en.2002-221099.

[23] Scarlett JM, Jobst EE, Enriori PJ, Bowe DD, Batra AK, Grant WF, et al. Regulation of central melanocortin signaling by interleukin-1 beta. Endocrinology. 2007;**148**(9):4217-4225. DOI: 10.1210/en.2007-0017.

[24] Suzuki H, Asakawa A, Amitani H, Fujitsuka N, Nakamura N, Inui A. Cancer cachexia pathophysiology and translational aspect of herbal medicine. Japan J. Clin. Oncol. 2013; 43(7):695-705. DOI: 10.1093/jjco/hyt075.

[25] Tuca A., Jimenez-Fonseca P, Gascón P. Clinical evaluation and optimal management of cancer cachexia. Crit. Rev. Oncol. Hematol. 2013;88(3):625-636. DOI: 10.1016/j. critrevonc. 2013.07.015.

[26] Wigmore SJ, Plester CE, Ross JA, Fearon KC. Contribution of anorexia and hypermetabolism to weight loss in anicteric patients with pancreatic cancer. Br. J. Surg. 1997b;**84**(2):196-197. DOI: 10.1002/bjs.18008 40214.

[27] Deutsch J, Kolhouse JF. Assessment of gastrointestinal function and response to megesterol acetate in subjects with gastrointestinal cancers and weight loss. Support. Care Cancer. 2004;**12**(7):503-510. DOI: 10.1007/s00520-004-0615-4.

[28] Phillips ME. Pancreatic exocrine insufficiency following pancreatic resection. Pancreatology. 2015;**15**(5):449-455. DOI: 10.1016/j.pan.2015.06.003.

[29] Malleo G, Crippa S, Butturini G, Salvia R, Partelli S, Rossini R, Bacchion M, Pederzoli P, Bassi C. Delayed gastric emptying after pylorus-preserving pancreaticoduodenectomy: validation of International Study Group of Pancreatic Surgery classification and analysis of risk factors. HPB (Oxford). 2010;**12**(9):610-618. DOI: 10.1111/j.1477-2574.2010.00203.x.

[30] Ebrahimi B, Tucker SL, Li D, Abbruzzese JL, Kurzrock R. Cytokines in pancreatic carcinoma: correlation with phenotypic characteristics and prognosis. Cancer. 2004;**101**(12): 2727-2736.

[31] Laviano A, Meguid MM, Rossi-Fanelli F. Cancer anorexia: clinical implications, pathogenesis, and therapeutic strategies. Lancet Oncol. 2003;**4**(11):686-694. DOI: 10.1016/S1470-2045 (03)01247-6.

[32] Fearon K, Arends J, Baracos V. Understanding the mechanisms and treatment options in cancer cachexia. Nat. Rev. Clin. Oncol. 2013;**10**(2):90-99. DOI: 10.1038/nrclinonc.2012.209.

[33] Grunfeld C, Zhao C, Fuller J, Pollack A, Moser A, Friedman J, et al. Endotoxin and cytokines induce expression of leptin, the ob gene product, in hamsters. J. Clin. Invest. 1996;**97**(9):2152-2157. DOI: 10.1172/JCI118653.

[34] Janik JE, Curti BD, Considine RV, Rager HC, Powers GC, Alvord WG. Interleukin 1 alpha increases serum leptin concentrations in humans. J. Clin. Endocrinol. Metab. 1997;**82**(9):3084-3086.

[35] Sarraf P, Frederich RC, Turner EM, Ma G, Jaskowiak NT, Rivet DJ 3rd. Multiple cytokines and acute inflammation raise mouse leptin levels: potential role in inflammatory anorexia. J. Exp. Med. 1997;**185**(1):171-175. DOI: 10.1084/jem.185.1.171.

[36] Finck BN, Kelley KW, Dantzer R, Johnson RW. *In vivo* and *in vitro* evidence for the involvement of tumor necrosis factor-alpha in the induction of leptin by lipopolysaccharide. Endocrinology. 1998;**139**(5):2278-2283.

[37] Faggioni R, Fuller J, Moser A, Feingold KR, Grunfeld C. LPS-induced anorexia in leptin-deficient (ob/ob) and leptin receptor-deficient (db/db) mice. Am. J. Physiol. 1997;**273**(1): R181–R186.

[38] Simons JP, Schols AM, Campfield LA, Wouters EF, Saris WH. Plasma concentration of total leptin and human lung-cancer-associated cachexia. Clin. Sci. (Lond.). 1997;**93**(3): 273-277.

[39] Wallace AM, Sattar N, McMillan DC. Effect of weight loss and the inflammatory response on leptin concentrations in gastrointestinal cancer patients. Clin. Cancer Res. 1998;**4**(12):2977-2979.

[40] Mantovani G, Macciò A, Mura L, Massa E, Mudu MC, Mulas C, et al. Serum levels of leptin and proinflammatory cytokines in patients with advanced-stage cancer at different sites. J. Mol. Med. (Berl.). 2000;**78**(10):554-561. DOI: 10.1007/s001090000137.

[41] Bing C, Taylor S, Tisdale MJ, Williams G. Cachexia in MAC16 adenocarcinoma: suppression of hunger despite normal regulation of leptin, insulin and hypothalamic neuropeptide. Y. J. Neurochem. 2001;**79**(5):1004-1012. DOI: 10.1046/j.1471-4159.2001.00639.x.

[42] Inui A. Cancer anorexia-cachexia syndrome: are neuropeptides the key?. Cancer Res. 1999;**59**(18):4493-4501.

[43] Shintani F, Kanba S, Nakaki T, Nibuya M, Kinoshita N, Suzuki E, et al. Interleukin-1 beta augments release of norepinephrine, dopamine, and serotonin in the rat anterior hypothalamus. J. Neurosci. 1993;**13**(8):3574-3581.

[44] Heisler LK, Cowley MA, Tecott LH, Fan W, Low MJ, Smart JL, et al. Activation of central melanocortin pathways by fenfluramine. Science. 2002;**297**(5581):609-611. DOI: 10.1126/science.1072327.

[45] Cangiano C, Cascino A, Ceci F, Laviano A, Mulieri M, Muscaritoli M, et al. Plasma and CSF tryptophan in cancer anorexia. J. Neural Transm. Gen. Sect. 1990;**81**(225):225-233. DOI: 10.1007/BF01245044.

[46] Cangiano C, Testa U, Muscaritoli M, Meguid MM, Mulieri M, Laviano A, et al. Cytokines, tryptophan and anorexia in cancer patients before and after surgical tumor ablation. Anticancer Res. 1994;**14**(3B):1451-1455.

[47] Li G, Klein RL, Matheny M, King MA, Meyer EM, Scarpace PJ. Induction of uncoupling protein 1 by central interleukin-6 gene delivery is dependent on sympathetic innervation of brown adipose tissue and underlies one mechanism of body weight reduction in rats. Neuroscience. 2002;**115**(3):879-889. DOI: 10.1016/S0306-4522(02)00447-5.

[48] Arruda AP, Milanski M, Romanatto T, Solon C, Coope A, Alberici LC, et al. Hypothalamic actions of tumor necrosis factor alpha provide the thermogenic core for the wastage syndrome in cachexia. Endocrinology. 2010;**151**(2):683-694. DOI: 10.1210/en.2009-0865.

[49] Oudart H, Calgari C, Andriamampandry M, Le Maho Y, Malan A. Stimulation of brown adipose tissue activity in tumor-bearing rats. Can. J. Physiol. Pharmacol. 1995;**73**(11): 1625-1631.

[50] Roe SY, Cooper AL, Morris ID, Rothwell NJ. Involvement of prostaglandins in cachexia induced by T-cell leukemia in the rat. Metabolism. 1997;**46**(4):359-365.

[51] Rydén M, Arvidsson E, Blomqvist L, Perbeck L, Dicker A, Arner P. Targets for TNF-alpha-induced lipolysis in human adipocytes. Biochem. Biophys. Res. Commun. 2004;**318**(1): 168-175. DOI: 10.1016/j.bbrc.2004.04.010.

[52] Zhang HH1, Halbleib M, Ahmad F, Manganiello VC, Greenberg AS. Tumor necrosis factor-alpha stimulates lipolysis in differentiated human adipocytes through activation of extracellular signal-related kinase and elevation of intracellular cAMP. Diabetes. 2002;**51**(10):2929-2935. DOI: 10.2337/diabetes.51.10.2929.

[53] Cawthorn WP, Heyd F, Hegyi K, Sethi JK. Tumour necrosis factor-alpha inhibits adipogenesis via a betacatenin/TCF4(TCF7L2)-dependent pathway. Cell Death Differ. 2007;**14**(7):1361-1373. DOI: 10.1038/sj.cdd.4402127.

[54] Hammarstedt A, Isakson P, Gustafson B, Smith U. Wntsignaling is maintained and adipogenesis inhibited by TNFalpha but not MCP-1 and resistin. Biochem. Biophys. Res. Commun. 2007;**357**(3):700-706. DOI: 10.1016/j.bbrc.2007.03.202.

[55] Llovera M, Carbó N, López-Soriano J, García-Martínez C, Busquets S, Alvarez B, et al. Different cytokines modulate ubiquitin gene expression in rat skeletal muscle. Cancer Lett. 1998;**133**(1):83-87. DOI: 10.1016/S0304- 3835(98)00216-X.

[56] Li YP, Reid MB. NF-kappaB mediates the protein loss induced by TNF-alpha in differentiated skeletal muscle myotubes. Am. J. Physiol. Regul. Integr. Comp. Physiol. 2000;**279**(4): R1165–R1170.

[57] Guttridge DC, Mayo MW, Madrid LV, Wang CY, Baldwin AS Jr. NF-kappaB-induced loss of MyoD messenger RNA: possible role in muscle decay and cachexia . Science. 2000;**289**(5488):2363-2366. DOI: 10.1126/science.289.5488.2363.

[58] Martignoni ME, Kunze P, Hildebrandt W, Künzli B, Berberat P, Giese T, et al. Role of mononuclear cells and inflammatory cytokines in pancreatic cancer-related cachexia. Clin. Cancer Res. 2005;**11**(16):5802-5808. DOI: 10.1158/1078-0432.CCR-05-0185.

[59] Tsoli M, Moore M, Burg D, Painter A, Taylor R, Lockie SH, et al. Activation of thermogenesis in brown adipose tissue and dysregulated lipid metabolism associated with cancer cachexia in mice. Cancer Res. 2012;**72**(17):4372-4382. DOI: 10.1158/0008-5472. CAN-11-3536.

[60] Strassmann G, Fong M, Kenney JS, Jacob CO. Evidence for the involvement of interleukin 6 in experimental cancer cachexia. J. Clin. Invest. 1992;**89**(5):1681-1684. DOI: 10.1172/ JCI115767.

[61] Martignoni ME, Dimitriu C, Bachmann J, Krakowski-Rosen H, Ketterer K, Kinscherf R, et al. Liver macrophages contribute to pancreatic cancerrelated cachexia. Oncol. Rep. 2009;**21**(2):363-369. DOI: 10.3892/or_00000231.

[62] Fearon KC, Barber MD, Falconer JS, McMillan DC, Ross JA, Preston T, et al. Pancreatic cancer as a model: inflammatory mediators, acute-phase response, and cancer cachexia. World J. Surg. 1999;**23**(6):584-588. DOI: 10.1007/PL00012351.

[63] Preston T, Slater C, McMillan DC, Falconer JS, Shenkin A, Fearon KC, et al. Fibrinogen synthesis is elevated in fasting cancer patients with an acute phase response. J. Nutr. 1998;**128**(8):1355-1360.

[64] Todorov PT, McDevitt TM, Meyer DJ, Ueyama H, Ohkubo I, Tisdale MJ, et al. Purification and characterization of a tumor lipid-mobilizing factor. Cancer Res. 1998;**58**(11): 2353-2358.

[65] Felix K, Fakelman F, Hartmann D, Giese NA, Gaida MM, Schnölzer M, et al. Identification of serum proteins involved in pancreatic cancer cachexia. Life Sci. 2011;**88**(5-6):218-225. DOI: 10.1016/j.lfs.2010.11.011.

[66] Hirai K, Hussey HJ, Barber MD, Price SA, Tisdale MJ. Biological evaluation of a lipid-mobilizing factor isolated from the urine of cancer patients. Cancer Res. 1998;**58**(11): 2359-2365.

[67] Khan S, Tisdale MJ. Catabolism of adipose tissue by a tumour-produced lipid-mobilising factor. Int. J. Cancer. 1999;**80**(3):444-447. DOI: 10.1002/(SICI)1097-0215(19990129) 80:3%3C444::AID-IJC18%3E3. 3.CO;2-L.

[68] Russell ST, Hirai K, Tisdale MJ. Role of beta3-adrenergic receptors in the action of a tumour lipid mobilizing factor. Br. J. Cancer. 2002;**86**(3):424-428. DOI: 10.1038/sj.bjc.6600086.

[69] Russell ST, Tisdale MJ. Effect of a tumour-derived lipid-mobilising factor on glucose and lipid metabolism *in vivo*. Br. J. Cancer. 2002;**87**(5):580-584. DOI: 10.1038/sj.bjc.6600493.

[70] Bing C, Russell ST, Beckett EE, Collins P, Taylor S, Barraclough R, et al. Expression of uncoupling proteins-1, -2 and -3 mRNA is induced by an adenocarcinoma-derived lipid-mobilizing factor. Br. J. Cancer. 2002;**86**(4):612-618. DOI: 10.1038/sj.bjc.6600101.

[71] Islam-Ali B, Khan B, Price SA, Tisdale MJ. Modulation of adipocyte G-protein expression in cancer cachexia by a lipid-mobilizing factor (LMF). Br. J. Cancer. 2001;**85**(5):758-763. DOI: 10.1054/bjoc.2001.1992.

[72] Todorov PT, Deacon M, Tisdale MJ. Structural analysis of a tumor-produced sulfated glycoprotein capable of initiating muscle protein degradation. J. Biol. Chem. 1997;**272**(19): 12279-12288. DOI: 10.1074/jbc.272.19.12279.

[73] Todorov P, Cariuk P, McDevitt T, Coles B, Fearon K, Tisdale M. Characterization of a cancer cachectic factor. Nature. 1996;**379**(6567):739-742. DOI: 10.1038/379739a0.

[74] Wigmore SJ, Todorov PT, Barber MD, Ross JA, Tisdale MJ, Fearon KC. Characteristics of patients with pancreatic cancer expressing a novel cancer cachectic factor. Br. J. Surg. 2000b;**87**(1):53-58. DOI: 10.1046/j.1365- 2168.2000.01317.x.

[75] Cabal-Manzano R, Bhargava P, Torres-Duarte A, Marshall J, Bhargava P, Wainer IW. Proteolysis-inducing factor is expressed in tumours of patients with gastrointestinal cancers and correlates with weight loss. Br. J. Cancer. 2001;**84**(12):1599-1601. DOI: 10.1054/bjoc.2001.1830.

[76] Cariuk P, Lorite MJ, Todorov PT, Field WN, Wigmore SJ, Tisdale MJ. Induction of cachexia in mice by a product isolated from the urine of cachectic cancer patients. Br. J. Cancer. 1997;**76**(5):606-613. DOI: 10.1038/bjc.1997.433.

[77] Lorite MJ, Cariuk P, Tisdale MJ. Induction of muscle protein degradation by a tumour factor. Br. J. Cancer. 1997;**76**(8):1035-1040. DOI: 10.1038/bjc.1997.504.

[78] Lorite MJ, Smith HJ, Arnold JA, Morris A, Thompson MG, Tisdale MJ. Activation of ATP-ubiquitin-dependent proteolysis in skeletal muscle *in vivo* and murine myoblasts *in vitro* by a proteolysis-inducing factor (PIF). Br. J. Cancer. 2001;**85**(2):297-302. DOI: 10.1054/bjoc.2001.1879.

[79] Whitehouse AS, Tisdale MJ. Increased expression of the ubiquitin proteasome pathway in murine myotubes by proteolysis-inducing factor (PIF) is associated with activation of the transcription factor NF-kappaB. Br. J. Cancer. 2003;**89**(6):1116-1122. DOI: 10.1038/sj.bjc.6601132.

[80] Wyke SM, Tisdale MJ. NF-kappaB mediates proteolysis-inducing factor induced protein degradation and expression of the ubiquitin-proteasome system in skeletal muscle. Br. J. Cancer. 2005;**92**(4):711-721. DOI: 10.1038/sj.bjc.66 02402.

[81] Smith HJ, Tisdale MJ. Signal transduction pathways involved in proteolysis-inducing factor induced proteasome expression in murine myotubes. Br. J. Cancer. 2003;**89**(9):1783-1788. DOI: 10.1038/sj.bjc.6601328.

[82] Wyke SM, Khal J, Tisdale MJ. Signalling pathways in the induction of proteasome expression by proteolysis-inducing factor in murine myotubes. Cell Signal. 2005;**17**(1):67-75. DOI: 10.1016/j.cellsig. 2004.05.015.

[83] Russell ST, Eley H, Tisdale MJ. Role of reactive oxygen species in protein degradation in murine myotubes induced by proteolysis-inducing factor and angiotensin II. Cell Signal. 2007;**19**(8):1797-1806. DOI: 10.1016/j.cellsig.2007.04.003.

[84] Smith HJ, Wyke SM, Tisdale MJ. Role of protein kinase C and NF-kappaB in proteolysis-inducing factor-induced proteasome expression in C(2)C(12) myotubes. Br. J. Cancer. 2004;**90**(9):1850-1857. DOI: 10.1038/sj.bjc.6601767.

[85] Eley HL, Tisdale MJ. Skeletal muscle atrophy, a link between depression of protein synthesis and increase in degradation. J. Biol. Chem. 2007;**282**(10):7087-7097. DOI: 10.1074/jbc.M610378200.

[86] Zamanian-Daryoush M, Mogensen TH, DiDonato JA, Williams BR. NF-kappaB activation by double-stranded-RNA-activated protein kinase (PKR) is mediated through NF-kappaB-inducing kinase and IkappaB kinase. Mol. Cell Biol. 2000;**20**(4):1278-1290. DOI: 10.1128/MCB.20.4.1278-1290. 2000.

[87] Watchorn TM, Waddell I, Dowidar N, Ross JA. Proteolysisinducing factor regulates hepatic gene expression via the transcription factors NF-(kappa)B and STAT3. FASEB J. 2001;**15**(3):562-564.

[88] Watchorn TM, Dowidar N, Dejong CH, Waddell ID, Garden OJ, Ross JA. The cachectic mediator proteolysis inducing factor activates NF-kappaB and STAT3 in human Kupffer cells and monocytes. Int. J. Oncol. 2005;**27**(4):1105-1111.

[89] Olguin HC, Olwin BB. Pax-7 up-regulation inhibits myogenesis and cell cycle progression in satellite cells: a potential mechanism for self-renewal. Dev. Biol. 2004;**275**(2):375-388. DOI: 10.1016/j.ydbio.2004.08.015.

[90] He WA, Berardi E, Cardillo VM, Acharyya S, Aulino P, Thomas-Ahner J, et al. NF-κB-mediated Pax7 dysregulation in the muscle microenvironment promotes cancer cachexia. J. Clin. Invest. 2013;**123**(11):4821-4835. DOI: 10.1172/JCI68523.

[91] Imoto A, Mitsunaga S, Inagaki M, Aoyagi K, Sasaki H, Ikeda M, et al. Neural invasion induces cachexia via astrocytic activation of neural route in pancreatic cancer. Int. J. Cancer. 2012;**131**(12):2795-2807. DOI: 10.1002/ijc.27594.

[92] Bozzetti F, Group SW. Screening the nutritional status in oncology: a preliminary report on 1,000 outpatients. Support. Care Cancer. 2009;**17**:279-284. DOI: 10.1007/s00520-008-0476-3.

[93] Ottery F. Supportive nutritional management of the patient with pancreatic cancer. Oncology (Williston Park). 1996;**10**:26-32.

[94] Nitenberg G, Raynard B. Nutritional support of the cancer patient: issues and dilemmas. Crit. Rev. Oncol. Hematol. 2000;**34**:137-168. DOI: 10.1016/S1040-8428(00)00048-2.

[95] Jatoi A, Loprinzi CL. Current management of cancer-associated anorexia and weight loss. Oncology (Williston Park). 2001;**15**(4):497-502.

[96] el-Kamar FG, Grossbard ML, Kozuch PS. Metastatic pancreatic cancer: emerging strategies in chemotherapy and palliative care. Oncologist. 2003;**8**(1):18-34. DOI: 10.1634/theoncologist.8-1-18.

[97] Ovesen L, Allingstrup L, Hannibal J, Mortensen EL, Hansen OP. Effect of dietary counseling on food intake, body weight, response rate, survival, and quality of life in cancer patients undergoing chemotherapy: a prospective, randomized study. J. Clin. Oncol. 1993;**11**(10):2043-2049.

[98] Fearon KC, Von Meyenfeldt MF, Moses AG, Van Geenen R, Roy A, Gouma DJ, et al. Effect of a protein and energy dense N-3 fatty acid enriched oral supplement on loss of weight and lean tissue in cancer cachexia: a randomised double blind trial. Gut. 2003;**52**(10):1479-1486. DOI: 10.1136/gut.52.10.1479.

[99] Bauer JD, Capra S. Nutrition intervention improves outcomes in patients with cancer cachexia receiving chemotherapy–a pilot study. Support. Care Cancer. 2005;**13**:270-274. DOI: 10.1007/s00520-004-0746-7.

[100] Barber MD, Ross JA, Voss AC, Tisdale MJ, Fearon KC. The effect of an oral nutritional supplement enriched with fish oil on weight-loss in patients with pancreatic cancer. Br. J. Cancer. 1999;**81**(1):80-86. DOI: 10.1038/sj.bjc.6690654.

[101] Kraft M, Kraft K, Gärtner S, Mayerle J, Simon P, Weber E, et al. L-Carnitine-supplementation in advanced pancreatic cancer (CARPAN)–a randomized multicentre trial. Nutr. J. 2012;**11**:52. DOI: 10.1186/1475-2891-11-52.

[102] Pelzer U, Arnold D, Gövercin M, Stieler J, Doerken B, Riess H, et al. Parenteral nutrition support for patients with pancreatic cancer. Results of a phase II study. BMC Cancer. 2010;**10**:86. DOI: 10.1186/1471-2407-10-86.

[103] Nixon DW, Lawson DH, Kutner M, Ansley J, Schwarz M, Heymsfield S, et al. Hyperalimentation of the cancer patient with protein-calorie undernutrition. Cancer Res. 1981;**41**(6):2038-2045.

[104] Bruera E, Macmillan K, Kuehn N, Hanson J, MacDonald RN. A controlled trial of megestrol acetate on appetite, caloric intake, nutritional status, and other symptoms in patients with advanced cancer. Cancer. 1990;**66**(6):1279-1282. DOI: 10.1002/1097-0142(19900915)66:6%3C1279::AIDCNCR2820660630%3E3.0.CO;2-R.

[105] Loprinzi CL, Ellison NM, Schaid DJ, Krook JE, Athmann LM, Dose AM, et al. Controlled trial of megestrol acetate for the treatment of cancer anorexia and cachexia. J. Natl. Cancer Inst. 1990;**82**(13):1127-1132. DOI: 10.1093/jnci/82.13.1127.

[106] Loprinzi CL, Michalak JC, Schaid DJ, Mailliard JA, Athmann LM, Goldberg RM, et al. Phase III evaluation of four doses of megestrol acetate as therapy for patients with cancer anorexia and/or cachexia. J. Clin. Oncol. 1993;**11**(4):762-767.

[107] Westman G, Bergman B, Albertsson M, Kadar L, Gustavsson G, Thaning L, et al. Megestrol acetate in advanced, progressive, hormone-insensitive cancer. Effects on the quality of life: a placebo-controlled, randomised, multicentre trial. Eur. J. Cancer. 1999;**35**(4):586-595. DOI: 10.1016/S0959-8049(98)00398-0.

[108] Pascual López A, Roqué i Figuls M, Urrútia Cuchi G, Berenstein EG, Almenar Pasies B, Balcells Alegre M, Herdman M. Systematic review of megestrol acetate in the treatment of anorexia-cachexia syndrome. J Pain Symptom Manage. 2004;**27**(4):360-369. DOI: 10.1016/j.jpainsymman.2003.09.007.

[109] Leśniak W, Bała M, Jaeschke R, Krzakowski M. Effects of megestrol ′ acetate in patients with cancer anorexia-cachexia syndrome–a systematic review and meta-analysis. Pol. Arch. Med. Wewn. 2008;**118**(11):636-644.

[110] Loprinzi CL, Schaid DJ, Dose AM, Burnham NL, Jensen MD. Body-composition changes in patients who gain weight while receiving megestrol acetate. J. Clin. Oncol. 1993b;**11**(1):152-154.

[111] McCarthy HD, Crowder RE, Dryden S, Williams G. Megestrol acetate stimulates food and water intake in the rat: effects on regional hypothalamic neuropeptide Y concentrations. Eur. J. Pharmacol. 1994;**265**:99-102. DOI: 10.1016/0014-2999(94)90229-1.

[112] Mantovani G, Macciò A, Lai P, Massa E, Ghiani M, Santona MC. Cytokine activity in cancer-related anorexia/cachexia: role of megestrol acetate and medroxyprogesterone acetate. Semin Oncol. 1998a;**25**:45-52.

[113] Mantovani G, Macciò A, Lai P, Massa E, Ghiani M, and Santona MC. Cytokine involvement in cancer anorexia/cachexia: role of megestrol acetate and medroxyprogesterone

acetate on cytokine downregulation and improvement of clinical symptoms. Crit. Rev. Oncog. 1998b;**9**:99-106. DOI: 10.1615/CritRevOncog.v9.i2.10.

[114] Willox JC, Corr J, Shaw J, Richardson M, Calman KC, Drennan M. Prednisolone as an appetite stimulant in patients with cancer. Br. Med. J. (Clin. Res. Ed.). 1984;**288**(6410):27. DOI: 10.1136/bmj.288.6410.27.

[115] Bruera E, Roca E, Cedaro L, Carraro S, Chacon R. Action of oral methylprednisolone in terminal cancer patients: a prospective randomized double-blind study. Cancer Treat. Rep. 1985;**69**:751-754.

[116] Loprinzi CL, Kugler JW, Sloan JA, Mailliard JA, Krook JE, Wilwerding MB, et al. Randomized comparison of megestrol acetate versus dexamethasone versus fluoxymesterone for the treatment of cancer anorexia/cachexia. J. Clin. Oncol. 1999;**17**(10):3299-3306.

[117] Plata-Salamán CR. Dexamethasone inhibits food intake suppression induced by low doses of interleukin-1 beta administered intracerebroventricularly. Brain Res. Bull. 1991;**27**:737-738. DOI: 10.1016/0361-9230(91)90055-O.

[118] Nelson K, Walsh D, Deeter P, Sheehan F. A phase II study of delta- 9-tetrahydrocannabinol for appetite stimulation in cancer-associated anorexia. J. Palliat. Care. 1994;**10**:14-18.

[119] Jatoi A, Windschitl HE, Loprinzi CL, Sloan JA, Dakhil SR, Mailliard JA, et al. Dronabinol versus megestrol acetate versus combination therapy for cancer-associated anorexia: a North Central Cancer Treatment Group study. J. Clin. Oncol. 2002;**20**(2):567-573. DOI: 10.1200/JCO.20.2.567.

[120] McMillan DC, Leen E, Smith J, Sturgeon C, Preston T, Cooke TG. Effect of extended ibuprofen administration on the acute phase protein response in colorectal cancer patients. Eur. J. Surg. Oncol. 1995;**21**(5):531-534. DOI: 10.1016/S0748-7983(95)97157-2.

[121] Preston T, Fearon KC, McMillan DC, Winstanley FP, Slater C, Shenkin A, et al. Effect of ibuprofen on the acute-phase response and protein metabolism in patients with cancer and weight loss. Br. J. Surg. 1995;**82**(2):229-234. DOI: 10.1002/bjs.1800820233.

[122] Wigmore SJ, Falconer JS, Plester CE, Ross JA, Maingay JP, Carter DC, et al. Ibuprofen reduces energy expenditure and acute-phase protein production compared with placebo in pancreatic cancer patients. Br. J. Cancer. 1995;**72**(1):185-188. DOI: 10.1038/bjc.1995.300.

[123] Gelin J, Andersson C, Lundholm K. Effects of indomethacin, cytokines, and cyclosporin A on tumor growth and the subsequent development of cancer cachexia. Cancer Res. 1991;**51**(3):880-885.

[124] Gelin J, Moldawer LL, Lönnroth C, Sherry B, Chizzonite R, Lundholm K. Role of endogenous tumor necrosis factor alpha and interleukin 1 for experimental tumor growth and the development of cancer cachexia. Cancer Res. 1991;**51**(1):415-421.

[125] Lundholm K, Gelin J, Hyltander A, Lönnroth C, Sandström R, Svaninger G, et al. Anti-inflammatory treatment may prolong survival in undernourished patients with metastatic solid tumors. Cancer Res. 1994;**54**(21):5602-5606.

[126] McMillan DC, O'Gorman P, Fearon KC, McArdle CS. A pilot study of megestrol acetate and ibuprofen in the treatment of cachexia in gastrointestinal cancer patients. Br. J. Cancer. 1997;**76**(6):788-790. DOI: 10.1038/bjc.1997.463.

[127] Lai V, George J, Richey L, Kim HJ, Cannon T, Shores C, et al. Results of a pilot study of the effects of celecoxib on cancer cachexia in patients with cancer of the head, neck, and gastrointestinal tract. Head Neck. 2008;**30**(1):67-74. DOI: 10.1002/hed.20662.

[128] McMillan DC, Wigmore SJ, Fearon KC, O'Gorman P, Wright CE, McArdle CS. A prospective randomized study of megestrol acetate and ibuprofen in gastrointestinal cancer patients with weight loss. Br. J. Cancer. 1999;**79**:495-500. DOI: 10.1038/sj.bjc.6690077.

[129] Sampaio EP, Sarno EN, Galilly R, Cohn ZA, Kaplan G. Thalidomide selectively inhibits tumor necrosis factor alpha production by stimulated human monocytes. J. Exp. Med. 1991;**173**(3):699-703. DOI: 10.1084/jem.173.3.699.

[130] Bruera E, Neumann CM, Pituskin E, Calder K, Ball G, Hanson J. Thalidomide in patients with cachexia due to terminal cancer: preliminary report. Ann. Oncol. 1999;**10**(7):857-859. DOI: 10.1023/A:1008329821941.

[131] Gordon JN, Trebble TM, Ellis RD, Duncan HD, Johns T, Goggin PM. Thalidomide in the treatment of cancer cachexia: a randomised placebo controlled trial. Gut. 2005;**54**(4):540-545. DOI: 10.1136/gut.2004.047563.

[132] Meydani SN, Lichtenstein AH, Cornwall S, Meydani M, Goldin BR, Rasmussen H, et al. Immunologic effects of national cholesterol education panel step-2 diets with and without fish-derived N-3 fatty acid enrichment. J. Clin. Invest. 1993;**92**:105-113. DOI: 10.1172/JCI116537.

[133] Wigmore SJ, Fearon KC, Maingay JP, Ross JA. Downregulation of the acute-phase response in patients with pancreatic cancer cachexia receiving oral eicosapentaenoic acid is mediated via suppression of interleukin-6. Clin. Sci. (Lond.). 1997;**92**:215-221.

[134] Tisdale MJ, Beck SA. Inhibition of tumour-induced lipolysis *in vitro* and cachexia and tumour growth *in vivo* by eicosapentaenoic acid. Biochem. Pharmacol. 1991;**41**:103-107. DOI: 10.1016/0006-2952(91)90016-X.

[135] Tisdale MJ. Inhibition of lipolysis and muscle protein degradation by EPA in cancer cachexia. Nutrition. 1996;**12**:S31–S33. DOI: 10.1016/0899-9007(95)00066-6.

[136] Hussey HJ, Tisdale MJ. Effect of a cachectic factor on carbohydrate metabolism and attenuation by eicosapentaenoic acid. Br. J. Cancer. 1999;**80**:1231-1235. DOI: 10.1038/sj.bjc.6690490.

[137] Wigmore SJ, Ross JA, Falconer JS, Plester CE, Tisdale MJ, Carter DC. The effect of polyunsaturated fatty acids on the progress of cachexia in patients with pancreatic cancer. Nutrition. 1996;**12**:S27–S30. DOI: 10.1016/0899-9007(95)00078-X.

[138] Wigmore SJ, Barber MD, Ross JA, Tisdale MJ, Fearon KC. Effect of oral eicosapentaenoic acid on weight loss in patients with pancreatic cancer. Nutr. Cancer. 2000b;**36**(2):177-184. DOI: 10.1207/S1532791 4NC3602_6.

[139] Fearon KC, Barber MD, Moses AG, Ahmedzai SH, Taylor GS, Tisdale MJ, et al. Double-blind, placebo-controlled, randomized study of eicosapentaenoic acid diester in patients with cancer cachexia. J. Clin. Oncol. 2006a;**24**(21):3401-3407. DOI: 10.1200/JCO.2005.04.5724.

[140] Jatoi A, Rowland K, Loprinzi CL, Sloan JA, Dakhil SR, MacDonald N, et al. An eicosapentaenoic acid supplement versus megestrol acetate versus both for patients with cancer-associated wasting: a North Central Cancer Treatment Group and National Cancer Institute of Canada collaborative effort. J. Clin. Oncol. 2004;**22**(12):2469-2476. DOI: 10.1200/JCO.2004.06.024.

[141] Mantovani G, Macciò A, Madeddu C, Serpe R, Massa E, Dessì M, et al. Randomized phase III clinical trial of five different arms of treatment in 332 patients with cancer cachexia. Oncologist. 2010;**15**(2):200-211. DOI: 10.1634/theoncologist.2009-0153.

[142] Rigas JR, Schuster M, Orlov SV, Milovanovic B, Prabhash K, Smith JT, et al. Effect of ALD518, a humanized anti-IL-6 antibody, on lean body mass loss and symptoms in patients with advanced non-small cell lung cancer (NSCLC): results of a phase II randomized, double-blind safety and efficacy trial. J. Clin. Oncol. 2010;**28** (abstract 7622).

[143] Schuster M, Rigas JR, Orlov SV, Milovanovic B, Prabhash K, Smith JT. ALD518, a humanized anti-IL-6 antibody, treats anemia in patients with advanced non-small cell lung cancer (NSCLC): results of a phase II, randomized, double-blind, placebo-controlled trial. J. Clin. Oncol. 2010;**28** (abstract 7631.).

[144] Bayliss TJ, Smith JT, Schuster M, Dragnev KH, Rigas JR. A humanized anti-IL-6 antibody (ALD518) in non-small cell lung cancer. Expert Opin. Biol. Ther. 2011;**11**:1663-1668. DOI: 10.1517/14712598.2011.627850.

[145] Ando K, Takahashi F, Motojima S, Nakashima K, Kaneko N, Hoshi K, et al. Possible role for tocilizumab, an anti-interleukin-6 receptor antibody, in treating cancer cachexia. J. Clin. Oncol. 2013;**31**(6):e69–e72. DOI: 10.1200/JCO.2012.44.2020.

[146] Chasen M, Hirschman SZ, Bhargava R. Phase II study of the novel peptide-nucleic acid OHR118 in the management of cancer-related anorexia/cachexia. J. Am. Med. Dir. Assoc. 2011;**12**:62-67. DOI: 10.1016/j.jamda.2010.02.012.

[147] ClinicalTrials.gov. Open label study with OHR/AVR118 in advanced cancer patients with anorexia-cachexia [Internet]. Available from: http://clinicaltrials.gov/ct2/show/NCT01206335 [Accessed: December 2013].

[148] Zhou X, Wang JL, Lu J, Song Y, Kwak KS, Jiao Q, et al. Reversal of cancer cachexia and muscle wasting by ActRIIB antagonism leads to prolonged survival. Cell. 2010;**142**:531-543. DOI: 10.1016/j.cell.2010.07.011.

[149] ClinicalTrials.gov. Clinical study of BYM338 for the treatment of unintentional weight loss in patients with cancer of the lung or the pancreas [Internet]. Available from: http://clinicaltrials.gov/ct2/show/NCT01433263 [Accessed: December 2013].

[150] ClinicalTrials.gov. A Phase 2 study of LY2495655 in participants with pancreatic cancer [Internet]. Available from: http://clinicaltrials.gov/ct2/show/NCT01505530 [Accessed: December 2013].

[151] Bachmann J, Ketterer K, Marsch C, Fechtner K, Krakowski-Roosen H, Büchler MW, et al. Pancreatic cancer related cachexia: influence on metabolism and correlation to weight loss and pulmonary function. BMC Cancer. 2009;**9**:255. DOI: 10.1186/1471-2407-9-255.

9

Sarcopenia in Chronic Illness and Rehabilitative Approaches

Raoul Saggini, Simona Maria Carmignano, Lucia Cosenza, Tommaso Palermo and Rosa Grazia Bellomo

Abstract

Primary sarcopenia is considered to be age-related when no other cause is evident, other than aging itself. Secondary sarcopenia should be considered when one or more other causes are evident, such as multiple chronic conditions. Previous studies have reported that low muscle strength and impaired physical performance can be found in chronic diseases, including metabolic disease (diabetes, hypertension, and obesity), arthritis, osteoporosis, cancer, chronic kidney disease, chronic obstructive pulmonary disease, neuromuscular disease, and chronic infection. The development of preventive and therapeutic strategies against secondary sarcopenia and wasting disorders in general is an epidemiological need. The planning of a complex rehabilitation program in sarcopenia associated to chronic conditions, in the context of a comprehensive treatment, is made up of a nutritional support, exercise, correction of lifestyles, and the use of advanced physical energies. Therefore, for the purposes of the optimal management, it is essential to identify the pathogenesis and clinical characteristics that can affect the different rehabilitative treatment.

Keywords: secondary sarcopenia, chronic illness, rehabilitative approaches

1. Introduction

Many definitions available on sarcopenia agree on to define it as paraphysiological phenomenon, characterized by loss of muscle mass that occurs with aging.

Some authors emphasize the histopathology defining sarcopenia as an increase of the adipose and connective component within the muscle itself, whereas others focus on the reduction of muscle strength and physical function [1, 2].

Cachexia is a composite word from the Greek words "kakos" (bad) and "hexis" (condition) and refers to the prognosis and functionality of patients suffering from cachexia. The characteristic of this complex metabolic disturbance is weight loss due to an underlying cause disease, such as heart failure, chronic pulmonary diseases, or cancer. According to the definition given by Cruz-Jentoft et al. in 2010, cachexia is found in patients with unintentional weight loss of 5% in the past year, a body mass index (BMI) lower than 20, decreased muscle mass as shown with bioimpedance analysis (BIA) or dual-energy X-ray absorptiometry (DEXA), low muscle strength, low serum albumin levels, anemia, and elevated biomarkers of inflammation [2].

Weight loss becomes a clinical sign of any progressive acute or chronic disease state. In its extreme form, it involves a significant lean body mass (including skeletal muscle) and fat loss. Skeletal muscle provides a fundamental basis for human function, enabling locomotion, and respiration. Muscle wasting is related to a poor quality of life and increased morbidity/mortality [3].

2. Sarcopenia in chronic illness

Sarcopenia can be defined as primary sarcopenia when due to the aging process and secondary when due to comorbidities, malnutrition, or immobility (**Figure 1**).

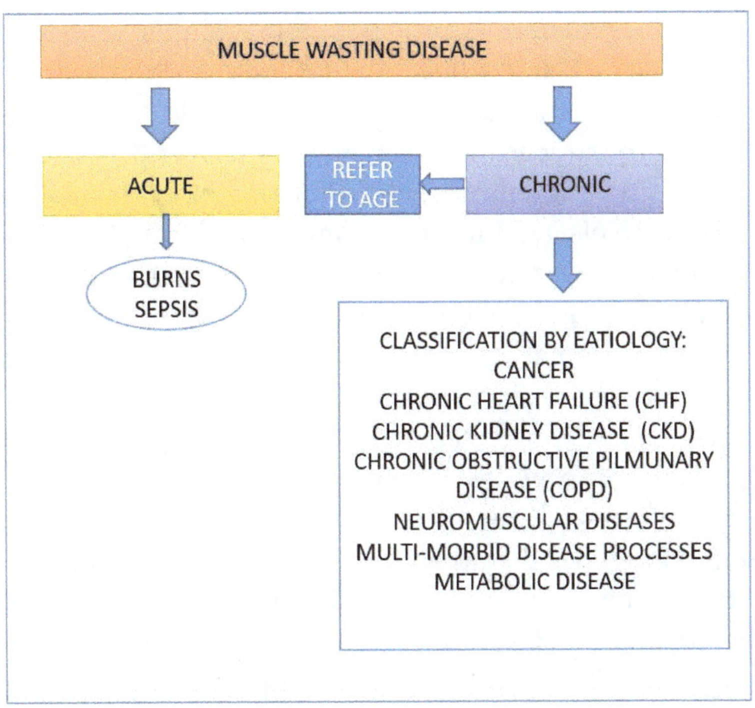

Figure 1. Classification of sarcopenia.

- Comorbidities that induce sarcopenia are organ failure (e.g. heart, kidneys, lungs, brain and liver), inflammatory diseases, cancer, and endocrine diseases.
- Malnutrition due to gastrointestinal disorders, anorexia in cases of polypharmacy, and inadequate intake due to psychosocial disorders lead to secondary sarcopenia.
- Inactivity as a result postoperative deconditioning or prolonged rehabilitation is the reason for activity-related secondary sarcopenia [4].

It has been known for millennia that muscle and fat wasting leads to poor outcomes, including deaths in chronic disease states. It is usually accompanied by physical inactivity, decreased mobility, slow gait, and poor physical endurance, which are also common features of the frailty syndrome. Although the specific contribution of each of these factors is unknown, there are more and more convincing evidence of chronic low-grade inflammation prominent role in the development of sarcopenia. According to recent studies, chronic inflammation is associated with many degenerative diseases [5]. Systemic inflammation is thus dependent on many factors that include diseases such as obesity, type 2 diabetes, dementia [5, 6], heart failure, and rheumatic diseases [7, 8], which can then be the result of this inflammatory condition and/or themselves can be the cause of the increase of inflammation. The impact of inflammation on the development of sarcopenia is supported by many studies. Animal studies show that low-grade inflammation reduction following the administration of ibuprofen in rats have determined a significant decrease in the loss of muscle mass [9]. Other studies, always conducted on animals, have shown that administration of interleukin-6 (IL-6) or tumor necrosis factor alpha (TNF-α) increases the skeletal muscle degradation, decreases protein synthesis, and reduces plasma concentrations of insulin-like growth factor (IGF) [10]. However, considering the studies of healthy elderly people living in the community, it was confirmed that one pro-inflammatory state produces, in the long-term, negative effects on sarcopenia. In the study "Longitudinal Aging Study Amsterdam," high levels of IL-6 and C-reactive protein (CRP) were associated with a double or triple risk of losing more than 40% to the hand grip (strength of the handshake) over 3 years. TNF-α, IL-1a, IL-6, IL-18, C-reactive protein (CRP) and fibrinogen are among the cytokines and acute phase proteins, that result to be more elevated in pro-inflammatory state [11]. Moreover, high levels of muscle catabolic biomarkers, which include IL-6, are important predictors of the decline in muscle strength [12]. Other authors report that IL-6 is a multifunctional cytokine because it has both pro and anti-inflammatory effects by determining muscular growth or atrophy, and according to different conditions, its effect is anabolic or catabolic. Several different pathophysiological processes induce sarcopenia following distinct pathways: neurological diseases produce sarcopenia by loss of motor neurons. Malabsorption leads to protein deficits and muscle catabolism. Disuse of muscles due to physical inactivity is followed by muscle degeneration. Hormonal disturbances of the thyroid, hypercortisolism, and insulin resistance lead to sarcopenia resulting from protein deficiency [13, 14]. These processes are found in combination or alone in many acute and chronic diseases above all in elderly patients, for example heart failure, chronic obstructive pulmonary disease (COPD), diabetes, neurological diseases, musculoskeletal diseases, as well as post-traumatic or postoperative conditions [15].

2.1. Sarcopenia: obesity and diabetes

Although the mechanism by which the potential TNF-α and IL-6 increase and the relationship with sarcopenia is not yet well defined, they may be related to the increase of the intramuscular adipose tissue. Under the pro-inflammatory stimulus, the intramuscular contents and intra-myocellular fat deposits increase creating a vicious circle where adipocytes, which secrete IL-6 and TNF-α as well as adipocines such as leptin and adiponectin, further promote inflammation [16].

More recently, Newman et al. have shown that it is important to consider in sarcopenia the percentage of fat mass. These authors have shown that people with higher body weight is not classified as suffering from sarcopenia, though their lean mass is sufficient compared to the total body weight [17]. Both sarcopenia and obesity represent, as the individual factors, a risk for adverse events, it has been shown that if present in combination, act synergistically increasing the earlier onset of disability [18]. For example, Rolland et al. found in a cohort study of women with sarcopenia, decreased physical performance (climbing stairs) compared to a group of healthy same aged, the worse performance was related to sarcopenia associated with obesity [19].

2.2. Chronic obstructive pulmonary disease

Chronic obstructive pulmonary disease (COPD) is a common cause of morbidity and mortality worldwide. The burden of disease is induced to a great extent by extrapulmonary symptoms, such as osteoporosis, heart failure, and sarcopenia. Using only BMI as a predictor of muscle mass or sarcopenia is misleading in these patients because the combination of abdominal obesity and sarcopenia is often present [20]. Sarcopenia affects 15% of patients with chronic obstructive pulmonary disease (COPD) stable and compromises the independence and the functional state of the musculoskeletal system. This loss of muscle mass does not seem to affect the outcome of pulmonary rehabilitation, which can lead to remission of the syndrome in selected patients. Pulmonary rehabilitation can improve symptoms and quality of life of patients with respiratory disease. It releases dyspnea and fatigue, as well as increasing exercise tolerance, emotional function so in indirect way it decreases frailty such as weakness, inactivity and fatigue, and then sarcopenia [21, 22].

It has been reported that patients with COPD and sarcopenia have nearly overlapping results after pulmonary rehabilitation compared to patients with COPD without sarcopenia, in terms of upper and lower limb strength, exercise capacity and health status [23].

Another important data are the absence of statistical differences about the body composition, functional performance, or health status between patients with and patients without sarcopenia undergone to pulmonary rehabilitation [24].

Musculoskeletal dysfunction is a recognized manifestation of COPD whose characteristics include the weakness of the quadriceps, the atrophy, and the change of type II fibers, all associated with a poor prognosis independent from lung function [25]. COPD determines an imbalance favoring protein breakdown over synthesis, apoptosis, sarcomere and sarcolemma damage, reduced myosin heavy chain-I isoform type I [slow twitch/endurance] muscle fibers, and a decreased density of capillaries and mitochondria [26–28]. This chronic disease is related to abnormalities of oxidative enzymes, mitochondrial activity, and expression of myogenin and m-cadherin—key molecules required for muscle growth and repair [29]. In chronic conditions, the poor peripheral oxygenation linked to abnormalities of gas exchange typical of COPD and anemia, as well as increased oxidation processes [30–32] associated with hypercapnia, create an acidosis condition that alters muscle proteases [33, 34], increasing catabolic activity in the muscle [35]. In addition, the effect of tobacco is associated with the [36] myopathy induced by corticosteroid use (especially systemic steroids) [37, 38], malnutrition that has a negative balance of energy [39], and reduction of physical activity leading sarcopenia [40]. The other mechanism involved in the genesis of sarcopenia is a sedentary lifestyle due not only to previous habits but also to reduced exercise tolerance. This was highlighted by disproportionate impairment of lower limb musculature in comparison to the upper limbs (that are subjected to a lesser degree of physical inactivity than the legs) [41] and by similarity in the structural changes seen in the sarcopenia of COPD and atrophy due to muscle disuse [42]. Furthermore, recovery of strength is possible with muscle training and conditioning [43, 44], and the apparent lack of correlation between the severity of airflow limitation and extent of muscle dysfunction [45]. Rehabilitation would therefore be expected to improve frailty and sarcopenia, but there are little published data on this as an intervention.

2.3. Sarcopenia: chronic renal failure

Patients with end-stage renal disease (ESRD) and chronic renal failure (CRF) receiving dialysis can have altered nutritional status and body composition due to dietary restrictions, level of physical activity, co-morbidities, metabolic alterations, and inflammation. Fatigue and immobility due to low muscle function are frequent symptoms reported by patients with chronic kidney disease. Sarcopenia is found in all stages of the disease and more distinctly in patients with high grades of renal function impairment. Pereira et al. found a significantly higher association of sarcopenia, diagnosed by BPA and hand grip strength measurements and mortality [46]. The degradation of proteins is an important energy production mechanism since the amino acids are rapidly converted to glucose. In conditions of catabolism generates an imbalance in favor of the degradation compared to the synthesis of proteins and, not existing a storage of the same, the muscle proteins are degraded and, if not additional sufficiently, develop muscle atrophy that determines a condition of sarcopenia [47, 48].

Many diseases promote protein catabolism, including the IRC; in particular, it was noted that during and after the hemodialysis session protein degradation is significantly accelerated. Several studies have shown that the ubiquitin-proteasome system (UPS) is the major proteolytic system in renal patients (**Figure 2**); despite prove even other hyperactive pathways (lysosomal cathepsin and calpain-gated calcium), caspase is a protease involved in cell apoptosis process that accelerates the degradation of the muscle through the reduction of complex protein structures in simple proteins, useful substrates for the UPS [49].

Several evidences have shown that patients with CRF, insulin resistance, inflammation, metabolic acidosis, and excess of angiotensin II determine high levels of caspase 3 and

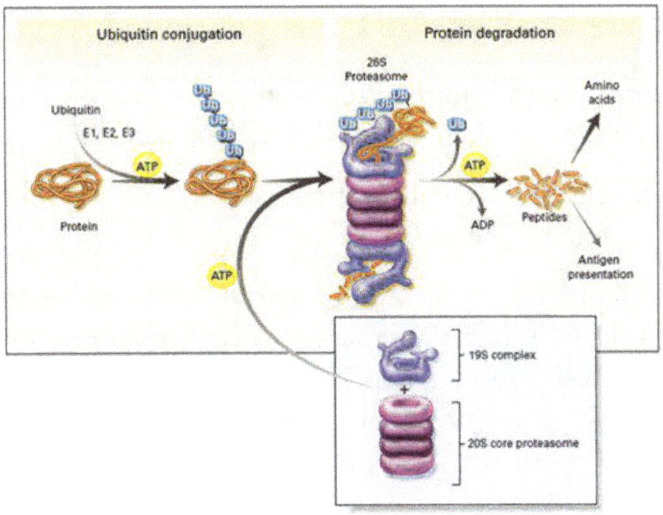

Figure 2. The proteins responsible for muscle degradation are first of all ubiquitin: the enzyme activates the ubiquitin E1, activating a cascade of ATP-dependent events. The ubiquitin chain is recognized by the proteasome 19S, which catalyzes entrance of the protein substrate in the proteasome core 20S, which is cleaved to peptides of the 26S proteasome. The peptides are degraded into amino acids to build cellular proteins or are released from the cells. From: Workeneh BT, Mitch WE. Review of muscle wasting associated with chronic kidney disease. The American Journal of Clinical Nutrition 2010;**91(suppl)**:1128S-1132S.

a significant increase of catabolic processes. These conditions promote the degradation of muscle protein, itself CRF can induce and enhance insulin resistance, encouraging the development of sarcopenia [50–52]. Another consequence of CRF, even more, of the hemodialysis treatment, is the presence of a chronic inflammatory state that, through different modulators, including TNF-alpha, suppresses the action of insulin, increases blood cortisol levels, and activates caspase-3. Glucocorticoids enhance degradation of muscle proteins by upregulation of UPS system. Metabolic acidosis, that is very common, especially in the case of dialysis treatment, determines sarcopenia through multiple mechanisms: induces a negative nitrogen balance and protein synthesis, promotes protein degradation by the UPS system and caspase 3 and alteration of pathway PI3K/Akt, which is a critical transduction signal in cell proliferation and cell cycle progression, apoptosis, and cellular metabolism. It reduces blood levels of IGF-1 and increases those of glucocorticoids. It is probably the main cause of the high prevalence of sarcopenia CFR [53]. The dialysis treatment, by itself, may determine, during each session, a damage to the protein metabolism, with the loss of amino acids and proteins in the dialysate, which reduces the availability of nutrients for muscle synthesis [54]. Many studies, in fact, show that the dialysis catabolic effects induce negative impact on the homeostasis of skeletal muscle protein with reduction of their synthesis and increase of their degradation [55]. Other authors noted that the increased protein lysis persists up to 2 hours after the end of hemodialysis session [56].

The mechanisms underlying this alteration of protein turnover were due not only to the reduction of circulating levels of amino acids and proteins but also to alterations of the factor and EIF2B (eukaryotic translation initiation factor 2 subunit B), which acts in the early steps of protein synthesis and activation of the inflammatory cascade [57].

2.4. Sarcopenia: chronic heart failure (CHF)

Heart dysfunction is a major factor limiting physical performance and skeletal muscle abnormalities, which often accompany CHF, may also contribute to fatigue and dyspnea (**Figure 3**).

Heart dysfunction is associated by metabolic changes that implicate inflammatory and endocrine disorders that determine muscle atrophy and weakness [58].

Cardiac myopathy is defined as muscle fiber atrophy, decreased capillary density, and a low number of type I fibers (fast) compared to type 2, with alteration of the normal ratio between type 1 fibers and type 2 fibers, changes that are responsible for intolerance to physical exercise [59]. Mechanism involved is the ubiquitin-mediated proteolysis and anorexia that exacerbate the weight loss process.

The UPS involves a multi-subunit protease that specifically degrades ubiquitin-conjugated proteins through the action of three enzymes, the ubiquitin-activating enzyme, the ubiquitin-conjugating enzyme, and ubiquitin ligases (atrogin-1 and MuRF-1). A higher frequency of myonuclear apoptosis has also been found in the muscle of patients with CHF relative to age-matched healthy controls [60].

In fact, patients develop anorexia that is secondary to intestinal edema with symptoms like dysgeusia, nausea, and gastroenteropathy and it is also mediated by several drugs such as digoxin, angiotensin-converting enzyme (ACE) inhibitors, β-blockers, and diuretics that favor a loss of nutrients. So, an insufficient intake or absorption of primary nutritional elements, or their loss, determines a malnutrition condition and muscle depletion.

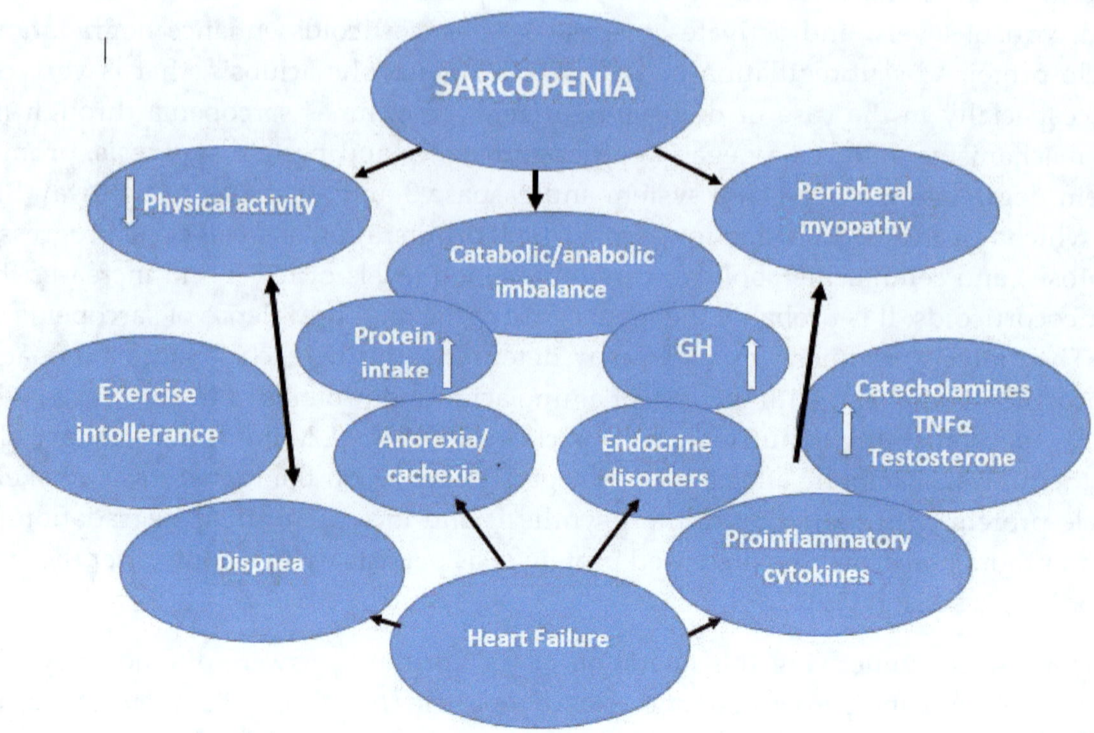

Figure 3. Pathophysiology of secondary sarcopenia.

Furthermore, elevation of angiotensin II levels aggravates these mechanisms. High levels of angiotensin II increase cytokines, such as TNF-alpha, interleukin 6, and glucocorticoids, which induce muscle protein degradation. TNF-α and its soluble receptors have been associated with declines in muscle mass and strength [61]. Another pathophysiological process is related to the decrease of expression of growth hormone (GH) and IGF-1 (anabolic hormones) in muscle, possibly contributing to muscle mass loss [62].

2.5. Sarcopenia: cancer

Within neoplastic sarcopenia definition (often described as cachexia), are included both the real cases of primary cachexia and the cases of nutritional deterioration secondary to obstruction of the digestive tract, chemo-radiotherapy toxicity, and post-surgical intestinal malabsorption syndromes (secondary cachexia). Cachexia is, regardless of the histology and location of the primary tumor, the most common paraneoplastic syndrome in patients with advanced cancer. Over 70% of cancer patients, especially in advanced stages, develop signs and symptoms of cachexia, and about 20% die because of its consequences [63].

Cachexia is characterized by alterations of all metabolic systems, production of circulating factors in part produced by the tumor, in part by the host cells, mainly macrophages, in response to the tumor, and reduced caloric intake.

Some of these alterations appear early in the natural history of neoplastic disease:

a. **Glucose metabolism**: Increased gluconeogenesis from lactate, amino acids, and free fatty acids with loss of protein and lipid reserves.

b. **Protein metabolism**: Increased turnover with decreased muscle and hepatic protein synthesis, increased hepatic synthesis of acute phase proteins, increased serum levels of proteolysis-inducing factor (PIF), and increased protein degradation from muscle tissue. The activation of muscle proteolytic systems, such as that of the ubiquitin-proteasome, is present even before there has been weight loss, suggesting that biomolecular alterations responsible for muscular loss are highlighted early in the natural history of neoplastic disease. Other proteolytic mechanisms provide the activation of calcium-dependent systems, such as that of calpain (regulated by a kinase ATP-dependent and an inhibitor, calpastatin).

c. **Lipid metabolism**: Increased beta-oxidation of fatty acids and the turnover of free fatty acids, increased serum lipoprotein, triglycerides, and production of lipid mobilizing factor (LMF), which induces lipolysis [64].

Some systemic effects of cancer cachexia, such as anorexia, "fatigue," and increased resting energy expenditure, are the result of circulating factors' action in part produced by the tumor and in part by the host cells, mainly macrophages, in response to the tumor. Among them, a central role is given by the pro-inflammatory cytokines (IL-1, IL-6, TNF-α, IFN-γ), which trigger the acute phase response with reduced synthesis of proteins (albumin, prealbumin, and transferrin) [65]. Cytokines such as interleukin-1 (IL-1) and tumor necrosis factor-α (TNF-α) have been suggested as involved in cancer-related anorexia, possibly by increasing the levels of corticotropin-releasing hormone (CRH), a central nervous system neurotransmitter that suppresses food intake, and the firing of glucose-sensitive neurons, which would also decrease food intake [66].

2.6. Secondary sarcopenia: assessment

The variability of weight, even when expressed as body mass index (BMI), is very wide in patients with chronic conditions. There is a correlation between the amount of weight loss and survival. The weight loss cannot be explained only by the decreased supply of food. In fact, it may be related to the size of the increase in basal metabolic rate (resting energy consumption). It is important at the same time in particular for patients suffering from metabolic syndrome and respiratory problems to assess the degree of overweight and obesity.

Therefore, it is necessary to investigate:

- Weight and height (BMI body mass index), and weight loss percentage in the previous period (2 weeks, 1 month, or 6 months).
- Assessment of the quantity and quality of food intake (presence or not of dysphagia). The term sarcopenic dysphagia means a condition characterized by the presence of dysphagia due to sarcopenia of swallowing muscles associated with secondary sarcopenia. Unlike in the elderly dysphagia in stroke outcome, the sarcopenic dysphagia is rarely acknowledged, probably due to the fact that the definition and diagnostic criteria of this condition have not yet been clearly established. According to Butler et al., muscle strength, measured with handgrip, correlates directly with the isometric strength of posterior tongue. This observation indicates that the muscle strength of tongue can be reduced with the generalized deficit in skeletal muscle force, like in sarcopenia [67].

The 10-item Eating Assessment Tool (EAT-10) and a water test (e.g. Toronto Bedside Swallowing Screening Test) or different viscosities (e.g. Volume-Viscosity Swallowing Test) combined with pulse oximetry are useful for dysphagia screening, and if it is confirmed, it requires further secondary clinical evaluations (speech therapist) and possibly instrumental study (Videofluoroscopic Swallowing Study) [68].

The Mini Nutritional Assessment (MNA) [68] is a multidimensional assessment tool, which is easy to complete and allow an easy and feasible large-scale use. The MNA includes 18 items divided into three main sectors (anthropometry and variations in weight, measuring quantitative and qualitative food intake, and disability status and cognitive status); the maximum score is 30. A score below 17 is indicative of malnutrition, a score between 17 and 23.5 is indicative of risk of malnutrition, and a score greater than 24 indicates a normal nutritional status.

The questionnaire allows to classify the nutritional state in an univoque way and has high interpersonal reliability and clearly defined thresholds. It has been validated in several ethnicities and ethnic-specific anthropometric cut-off has been set up [69].

The MNA is also a nutrition guide. Timely intervention blocks the weight loss in people who are at risk of malnutrition or undernourished. It takes in regard anthropometric, global, dietary, and subjective assessment, and it gives to this tool high sensitivity (96%) and specificity (98%) [70].

The scale allows to global assessment of patient as the prevalence of malnutrition increases significantly among hospitalized and institutionalized patients and those with cognitive impairment. The connection is simple enough to guess, the inability to feed on their own, the choice of foods, and the long-lasting immobility.

Perhaps less intuitive, chronic protein energy malnutrition affects the ongoing development of higher cognitive processes rather than simply showing a generalized cognitive and motor impairment.

Deficits of cognitive, emotional, and behavioral functioning are linked to structural abnormalities of different regions of the brain. Brain structures and brain circuits calculate different components of cognitive processes. Malnutrition has long-lasting effects in the processes of cognition and behavior [71].

According to the consensus conference of EWGSOP of 2009, the main parameters to be evaluated in the course of sarcopenia relate to muscle mass, muscle strength, and physical performance of the subject. Based on these three parameters, sarcopenia can be classified into three stages: pre-sarcopenia, sarcopenia, and its severe form [72].

Muscle mass can be assessed by magnetic resonance imaging (MRI) and computed tomography (CT); their use is limited in primary care settings by difficulties in access, costs, the lack of portable equipment, and the requirement of highly specialized personnel [73].

Dual-energy X-ray absorptiometry (DXA) is used to assess body composition and provides reproducible estimates of appendicular skeletal lean mass but it is known that the accuracy of DXA for assessing muscle mass in people of different ages and different pathological conditions may vary [74]. Bio-electrical impedance analysis (BIA) estimates the volume of fat and lean body mass based on the relationship between the volume of a conductor and its electrical resistance. It is not expensive, it can be used easily in clinical practice, both on ambulatory subjects and on hospitalized patients [75, 76]. A still not widely used method, but of extreme interest for the estimation muscular mass, it is represented by the ultrasounds.

Ultrasound allows to explore parenchymas and soft tissue of the human body, responding to all the ideal requirements of a diagnostic method: the almost absolute harmlessness, practicity, rapidity of implementation, and cost contents. According to Fanelli and Kuczmarski, ultrasound application represents a prediction system of body fat that is valid at least as far as plicometry [77], but there are still many limitations related to the application of the method: there is no conventional choice of best frequency to apply, body position, and probe pressure on the surface to be evaluated (**Table 1**).

This method, by measuring thickness of the muscular layers, visceral and subcutaneous fat, was useful in evaluating the regional body composition and where the plicometry is limited [78]. In 2012, Leahy et al. [79] took ultrasound and DXA measurements with good predictive accuracy. In addition, others have used ultrasound to predict the body density of lean men [77], lean women [80], obese adult, Japanese men and women [81], sumo wrestlers [82], the body fat percentage of physically active British and Chinese men [83], and the fat mass of pre-pubertal Japanese children. A new technology, a small, portable, hand-held 2.5 MHz A-mode ultrasound transducer designed specifically for the purpose of body composition assessment; it is connected to a laptop computer using a USB cable, the software assumes the acoustic reflections of the fat-muscle and muscle bone interfaces (Body View, IntelaMetrix, Inc., Livermore, CA) [84].

Advantages	Limitations
Lower cost than laboratory methods	Higher cost than field methods
High accuracy and precision in the hands of an experienced technician	Requires experienced technician, considerable skill is necessary
Capable of regional and segmental measurements	Measurement procedures and techniques are not yet standardized
Minimal tissue compression	Inherent artifacts (fascia etc.)
Noninvasive and no ionizing radiation	
Applicable for testing in the field	
Can measure other tissue thicknesses (muscle and bone)	
Short testing time, rapid procedure	

Table 1. Advantages and limitations of ultrasound application.

Studies reported qualitative changes in muscle related to sarcopenia (e.g. atrophy of type II muscle fibers, increase of intramuscular fat, increase of extracellular water relative to muscle volume) and that these abnormalities can be linked to differences in echo intensity obtained from ultrasonography images.

Enhanced echo intensity (EI) represents changes caused by increase of intramuscular fat and fibrous tissue: an increase of echogenicity indicates greater fibrous tissue and fat between muscular fibers (**Figure 4**) [85]. The simplicity of execution, the low cost, and wide availability make them ideal in the evaluation also for bedridden patients.

Muscle strength was assessed by functional tests: handgrip strength, the walking speed, flexion/extension of the thigh muscles, and forced expiratory flow. Handgrip strength appears to be the most widely used method for the measurement of muscle strength. Isometric handgrip strength shows a good correlation with leg strength and also with lower extremity power, knee extension torque, and calf cross-sectional muscle area [86, 87]. Standardized conditions for the test [88] include seating the subject in a standard chair with their forearms resting flat on the armchairs. Six measures should be taken, three with each arm. Ideally, the patients should be encouraged to squeeze as hard and as tightly as possible for 3–5 seconds for each of the six trials; usually, the highest reading of the six measurements is reported as the final result [89].

The most widely used tool in clinical practice for the assessment of physical performance is measured by gait speed alone or as part of a test battery such as short physical performance battery (SPPB). The SPPB is a test scored to a maximum of 12 points comprising an assessment of gait speed (over 3–4 m), a balance test, and a repeated chair stand test. These tests focus on lower extremity function, as the latter has been shown to correlate with mobility, disability, and patient outcomes, including hospitalization, institutionalization, and mortality. The SPPB takes about 10 min to complete. Participants presenting a score ≤8 points have been described as having a poor physical performance [90]. Other standalone tests can be performed to assess

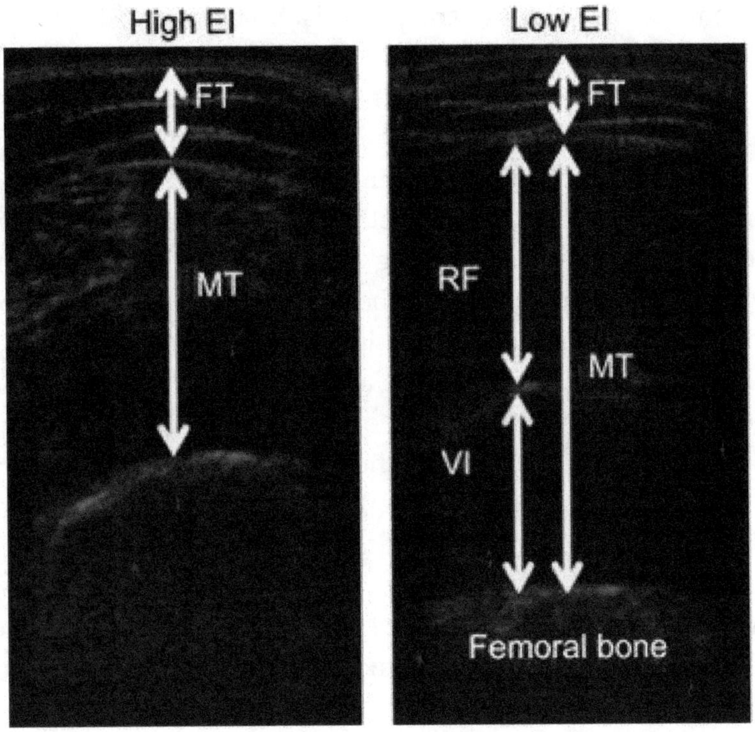

Figure 4. Echo intensity of the rectus femoris muscle. Left: High echo intensity; Right: low echo intensity. EI, echo intensity; FT, subcutaneous fat thickness; MT, muscle thickness; RF, rectus femoris muscle; VI, vastus intermedius muscle. From Watanabe et al. [85].

physical performance. In the Timed Up and Go (TUG) test, individuals are asked to rise from a standard armchair, walk to a marker 3 m away, turn, walk back, and sit down again. The 6-min walk distance or 400 m walk time can be used to measure aerobic capacity. The stair climb power test also shows good correlation with other measures of leg power and physical performance but is mostly restricted to use in research settings [91].

They have been proposed numerous biomarkers to evaluate the catabolic/anabolic balance of skeletal muscle: inflammation biomarkers, such as C-reactive protein, interleukin-6, and tumor necrosis factor-α, and other clinical parameters that express the general state of health like hemoglobin, serum albumin, and urinary creatinine. In the overall evaluation, it is important to measure, also, hormones: dehydroepiandrosterone sulfate, testosterone, insulin-like growth factor-1, and vitamin D, products of oxidative damage like advanced glycation end-products, protein carbonyls, and oxidized low-density lipoproteins, or antioxidants and finally α-tocopherol [92].

3. Rehabilitative approach

3.1. Nutritional-supplementary-integrative—intervention

Malnutrition and peripheral insulin resistance, which increases glucose levels in peripheral blood, are frequent alterations in pathologies that may cause sarcopenia.

The feeding of patient suffering from sarcopenia is essential, mostly the intake of essential amino acids. It should be reminded the importance of 3 protein meals intake and/or supplementation, better if it is given immediately after exercise. The reduced response to the protein synthesis after ingestion of small amounts of essential amino acids can be increased by the ingestion of a mixture with a greater amount of leucine (essential branched-chain amino acid) or a supplementation with hydroxy-methyl butyrate (HMB), a metabolite of leucine; it promotes protein synthesis by preventing protein breakdown. Hormone replacement therapy, if there are no contraindications can be used. According to the recommendations of the European Society for Clinical and Economic Aspects of Osteoporosis, Osteoarthritis and Musculoskeletal Diseases (ESCEO), it must be associated to physical exercise, a high protein diet (1–1.2 g/kg per day with at least 20–25 g of high quality protein, such as those derived from milk) [93]. Rizzoli et al. reported that the recommendations for optimal dietary protein intake are daily 1.0–1.2 g/kg (body weight) with an optimal repartition over each daily meal to prevent sarcopenia [94]. Paddon-Jones et al. proposed a dietary plan that includes 25–30 g of high quality protein per meal as dietary protein recommendations for the prevention of sarcopenia [95]. A protein-enriched diet equivalent to 1.3 g/kg/day achieved through lean red meat is safe and effective for enhancing the effects of progressive resistance training. Carnitine plays a decisive role in the metabolism of long-chain free fatty acids, thus affecting lipid metabolism and energy reserves within the cells. Carnitine is a necessary cofactor for the transport of long-chain fatty acids within the mitochondrial matrix, where they are subjected to oxidation for the production of cellular energy. A clinical study has shown that administration of 6 g/day of L-carnitine for the duration of 30 days was able to significantly improve the symptom "fatigue," appetite, and lean body mass of patients. Therefore, the administration of L-carnitine should be recommended in cachectic patients at a dose of 4–6 g/day orally for a period of time of 3-4 months being usually well tolerated by the patient. Occasional side effects of L-carnitine include epigastralgia and, more rarely, diarrhea [96].

In addition to the now well-known beneficial effects on bone, the vitamin D has positive extraskeletal effects; it acts on the muscle directly (receptor have been identified in skeletal muscle) and indirectly, through increasing of calcium that is essential for muscle contraction; and finally, it promotes the synthesis of contractile proteins [94]. Even supplements, such as omega-3 and carnitine, are widely recommended in this area [96, 97].

Creatine is a molecule produced in the body, and it is a natural amine endogenously synthesized by the liver, kidney, and pancreas from the amino acids arginine, glycine, and methionine. It stores high-energy phosphate groups in the form of phosphocreatine that releases energy to aid cellular function in brain, bones, muscles, and liver. It can be found in some foods, mostly meat, eggs, and fish [98]. Creatine supplementation became popular in the 1990s for enhancing athletic performance and building lean body mass [99]. It has also been used in the treatment of chronic heart failure and mitochondrial disorders. Recent findings have confirmed the potential therapeutic effects of creatine supplementation and have demonstrated that in the elderly, it improves the quality of life by increasing muscle strength and resistance to fatigue, improving performance in daily activities, and preventing bone loss [100, 101]. As a supplement, it is most commonly available as a monohydrate in powder, candy, gum, and liquid. Many synthetic derivatives are available, including creatine malate, creatine pyruvate, creatine citrate, creatine-magnesium chelate, and creatine ethyl ester. Studies with older people have used this regimen 2–5 g per day to ensure the saturation of muscle compound [102], and when it is associated with resistance training, training volume is increased, thereby enhancing strength and muscle mass [103].

The quality of proteins is paramount. A major stimulus in muscle anabolism has been reported as a result of an increase in circulating leucine levels. This was inferred from the observation that the ingestion of whey protein causes even more postprandial muscle protein synthesis rates relative to the ingestion of the intact or hydrolyzed casein and the difference is in the leucine content that has a key role in increasing muscle protein synthesis [104].

Whey protein can be considered a high quality protein, due to the anabolic properties attributed to the faster digestion and absorption of essential amino acids, such as leucine [105].

The mechanism of action of whey proteins is linked to the phosphorylation of p70S6K, which targets the ribosomal subunit S6 and thus promotes protein synthesis. It has been seen that its levels remain elevated even 2 hours after ingestion of whey proteins [106]. In association with amino acid supplementation, it is helpful to administer omega-3 fatty acid because these affect the membrane fluidity, endocytosis, exocytosis, absorption, and release of neurotransmitters such as acetylcholine involved in muscle contraction. They also stimulate the pathway of protein kinase C, enhancing muscle protein synthesis [107].

A recent integrative approach is the use of melatonin. Melatonin, also known as N-acetyl-5-methoxytryptamine, is a derivative of tryptophan, an essential amino acid [108]. It is well known for its role in synchronization of circadian rhythms such as sleep timing, blood pressure, and seasonal reproduction [109, 110], but it is also an antioxidant molecule since it seems to be essential regulator of homeostasis.

Lee et al. found an inverse association between urine melatonin and sarcopenia, suggesting that melatonin may have a protective role in the pathophysiology of sarcopenia. Aging and age-related conditions show an association with low melatonin level. Considering that melatonin has anti-apoptotic effects and attenuates autophagic pathways, its decrease may have a role in the pathogenesis of sarcopenia. Muscle is one of the systems that requires more oxygen and consequently generates more reactive species. Melatonin is a protective factor against this damage, scavenging free radicals, enhancement of antioxidant enzymes, and inhibition of pro-oxidant enzymes [111, 112].

Its antioxidant function is expressed by protection of the electron transport chain and mitochondrial DNA from oxidative damage more efficiently than other conventional antioxidants. So, it increases ATP production in mitochondria [113]. For example, melatonin induces autophagy in myoblast cells collaborating in myogenic differentiation degradation [88], but it inhibits autophagy in muscles from carbon tetrachloride-treated mice by reducing oxidative stress-induced damage. Melatonin reduces endoplasmic reticulum stress in skeletal muscle by increasing the expression of several proteins as well as mRNA levels [114]; this improves protein synthesis. It reduces inflammation in muscle cells, acting specifically against these cytokines in rats [115] and also in humans [116].

Melatonin is more than a regulator of circadian rhythm, it is an antioxidant molecule, and it seems to be essential as a physiological regulator of homeostasis. So, its supplementation may be useful to prevent or treat sarcopenia-associated diseases, including osteoporosis and neuromuscular dysfunction [117].

The management of weight loss in secondary sarcopenia must be evaluated with extreme care since it is known that any treatment of obesity is diet therapy which affects the loss of fat mass and lean mass. This loss of muscle mass is greater when they are prescribed diets with a very low calorie intake or less than 1000 kcal/day, which should be strongly discouraged in chronic diseases. In the management, it is necessary to ensure a moderate caloric restriction ensuring a gradual weight loss, from 0.5 to 1 kg per week, or a decline of 8–10% compared to the initial weight in 6 months. It is also necessary to ensure proper protein intake. Metabolic and epidemiological studies suggest that the current intake recommendations for protein in elderly may not be sufficient.

3.2. Reduction of chronic inflammation

Despite the different chronic conditions can lead to secondary sarcopenia, one of the factors underlying the development and progression is the state of chronic inflammation. The pronounced anti-inflammatory effects of extremely low frequency (ELF) magnetic fields may improve the well-being of patients suffering from illnesses of different etiology. Human studies regarding ultralow frequency magnetic field effects have been carried out in several clinical settings over the past 20 years for treating bone and joint diseases, neuropathies, spinal cord injury, diabetic neuropathy, immune disorders, and cardiomyopathy. Properly configured signals have been demonstrated to regulate major cellular functions, including cell proliferation, differentiation, apoptosis, cell cycle, DNA replication, and cytokine/chemokine expression [118, 119].

The anti-inflammatory effects have demonstrated a decrease in pro-inflammatory cytokines and increase in anti-inflammatory cytokines after traumatic brain injury. Several metabolic parameters change in consequence of exposure to electromagnetic field, as observed in injured rats [120], stroke, decreased pain in osteoarthritis [121], wound healing [122] and postsurgical recovery [123].

Saggini et al. show inflammatory effects of external pulsed electromagnetic fields in the treatment of low back pain with a decrease of pro-inflammatory cytokines (IL-6) after 40 minutes to a sequence of electromagnetic fields of low intensity with inferior frequencies at 100 KHz for a number of 10 sessions in 3 weeks [124]. Furthermore, they allow, as a consequence, a ionic flow capable of optimizing the intrinsic capacity of maintaining the intra and extracellular potential difference essential for the cellular metabolism and homeostasis [125].

The frequency of the field was such to "stimulate" several ions in the sense of the cyclotron frequency. These ions may be involved in the enzymatic chains experimentally affected. This issue needs to be analyzed in detail in the future through well-designed experiments [125].

The term cyclotron frequency points to the form of resonance, which is established at the level of cell membranes, using electromagnetic fields at a very low intensity and at a specific frequency (cyclotron), able to influence and stimulate the metabolism of human cells. It acts to adjust the ordered traffic of selected ions between the internal and external environments of the cell; it stimulates the activity of those ion-dependent enzymes allowing the occurrence of several biological reactions [126].

The bioresonance cyclotron technology (**Figure 5**) (Quantum Electrodynamic Catalysis) is able to provide magnetic fields that respond to the laws of quantum electrodynamics consistency (QUEC), i.e. fields that interact with the "Domains of Consistency" of water, contained in every living being, animal, and plant. The advantage of quanto-elettrodinamica (QUEC) technology is to be able to influence the movement of different ion species to the cell membranes and stimulate the formation of coherent structures by strengthening the metabolism and cell cooperation (homeostasis) [125, 126].

Exposure to bio-cyclotron resonance technology determines: a change of configuration of the water; the normalization of the ion concentration in intracellular and extracellular fluid; the biocatalytic stimulation of intracellular enzymatic functions [127, 128].

With ion cyclotron resonance, we have the possibility to intervene in noninvasive, natural and precise way, on body's homeostasis adjustment mechanisms, where the only pharmacological support can be incomplete.

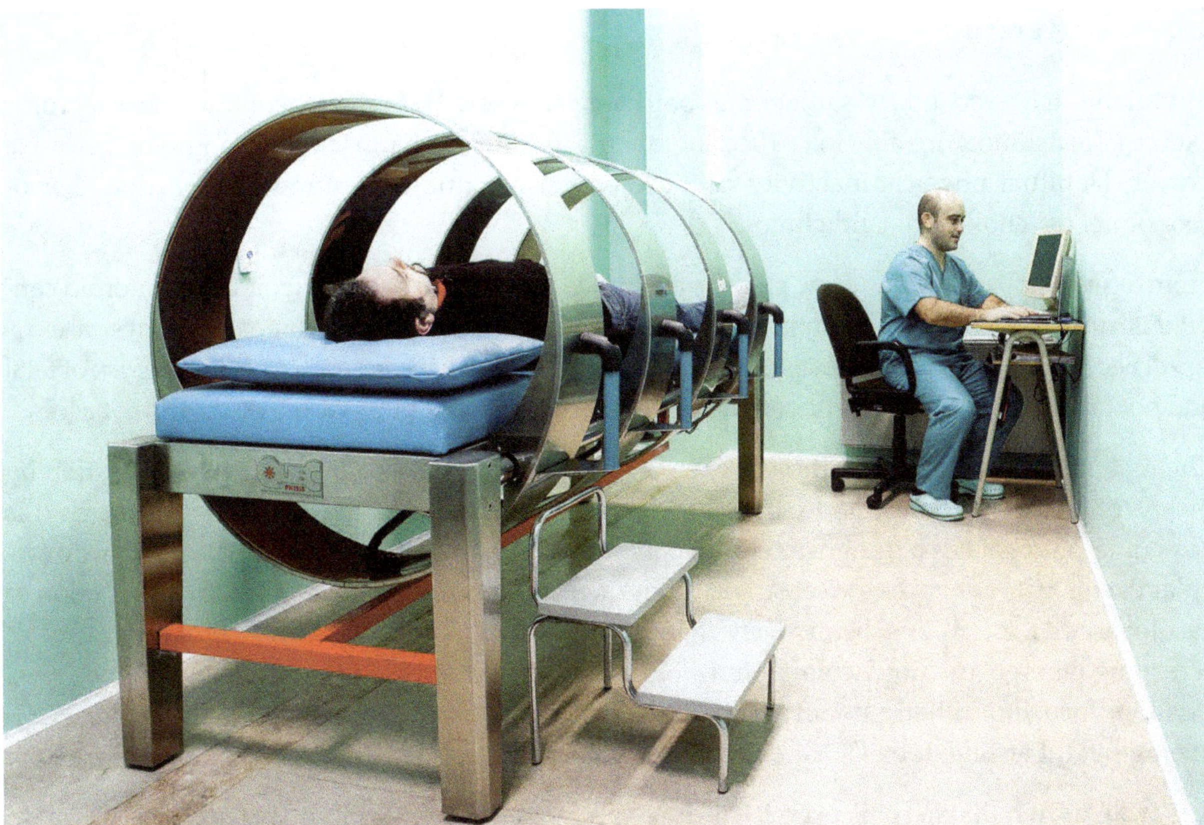

Figure 5. Ion cyclotron resonance with QUEC PHISIS QPS1.

Therefore, it is possible to:

1. Rebalance subjective metabolism
2. Adjust the enzyme functions, the ion channels, and the body pH3.
3. Strengthen the immune system
4. Encourage the bioavailability and absorption of nutrients for cell metabolism
5. Treat neuralgia, headaches, and migraines
6. Stimulate healing in all kinds of wounds, even after surgery
7. Balance the water retention
8. Enhance the effect of drugs and supplements
9. Detoxify and to allow antioxidant function against free radicals, metabolites, and toxins 10.
10. Stimulate a painkiller function (acute and chronic)
11. Get muscle relaxation, from anxiety and stress
12. Improve the homeostasis recovery under stress (physiological microtrauma and muscle protein catabolism).

3.3. Physical exercise

In patients with secondary sarcopenia, both aerobic exercise (endurance) and the anaerobic exercise (resistance) are able to reduce sarcopenia and increase muscular strength and muscle power. Habitual physical inactivity of these patients is due to a number of barriers: socio-economic, psychological, and clinics.

From a clinical point of view, these patients are fragile and sedentary with significant comorbid conditions, such as osteoporosis, anemia, and heart failure, which often limit their access to physical exercise. Theoretically, a physical exercise could be harmful as it may increase temporarily the risk of fatal and nonfatal cardiovascular events, especially if in the presence of other cardiovascular risk factors.

The recommends pre-participation of exercise protocols, provide cardiovascular evaluation by means of history (personal and family history) and physical examination alone, although this screening protocol has a recognized limited power (<10%) to detect potentially lethal cardiovascular event. ECG enhances the sensitivity of the screening process by allowing early detection of cardiovascular conditions distinctively manifesting with ECG abnormalities. If in the course of screening emerge, cardiovascular abnormalities should be assessed the need for further investigation, focusing initially noninvasive, such as echocardiography, Holter monitoring, ECG-averaging, tilt testing, the ECO-stress, myocardial scintigraphy, MRI, and cardiac CT (**Table 2**).

It is well known that aerobic exercise induces an increase in skeletal muscle mitochondria. In fact, adaptations to aerobic training appear to be the result of exercise-induced increases in the transcription of mitochondrial genes.

Absolute	Relative
Unstable coronary heart disease	Major risk factors for coronary heart disease
Decompensated heart failure	Decompensated diabetes
Severe pulmonary arterial hypertension (mean arterial pressure >55 mmHg)	Hypertension above 160/100 mmHg
Uncontrolled arrhythmias	Patients with pacemakers or defibrillators
Uncontrolled high blood pressure (>180/110 mmHg)	
Marfan's syndrome	
Severe symptomatic aortic stenosis, aortic dissection	

Table 2. Contraindications to exercise training.

Many studies have shown an improvement of muscle function even with aerobic or combined aerobic and anaerobic exercises. Aerobic training can include multiple sporting activities, such as stretching, walking, jogging, bicycle ergometer, and aerobic exercises. The latter often based on different tools: weights, elastic bands, rubber balls, rollers, and treadmill. A typical aerobic workout session could last about 90 minutes and be divided as follows: 15–20 minutes of stretching exercises, 20–50 minutes pedaling bicycle ergometer, and 20 minutes of recovery phase [129]. It should start with a lower intensity of training, with the shortest duration and for a few days a week [130]. Several authors showed a significant improvement in aerobic exercise capacity and muscle strength; an improvement in insulin resistance and anorexia; and an increase in ejection fraction, cardiac output, and stroke volume after 6 months of training. Aerobic exercise is related to significant reduction of systolic and diastolic pressure values [108] and an improvement in strength and muscle power [131]. It is well established that traditional, slow-velocity resistance exercise (RE) performing the concentric and eccentric phase of each muscle contraction in 2–3 s is a safe, feasible, and effective intervention to induce muscle hypertrophy and increase strength. It seems to increase muscle protein synthesis [132], satellite cell activation and proliferation [133], anabolic hormone production, and decrease in catabolic cytokine activity [134]. RE has been shown to increase both type I and II muscle fiber cross-sectional areas and whole body leading to an increase in muscle strength. Resistance training needs to use a progressively increasing load to maintain the desired range of repetitions per set of exercise (**Table 3**).

Fast-velocity RE (performing the concentric phase as quickly as possible and taking 2 sec to perform the eccentric phase of each muscle contraction) appears to be a novel intervention for older adults to enhance muscle power. With the subsequent atrophy of type II fibers with aging, fast-velocity movements are important for preserving aging muscle health. Several studies have shown a significant increase in muscle power with fast velocity RE in older adults, because of greater motor unit recruitment of type II fibers [135].

Physical training can improve balance and stability and thus has been recommended as part of rehabilitative exercise protocols. Studies demonstrate significant flexibility improvements (some joints show range of motion improvements of greater than 40%) with supervised exercise programs, including static stretching or a combination of stretching and movements

Type of training	Frequency	Intensity	Duration/set
Aerobic exercise	A minimum of 5 days/week for moderate intensity or 3 days/week for vigorous intensity	Moderate intensity 40–60% VO_2 max 40–60% VO_2 max 40–60% VO_2 max 3–6 METS	Accumulate at least 30 min/day of moderate-intensity activity, in bouts of at least 10 min each; continuous vigorous activity for at least 20 min/day
Resistance exercise involving the major muscle groups (free weights and machines)	At least 2 days/week	Slow-to-moderate lifting velocity 60–80% of 1 RM	8–10 exercises 1–3 sets per exercise 8–12 repetitions (1–3 min of rest among set)
Power training to practice only after the resistance training	2 days/week	Light-to-moderate loading (30–60% of 1 RM) High repetition velocity	1–3 sets per exercise, 6–10 repetitions

HR, heart rate; RM, repetition maximum; and METS, metabolic equivalents.

Table 3. Physical exercise indications.

through a full range of motion [136]. The recovery of proprioception is an essential part of the recovery of sarcopenia for the recovery the motor task is to be made through advanced systems for muscle strength and balance. I-Moove (**Figure 6**) has a balancing platform with helispheric movement and continuous realignment of spatial plans and subsystems of the body in order to maintain an optimal posture in open chain or to exert a tensile force. It also provides a real-time visual feedback that allows to monitor corrections [137].

It is possible to use whole body vibration and focal vibration system that is an effective method to activate the proprioceptive sensory system. It consists of the excitation of the afferents coming from the neuromuscular spindle. This causes the activation of a large number

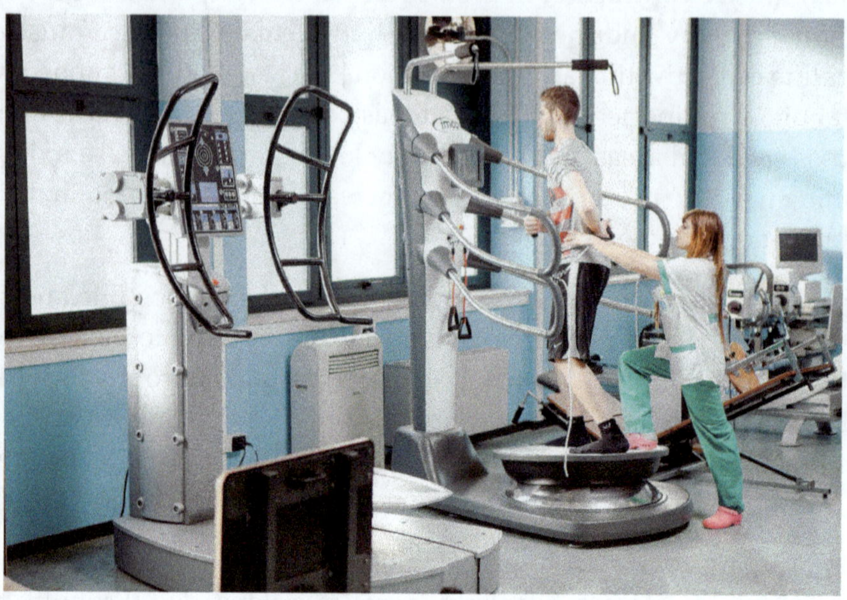

Figure 6. I-Moove and rehabilitative gym at University Centre of Physical Medicine and Rehabilitation University G. d' Annunzio- Chief R. Saggini.

of alpha-motor neurons, leading to the recruitment of muscle fibers, previously inactive, to contribute to muscle contraction. It has been demonstrated that mechanical vibration on a single muscle is able to activate Ia and II afferent nerve fibers of the muscle spindle, and hence the alpha motor neurons: this elicits the so-called Tonic Vibration Reflex (TVR), consisting in sustained contraction of the muscle vibrated and simultaneous relaxation of its prime antagonists. Neuromuscular electrical stimulation (NMES) is an alternative and potentially more effective mean than exercise alone of increasing the force of muscles. These alternative approaches to exercise offered a safe addition to a traditional, high-intensity volitional strengthening program with the aim to implement muscular mass and strength (as described in chapter *Rehabilitation in sarcopenic elderly*)

4. Dynamic antigravity postural system (SPAD)

SPAD®, a device for body weight relief, consisting of a machinery designed to reduce, modify, and condition the force of gravity acting on the body structures of movement during the act of rectilinear motion (**Figure** 7). The system is based on the rational that gait training can be made combining the motor task to sensory feedback, in line with the multisensory approach to postural balance. The system consists of a treadmill on which the patient carries out training in body weight support and of a structure to which the patient is harnessed by means of a pneumatic belt placed between the iliac crests and the costal arches, connected to lifting system with four tie rods attached to the body and to the pelvic girdle. Equipment is completed by four front pads (two on the humeral heads for the shoulder girdle and two on the anterior superior iliac spine for the pelvis), which act as stabilizers (as they prevent possible twisting of the pelvis or shoulder during movement on the treadmill), and at the same time as informants proprioceptive. Two rear pads can be placed on the interscapular region and on the sacral area; according to the characteristics of

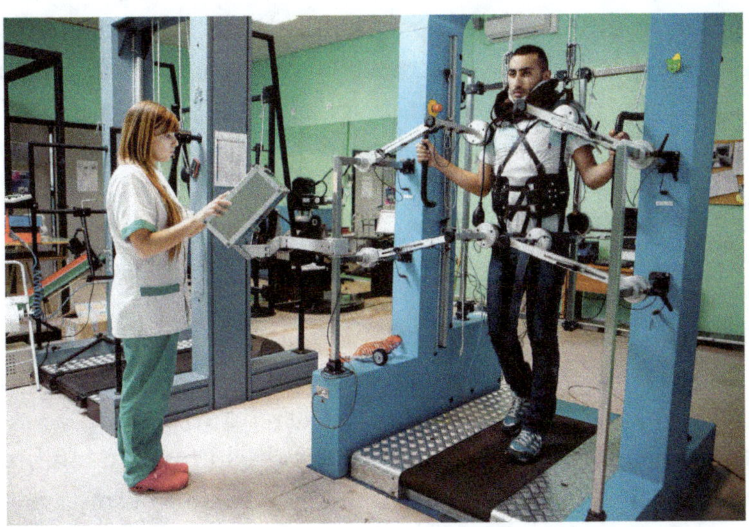

Figure 7. Dynamic antigravity postural system (SPAD).

the patient, an inflatable collar can also be used. Each session of SPAD® provides a 30–50% mean body weight relief and a training on the treadmill with adjustable speed (down to 0.01 km/h during the first session, allowing to become familiar with the machine and thus obtaining a higher compliance). The harnessing in body weight support allows the vertical excursion of the center of gravity of the subject, facilitating the execution of longer steps, according to the possibilities of the individual patient; the step performing is corrected continuously by the operator, inviting the patient to get an ordered cadence with sequential placement of heel-plant-toe. In this way, session after session, SPAD® allows to change asymmetrical gait adaptations, working with a dual action: a mechanical one, which allows a neuromotor retraining with cortical-subcortical learning aimed to the reacquisition of a balanced body schema that minimizes the energy consumption needed to maintain the posture, and a proprioceptive one, which acts on the maintenance of automatic and induced over time walking adaptations. The last part of the session provides for the reduction of body weight relief gradually to 0% and the reduction of the speed of the treadmill until the stop; in this way, in the last part of the session, the patient continuing to maintain the proprioceptive stimulus [138–140].

5. Exercises in virtual reality

Virtual reality exercises in the proposed protocol are based on the most recent findings about the neurophysiology of learning processes and movement memorization. The virtual reality system Riablo® is based on the use of sensors connected to a screen, which in real time sent the exact awareness of the carried out motor task to the patient, with the possibility to focus attention only on the fundamental elements of the movement reducing distracting stimuli from the surrounding real environment. It is possible to set a series of exercises: stand up from the chair; displacement of the load with bending knees; displacement of the load on the sagittal plane; displacement of the load on the sagittal and frontal planes; and bilateral squats with back support. The resulting motor performances and the collected kinematic data are entirely analyzed and recorded in the system, which calculate a score. This motivational input rewards the patient's efforts, ensuring faster progress [141].

6. Microgravity aquatic therapy

Aquatic therapy is based upon several important bioengineering properties. The basic forces acting upon the patient while in the water consist of buoyancy, drag, and inertial forces. Additional factors affecting the patient include hydrostatic pressure and specific heat. Various properties of water contribute to therapeutic effects, including the ability to use water for resistance in place of gravity or weights. Thermal stability that permits maintenance of near-constant temperature; hydrostatic pressure that supports, stabilizes and influences heart and lung function; buoyancy that permits floatation and reduces the effects of gravity; and turbulence and wave propagation that allow gentle manipulation and movement. In our clinical experience, microgravity aquatic therapy can restore active range of motion. In the water, where resistance of water changes depending on walking speed, it is possible to adjust the exercise intensity. Compared to slow movements, such as walking, the body is subjected to greater levels of water resistance with movements that require use of great muscle strength in a short period of time. Previous studies have found that by exercising in the water, where buoyancy makes it difficult to support the body, people can experience postural instability and improve dynamic balance and muscle strength [142]. As far as exercise safety was concerned, in the water buoyancy and viscosity, lower forces applied to body mass-bearing joints, such as the knee, and as a result, the aquatic exercise did not damage muscles and joints. Moreover, in the present aquatic exercise training, the level of intensity can be defined as "moderately strong."

7. Resistance exercise with Kineo system

Changes related to sarcopenia have negative implications on metabolism, cardiovascular, and muscular function. Physical exercise is the most effective intervention to improve quality of life, physical, and psychological health [143].

Physical exercise acts on all the physiopathological mechanisms of sarcopenia: increases mTOR expression that controls protein synthesis in the muscle in response to exercise and nutrition; decreases fat infiltration and prevents lipotoxicity; and regulates oxidative stress through activation of mitochondrial genes and optimization of energy production, increase of capillary density, and muscle perfusion.

A training program that includes endurance and resistance exercises has more positive effects on sarcopenic muscle: resistance exercises are more effective in increasing muscle mass and strength, whereas endurance exercises are more effective for improving maximum aerobic power [144].

Increase of muscle strength and mass can be achieved with an innovative system, such as the KINEO system: a multitasking ergonomic robotic platform that will give you the opportunity to differentiate the activities of muscular work in a highly efficient and accurate way. It is the only robotic platform that allows to differentiate the workload in the two movement phases: concentric and eccentric. This allows to optimize the training of strength and also to work with maximum loads in the concentric phase, as it reduces the load in the return movement.

Kineo (**Figure 8**) is the only robotic platform that allows to differentiate the workload in the two movement phases: concentric and eccentric. This allows to optimize the training of strength and also to work with maximum loads in the concentric phase, as it reduces the load in the return movement.

The Kineo system makes it possible to perform the movement with or without inertia: in the latter case, the displacement of the load requires an application of muscle strength

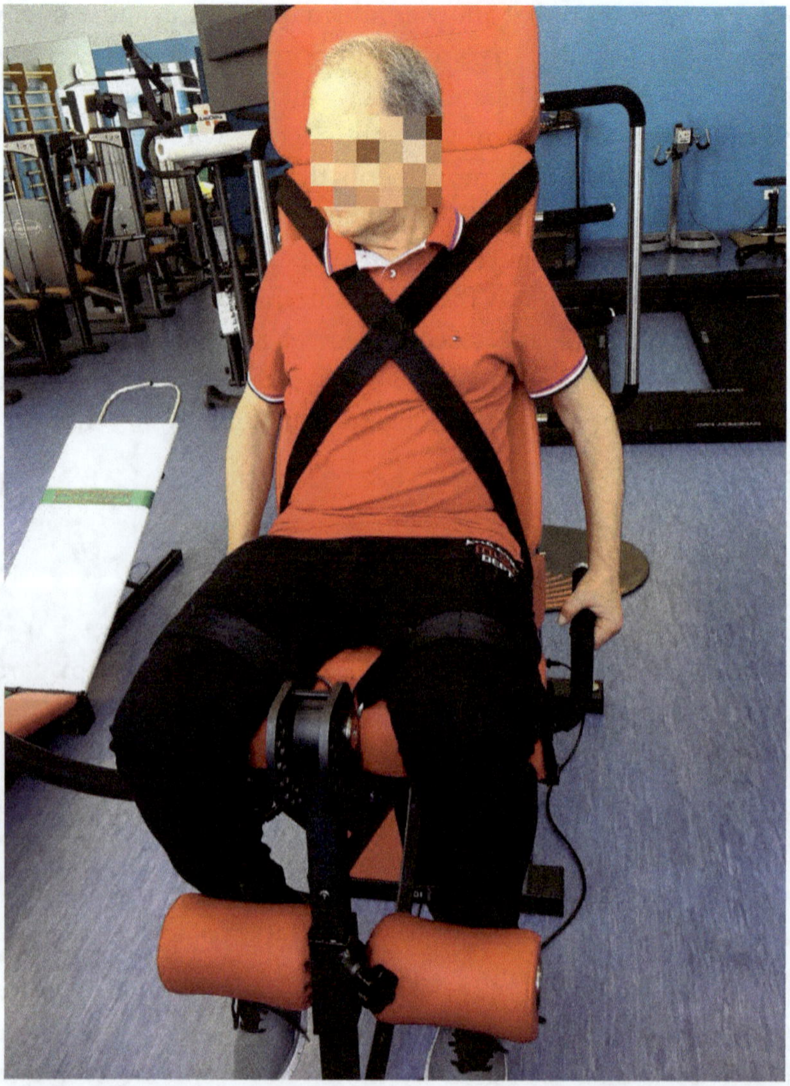

Figure 8. Kineo system.

throughout the movement, even in gestures characterized by great explosiveness. The set load remains constant in all angles and is not modified by inertia, as is the case with a traditional isotonic work. It is possible to differentiate the load between the concentric phase and the eccentric phase. It is possible to work in different conditions, such as elastic and "water viscous method." The elastic method uses resistance bands or springs as external resistance. The elongation of an elastic element depends on the strength applied to it by the subject and the nature of the elastic material (elastic constant). The advantage of the traditional elastic method is constituted by the gradual increase in the muscular effort while varying the workload is laborious.

Kineo elastic method is its ability to use differentiated loads between the concentric and eccentric phase to generate specific muscle adaptations and to use different methods in the concentric and eccentric phase.

Water workout is, universally, recognized as the most appropriate method for prevention and functional rehabilitation, because the load adapts exactly to the real strength of the subject. The "water viscous method," which can be considered as the most innovative, uses the principle of water workout and makes it available in a classic workout station. Kineo offers the possibility to use six levels (**Figure 9**) of viscosity simulating a workout in various fluids, such as water, oil, honey, and so on, which correspond to different levels of muscular effort. One of the most important applications of the water viscous method is the work for the stabilization of the joints, especially the knee joint, because the progressive increase in the viscous load involves the individual muscle groups according to physiologically correct models.

The water viscous method is characterized by the following features: the load increases or decreases depending on the speed of movement and level of viscosity; the speed is not constant but it depends on the level of applied force; and there is no inertia. When the movement stops, the load is immediately set to zero (maximum safety for the subject). Biphasic load: you can independently configure the level of viscosity in the concentric and eccentric phases (**Figure 10**). Unlike other methods, the progressive increase in the load according to the speed allows the subject to use a load that always respects his/her neuromuscular condition and prevents pain.

The training schedule with Kineo should involve two or three sessions a week in nonconsecutive days. The workload is related to the potentialities of the individual subject, which is analyzed with specific tests that evaluate strength, equilibrium, speed, and power. (see http://www.kineosystem.com/)

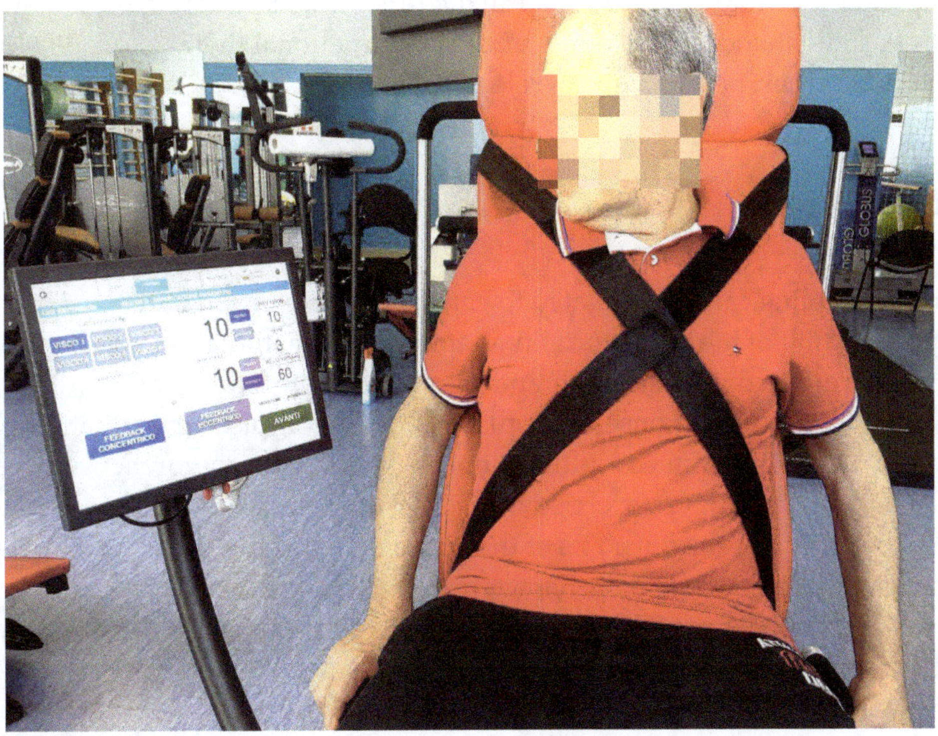

Figure 9. Kineo system, concentric vs. eccentric phase.

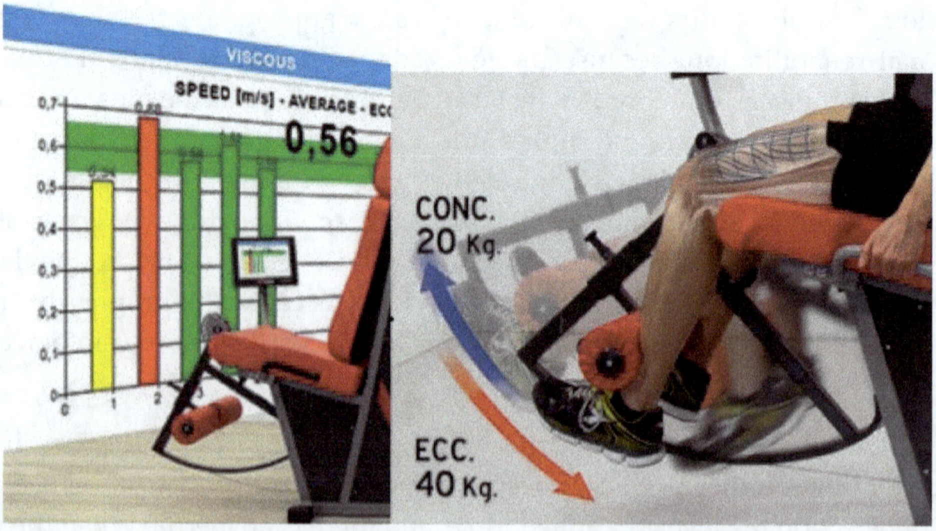

Figure 10. Kineo system, viscous method.

8. Quality of life improvement

The inclusive approach to improve the quality of life includes music therapy relaxation training, diaphragmatic breathing, guided imagery, self-hypnosis, mindfulness meditation, and distracting thoughts and activities outdoor exercises being perceived as energizing and indoor exercises being perceived as relaxing. Using methods deriving from cognitive therapy, patients are taught how to identify and change unhelpful or negative thoughts (cognitive restructuring) that contribute to psychological distress, while facilitating coping thoughts that reduce distress and enhance other coping efforts. Occupational therapists can help patient to maintain or resume their previous social role.

9. Conclusion

Sarcopenia is a disabling condition related to various adverse health outcomes such as mental disorders, poor quality of life, and mortality. Acting with rehabilitation goals is important for promoting positive functional (strength and power) and structural (hypertrophy and phenotypic changes) adaptive responses. The planning of a complex rehabilitation program in sarcopenia associated to chronic conditions, in the context of a comprehensive treatment, is made up of a nutritional support, exercise, correction of lifestyles, and use of advanced physical energies. Therefore, for the purposes of the optimal management, it is essential to identify the pathogenesis aspects and clinical characteristics, which can affect the different treatment choices in rehabilitation. A specialist in the identification, evaluation, and rehabilitation of neuromuscular, musculoskeletal, and functional disorders associated with chronic conditions and its treatment emphasizing the restoration and maintenance of function and quality of life. Future research should focus on better understanding the role of rehabilitation and on defining appropriate interventions for sarcopenia in chronic illness.

Author details

Raoul Saggini[1*], Simona Maria Carmignano[2], Lucia Cosenza[2], Tommaso Palermo[2] and Rosa Grazia Bellomo[3]

*Address all correspondence to: saggini@unich.it

1 Physical and Rehabilitation Medicine, Department of Medical Oral and Biotechnological Sciences, Director of the School of Specialty in Physical and Rehabilitation Medicine, "Gabriele d'Annunzio" University, National Coordinator of Schools of Specialty in Physical and Rehabilitation Medicine, Chieti-Pescara, Italy

2 School of Specialty in Physical and Rehabilitation Medicine, "Gabriele d'Annunzio" University of Chieti- Pescara, Italy

3 Physical and Rehabilitation Medicine, Department of Medicine and Sciences of Aging, "Gabriele d'Annunzio" University of Chieti-Pescara, Italy

References

[1] Morley JE, Anker SD, von Haehling S. Prevalence, incidence, and clinical impact of sarcopenia: Facts, numbers and epidemiology—update 2014. Journal of Cachexia, Sarcopenia and Muscle 2014;**5**:253-259. DOI: 10.1007/s13539-014-0161-y

[2] Cruz-Jentoft AJ, Baeyens JP, Bauer JM, Boirie Y, Cederholm T et al. European Working Group on Sarcopenia in Older People. Sarcopenia: European consensus on definition and diagnosis—Report of the European Working Group on Sarcopenia in Older People. Age and Ageing; 2010;**39:**412-413

[3] Kalantar-Zadeh K, Rhee C, Sim JJ, Stenvinkel P, Anker SD, Kovesdy CP. Why cachexia kills: Examining the causality of poor outcomes in wasting conditions. Journal of Cachexia, Sarcopenia and Muscle 2013;**4:**89-94

[4] Dovjak P. Sarcopenia in cases of cases of chronic and acute illness. Zeitschrift Fur Gerontologie Und Geriatrie. 2016;**9:**100-106. DOI: 10.1007/s00391-015-0986-9

[5] Berger MJ, Doherty TJ. Sarcopenia: Prevalence, mechanisms, and functional consequences. Interdisciplinary Topics in Gerontology 2010;**37:**94-114

[6] Bruunsgaard H, Andersen-Ranberg K, Jeune B, Pedersen AN, Skinhøj P, Pedersen BK et al. A high plasma concentration of TNF-alpha is associated with dementia in centenarians. The Journals of Gerontology. Series A, Biological Sciences and Medical Sciences. 1999;**54(7)**:M357-M364

[7] Toth MJ, Ades PA, Tischler MD, Tracy RP, LeWinter MM. Immune activation is associated with reduced skeletal muscle mass and physical function in chronic heart failure. International Journal of Cardiology 2006;**109**:179-187

[8] [8] Gratacós J, Collado A, Filella X, Sanmartí R, Cañete J, Llena J et al. Serum cytokines (IL-6, TNF-alpha, IL-1 beta and IFN-gamma) in ankylosing spondylitis: A close

correlation between serum IL-6 and disease activity and severity. British Journal of Rheumatology. 1994;**33(10)**:927-931

[9] Rieu I, Magne H, Savary-Auzeloux I, Averous J, Bos C, Peyron MA et al. Reduction of low grade inflammation restores blunting of postprandial muscle anabolism and limits sarcopenia in old rats. Journal of Physiology. 2009;**587(Pt 22):**5483-5492. DOI: 10.1113/jphysiol.2009.178319.

[10] Degens H. The role of systemic inflammation in age-related muscle weakness and wasting. Scandinavian Journal of Medicine and Science in Sports 2010;**20:**28-38

[11] Ferrucci L, Corsi A, Lauretani F, Bandinelli S, Bartali B, Taub DD et al. The origins of age-related proinflammatory state. Blood. 2005;**105(6)**:2294-2299

[12] Stenholm S, Maggio M, Lauretani F, Bandinelli S, Ceda GP, Di Iorio A et al. Anabolic and catabolic biomarkers as predictors of muscle strength decline: The InCHIANTI study. Rejuvenation Research 2010;**13**:3-11

[13] Ershler WB. Interleukin-6: A cytokine for gerontologists. Journal of the American Geriatrics Society 1993;**41:**176-181

[14] Sieber CC. Malnutrition in the elderly—when too much turns into too few. Zeitschrift für Gerontologie und Geriatrie. 2007;**40(1)**:1-2

[15] Miller MS, Callahan DM, Toth MJ. Skeletal muscle myofilament adaptations to aging, disease, and disuse and their effects on whole muscle performance in older adult humans. Frontiers in Physiology 2014;**5**:369

[16] Degens H. Age-related skeletal muscle dysfunction: Causes and mechanisms. Journal of Musculoskeletal & Neuronal Interactions 2007;**7**:246-252

[17] Mathus-Vliegen EM. Obesity and the elderly. Journal of Clinical Gastroenterology 2012;**46**:533-544

[18] Bouchonville MF, Villareal DT. Sarcopenic obesity: How do we treat it?. Current Opinion in Endocrinology, Diabetes, and Obesity 2013;**20**:412-419

[19] Rolland Y, Lauwers-Cances V, Cristini C, Abellan van Kan G, Janssen I, Morley JE et al. Difficulties with physical function associated with obesity, sarcopenia, and sarcopenic-obesity in community-dwelling elderly women: The EPIDOS (EPIDemiologie de l'OSteoporose) Study. American Journal of Clinical Nutrition. 2009;**89(6)**:1895-1900

[20] Tamene, A et al. Chronic obstructive pulmonary disease (COPD) is a common comorbidity and is independently associated with adverse outcomes in African-American patients with heart failure. Journal of the American College of Cardiology. 2013;**61(10)**:E728

[21] Fragoso CA, Enright PL, McAvay G, Van Ness PH, Gill TM. Frailty and respiratory impairment in older persons. The American Journal of Medicine 2012;125:79-86.

[22] Kon SS, Canavan JL, Nolan CM, Clark AL, Jones SE, Cullinan P et al. The 4-metre gait speed in COPD: Responsiveness and minimal clinically important difference. The European Respiratory Journal 2014;**43**:1298-1305

[23] Liu CK, Leng X, Hsu FC, Kritchevsky SB, Ding J, Earnest CP, et al. The Journal of Nutrition, Health & Aging 2014;**18**:59. DOI: 10.1007/s12603-013-0369-0

[24] Jones SE, Maddocks M, Kon SSC, Canavan JL, Nolan CM, Clark AL et al. Sarcopenia in COPD: Prevalence, clinical correlates and response to pulmonary rehabilitation. Thorax 2015;**70**:213-218

[25] Janssen I, Shepard DS, Katzmarzyk PT, Roubenoff R. The healthcare costs of sarcopenia in the United States. Journal of the American Geriatrics Society. 2004;**52(1)**:80-85

[26] Debigaré R, Marquis K, Côté CH, Tremblay RR, Michaud A, LeBlanc P, et al. Catabolic/anabolic balance and muscle wasting in patients with COPD. CHEST Journal. 2003;**124(1):**83-89

[27] Gosker H, Van Mameren H, Van Dijk P, Engelen M, Van der Vusse G, Wouters E, et al. Skeletal muscle fibre-type shifting and metabolic profile in patients with chronic obstructive pulmonary disease. European Respiratory Journal. 2002;**19(4)**:617-625

[28] Gosker H, Hesselink M, Duimel H, Ward K, Schols A. Reduced mitochondrial density in the vastus lateralis muscle of patients with COPD. European Respiratory Journal. 2007;**30(1)**:73-79

[29] Gea J, Agustí A, Roca J. Pathophysiology of muscle dysfunction in COPD. Journal of Applied Physiology. 2013;**114(9):**1222-1234

[30] Pitsiou G, Kyriazis G, Hatzizisi O, Argyropoulou P, Mavrofridis E, Patakas D. Tumor necrosis factor—alpha serum levels, weight loss and tissue oxygenation in chronic obstructive pulmonary disease. Respiratory Medicine. 2002;**96(8)**:594-598

[31] Brunelle J, Chandel N. Oxygen deprivation induced cell death: An update. Apoptosis. 2002;**7(6)**:475-482

[32] Gonzalez NC, Wood JG. Alveolar Hypoxia-Induced Systemic Inflammation: What Low PO2 Does and Does Not Do. Advances in experimental medicine and biology. 2010;662:27-32. doi:10.1007/978-1-4419-1241-1_3

[33] Rafferty GF, Lou Harris M, Polkey MI, Greenough A, Moxham J. Effect of hypercapnia on maximal voluntary ventilation and diaphragm fatigue in normal humans. American Journal of Respiratory and Critical Care Medicine. 1999;**160(5)**:1567-1571

[34] England BK, Chastain JL, Mitch WE. Abnormalities in protein synthesis and degradation induced by extracellular pH in BC3H1 myocytes. American Journal of Physiology. Cell Physiology. 1991;**260(2):**C277-C282

[35] Sanders KJ, Kneppers AE, van de Bool C, Langen RC, Schols AM. Cachexia in chronic obstructive pulmonary disease: New insights and therapeutic perspective. Journal of Cachexia, Sarcopenia and Muscle. 2016;**7(1)**:5-22

[36] Barreiro E, Peinado VI, Galdiz JB, Ferrer E, Marin-Corral J, Sánchez F, et al. Cigarette smoke-induced oxidative stress: A role in chronic obstructive pulmonary disease skeletal muscle dysfunction. American Journal of Respiratory and Critical Care Medicine. 2010;**182(4)**:477-488

[37] Ramsay D, Zochodne D, Robertson D, Nag S, Ludwin S. A syndrome of acute severe muscle necrosis in intensive care unit patients. Journal of Neuropathology and Experimental Neurology. 1993;**52(4)**:387-398

[38] Decramer M, De Bock V, Dom R. Functional and histologic picture of steroid-induced myopathy in chronic obstructive pulmonary disease. American Journal of Respiratory and Critical Care Medicine. 1996;**153(6)**:1958-1964

[39] Calvani R, Miccheli A, Landi F, Bossola M, Cesari M, Leeuwenburgh C, et al. Current nutritional recommendations and novel dietary strategies to manage sarcopenia. The Journal of Frailty & Aging. 2013;**2(1)**:38

[40] Landi F, Marzetti E, Martone AM, Bernabei R, Onder G. Exercise as a remedy for sarcopenia. Current Opinion in Clinical Nutrition and Metabolic Care. 2014;**17(1)**:25-31.

[41] Gea J, Orozco-Levi M, Barreiro E, Ferrer A, Broquetas J. Structural and functional changes in the skeletal muscles of COPD patients: The "compartments" theory. Monaldi Archives for Chest Disease. 2001;**56(3)**:214-224

[42] Chopard A, Hillock S, Jasmin BJ. Molecular events and signalling pathways involved in skeletal muscle disuse-induced atrophy and the impact of countermeasures. Journal of Cellular and Molecular Medicine. 2009;**13(9b)**:3032-3050

[43] Maltais F, LeBlanc P, Simard C, Jobin J, Bérubé C, Bruneau J, et al. Skeletal muscle adaptation to endurance training in patients with chronic obstructive pulmonary disease. American Journal of Respiratory and Critical Care Medicine. 1996;**154(2)**:442-447

[44] O'Shea SD, Taylor NF, Paratz JD. Progressive resistance exercise improves muscle strength and may improve elements of performance of daily activities for people with COPD: A systematic review. CHEST Journal. 2009;**136(5)**:1269-1283

[45] Seymour J, Spruit M, Hopkinson N, Natanek S, Man W-C, Jackson A, et al. The prevalence of quadriceps weakness in COPD and the relationship with disease severity. European Respiratory Journal. 2010;**36(1)**:81-88.

[46] Pereira RA, Cordeiro AC, Avesani CM, Carrero JJ, Lindholm B, Amparo FC et al. Sarcopenia in chronic kidney disease on conservative therapy: Prevalence and association with mortality. Nephrol Dial Transplant. 2015;**30(10)**:1718-1725

[47] Zha Y, Qian Q. Protein nutrition and malnutrition in CKD. Nutrients. 2017;**9**:208. DOI: 10.3390/nu9030208

[48] Du J, Wang X, Miereles C, Bailey JL, Debigare R, Zheng B, et al. Activation of caspase-3 is an initial step triggering accelerated muscle proteolysis in catabolic conditions. J Clin Invest. 2004;**113(1)**:115-123

[49] Chauveau P, Combe C, Laville M, Fouque D, Azar R, Cano N et al. Factors influencing survival in hemodialysis patients aged older than 75 years: 2.5-year outcome study. American Journal of Kidney Diseases. 2001;**37(5)**:997-1003

[50] Zhang L, Du J, Hu Z, Han G, Delafontaine P, Garcia G, Mitch WE. IL-6 and serum amyloid A synergy mediates angiotensin II-induced muscle wasting. Journal of the American Society of Nephrology. 2009;**20(3):**604-612

[51] Song YH, Li Y, Du J, Mitch WE, Rosenthal N, Delafontaine P. Muscle-specific expression of IGF-1 blocks angiotensin II-induced skeletal muscle wasting. Journal of Clinical Investigation. 2005;**115(2):**451-458

[52] Kuemmerle N, Krieg RJ Jr, Latta K, Challa A, Hanna JD, Chan JC. Growth hormone and insulin-like growth factor in non-uremic acidosis and uremic acidosis. Kidney International Supplements 1997;**58:**S102-S105

[53] Löfberg E, Essén P, McNurlan M, Wernerman J, Garlick P, Anderstam B et al. Effect of hemodialysis on protein synthesis. Clinical Nephrology. 2000;**54(4)**:284-294

[54] Lim VS, Ikizler TA, Raj DS, Flanigan MJ. Does hemodialysis increase protein breakdown? Dissociation between whole-body amino acid turnover and regional muscle kinetics. Journal of the American Society of Nephrology. 2005;**16(4)**:862-868

[55] Ikizler TA, Flakoll PJ, Parker RA, Hakim RM. Amino acid and albumin losses during hemodialysis. Kidney International. 1994;**46(3)**:830-837

[56] Kobayashi H, Børsheim E, Anthony TG, Traber DL, Badalamenti J, Kimball SR et al. Reduced amino acid availability inhibits muscle protein synthesis and decreases activity of initiation factor eIF2B. American Journal of Physiology. Endocrinology and Metabolism. 2003;**284(3)**:E488-E498

[57] Shyu KG, Lu MJ, Wang BW, Sun HY, Chang H. Myostatin expression in ventricular myocardium in a rat model of volume-overload heart failure. European Journal of Clinical Investigation. 2006;**36(10)**:713-719

[58] Cunha TF, Bacurau AV, Moreira JB, Paixão NA, Campos JC, Ferreira JC et al. Exercise training prevents oxidative stress and ubiquitin-proteasome system overactivity and reverse skeletal muscle atrophy in heart failure. PLoS One. 2012;**7(8)**:e41701

[59] Sakuma K, Yamaguchi A. Sarcopenia and cachexia: The adaptations of negative regulators of skeletal muscle mass. Journal of Cachexia, Sarcopenia and Muscle 2012;**3**:77-94

[60] Forbes SC, Little JP, Candow DG. Exercise and nutritional interventions for improving aging muscle health. Endocrine 2012;**42:**29-38

[61] Hambrecht R, Schulze PC, Gielen S, Linke A, Möbius-Winkler S, Yu J et al. Reduction of insulin-like growth factor-I expression in the skeletal muscle of noncachectic patients with chronic heart failure. Journal of the American College of Cardiology. 2002;**39(7)**:1175-1181

[62] Strasser F, Anker SD, Bosaeus I, Bruera E, Fainsinger RL, et al. Definition and classification of cancer cachexia: An international consensus. The Lancet Oncology 2011;**12**:489-495

[63] Busquets S, Felipe A, Lopez-Soriano, FJ. Molecular mechanisms involved in muscle wasting in cancer and ageing: Cachexia versus sarcopenia. The International Journal of Biochemistry & Cell Biology 2005;**37:**1084-1104

[64] Argiles JM, Busquets S, Lopez-Soriano FJ. The pivotal role of cytokines in muscle wasting during cancer. The International Journal of Biochemistry & Cell Biology. 2005;**37:**1609-1619

[65] Watanobe H, Takebe K. Intravenous administration of tumor necrosis factor-alpha stimulates corticotropin releasing hormone secretion in the push-pull cannulated median eminence of freely moving rats. Neuropeptides. 1992;**22:81-84**

[66] Butler SG, Stuart A, Leng X, Wilhelm E, Rees C, Williamson J. The relationship of aspiration status with tongue and handgrip strength in healthy older adults. The Journals of Gerontology. Series A, Biological Sciences and Medical Sciences. 2011;**66(4)**:452-458

[67] Wakabayashi H. Presbyphagia and sarcopenic dysphagia: Association between aging, sarcopenia, and deglutition disorders. The Journal of Frailty & Aging. 2014;**3(2)**:97-103

[68] Guidoz Y, Wellas BJ, Garry PJ. Mini Nutritional Assessment: A practical assessment tool for grading the nutritional state of elderly patient. In: Wellas BJ, Guidoz Y, Garry PJ, Albarede JL, eds. Nutrition in the Elderly, the Mini Nutritional Assessment (MNA). Facts and Research in Gerontology 1994/1995. 2nd ed. Paris: Serdi Publishing Company; 1995. pp. 15-60

[69] Kaiser MJ, Bauer JM, Ramsch C et al. The Journal of Nutrition, Health & Aging 2009;**13:**782. DOI: 10.1007/s12603-009-0214-7

[70] Kaur S, Miller MD, Halbert J, Giles LC, Crotty M. Nutritional status of adults participating in ambulatory rehabilitation. Asia Pacific Journal of Clinical Nutrition. 2008;**17(2)**:199-207

[71] Strupp BJ, Levitsky DA. Enduring cognitive effects of early malnutrition: A theoretical appraisal. Journal of Nutrition 1995;**125:2221S-2232S**.

[72] Jentoft AJ, Baeyens JP, Bauer JM et al. Sarcopenia: European consensus on definition and diagnosis: Report of the European Working Group on Sarcopenia in Older People. Age and Ageing. 2010;**39(4)**:412-423

[73] Mitsiopoulos N, Baumgartner RN, Heymsfield SB, Lyons W, Gallagher D et al. Cadaver validation of skeletal muscle measurement by magnetic resonance imaging and computerized tomography. Journal of Applied Physiology. 1998;**85(1)**:115-122

[74] Levine JA, Abboud L, Barry M, Reed JE, Sheedy PF, Jensen MD. Measuring leg muscle and fat mass in humans: Comparison of CT and dual-energy X-ray absorptiometry. Journal of Applied Physiology. 2000;**88(2)**:452-456

[75] Vona-Davis, Rose DP. Adipokines as endocrine, paracrine, and autocrine factors in breast cancer risk and progression. Endocrine-Related Cancer. 2007;**14(2)**:189-206

[76] Sullivan DH, Walls RC, Bopp MM. Protein energy undernutrition and the risk of mortality within one years of hospital discharge: A follow-up study. Journal of the American Geriatrics Society 1995b;**43**:507-512

[77] Fanelli MT, Kuczmarski RJ. Ultrasound as an approach to assessing body composition. American Journal of Clinical Nutrition1984;**39(5)**:703-709

[78] Kuczmarski RJ, Fanelli MT, Koch GG. Ultrasonic assessment of body composition in obese adults: Overcoming the limitations of the skinfold caliper. American Journal of Clinical Nutrition. 1987;**45(4)**:717-724

[79] Leahy S, Toomey C, McCreesh K, O'Neill C, Jakeman P. Ultrasound measurement of subcutaneous adipose tissue thickness accurately predicts total and segmental body fat of young adults. Ultrasound in Medicine and Biology. 2012;**38(1)**:28-34

[80] Volz PA, Ostrove SM. Evaluation of a portable ultrasonoscope in assessing the body composition of college-age women. Medicine & Science in Sports & Exercise. 1984;**16(1)**:97-102

[81] Abe T, Kondo M, Kawakami Y, Fukunaga T. Prediction equations for body composition of Japanese adults by B-mode ultrasound. American Journal of Human Biology. 1994;**6(2)**:161-170.

[82] Saito K, Nakaji S, Umeda T, Shimoyama T, Sugawara K, Yamamoto Y. Development of predictive equations for body density of sumo wrestlers using B-mode ultrasound for the determination of subcutaneous fat thickness. British Journal of Sports Medicine. 2003;**37(2)**:144-148.

[83] Eston R, Evans R, Fu F. Estimation of body composition in Chinese and British men by ultrasonographic assessment of segmental adipose tissue volume. British Journal of Sports Medicine. 1994;28(1):9-13.

[84] Silva L. An Introduction to Ultrasound and the BodyMetrixSystem. Livermore, California, USA: IntelaMetrix; 2010.

[85] Watanabe Y, Yamada Y, Fukumoto Y, Ishihara T, Yokoyama K, Yoshida T et al. Echo intensity obtained from ultrasonography images reflecting muscle strength in elderly men. Clinical Interventions in Aging 2013;**8**:993-998

[86] Lauretani F, Russo CR, Bandinelli S, Bartali B, Cavazzini C, Di Iorio A,. Age-associated changes in skeletal muscles and their effect on mobility: An operational diagnosis of sarcopenia. Journal of Applied Physiology. 2003;**95(5)**:1851-1860

[87] Roberts HC, Denison HJ, Martin HJ, Patel HP, Syddall H, Cooper C, Sayer AA. A review of the measurement of grip strength in clinical and epidemiological studies: Towards a standardised approach. Age and Ageing. 2011;**40(4)**:423

[88] Magasi SR, Bubela DJ, Wang Y-C, Gershon RC. Grip and knee extension muscle strength reflect a common construct among adults. Muscle and Nerve 2012; **46**:555-558.

[89] Bean JF, Kiely DK, Herman S, Leveille SG, Mizer K, Frontera WR, Fielding RA. The relationship between leg power and physical performance in mobility-limited older people. Journal of the American Geriatrics Society. 2002;**50(3)**:461-467

[90] National Institute on Aging, Laboratory of Epidemiology, Demography, and Biometry. https://www.nia.nih.gov/

[91] Kiely DK, LaRose S, Alian J, Frontera WR. Is stair climb power a clinically relevant measure of leg power impairments in at-risk older adults? Archives of Physical Medicine and Rehabilitation 2007;**88**:604-609.

[92] Cesari M, Roger A, Pahor M, Goodpaster B, Hellerstein M, Gabor A. Biomarkers of sarcopenia in clinical trials—recommendations from the International Working Group on Sarcopenia. Journal of Cachexia, Sarcopenia and Muscle 2012;**3(3)**:181-190.

[93] Bukhari SS, Phillips BE, Wilkinson DJ, Limb MC, Rankin D, Mitchell WK, et al. Intake of low-dose leucine-rich essential amino acids stimulates muscle anabolism equivalently to bolus whey protein in older women at rest and after exercise. American Journal of Physiology. Endocrinology and Metabolism. 2015;**308(12)**:E1056-E1065.

[94] Rizzoli R. Nutrition and Sarcopenia. Journal of Clinical Densitometry. 2015;**18(4)**:483-487.

[95] Paddon-Jones D, Rasmussen BB. Dietary protein recommendations and the prevention of sarcopenia. Current Opinion in Clinical Nutrition and Metabolic Care. 2009;**12(1)**:86-90

[96] Saggini R, Calvani M. The treatment of cancer: a comprehensive therapeutic model entailing a complex of interaction modalities. DOI: 10.5772/55696

[97] Saggini R, Bellomo RG, Carmignano SM, Saggini A. Cancer pain—The role of an integrated, comprehensive rehabilitation program in its management. In: Rangel LBA, Silva IA, editors. Updates on Cancer Treatment. Rijeka, Croatia, InTech; 2015

[98] Wyss M, Kaddurah-Daouk R. Creatine and creatinine metabolism. Physiological Reviews 2000;**80**:1107-1213.

[99] Candow DG. Sarcopenia: Current theories and the potential beneficial effect of creatine application strategies. Biogerontology. 2011;**12**:273-281.

[100] Gualano B, Artioli GG, Poortmans JR, Lancha Junior AH. Exploring the therapeutic role of creatine supplementation. Amino Acids 2010;**38**:31-44.

[101] Rawson ES, Wehnert ML, Clarkson PM. Effects of 30 days of creatine ingestion in older men. European Journal of Applied Physiology and Occupational Physiology 1999;**80**:139-144.

[102] Hultman E, Söderlund K, Timmons JA, Cederblad G, Greenhaff PL. Muscle creatine loading in men. Journal of Applied Physiology 1996;**81**:232-237.

[103] Gualano B, Roschel H, Lancha-Jr AH, Brightbill CE, Rawson ES. In sickness and in health: The widespread application of creatine supplementation. Amino Acids 2012;**43**:519-529.

[104] Pennings B, Boirie Y, Senden J, Gijsen AP, Kuipers H, van Loon LJ. Whey protein stimulates postprandial muscle protein accretion more effectively than do casein and casein hydrolysate in older men. The American Journal of Clinical Nutrition 2011;**93**:997-1005.

[105] Burd NA, Yang Y, Moore DR, Tang JE, Tarnopolsky MA, Phillips SM. Greater stimulation of myofibrillar protein synthesis with ingestion of whey protein isolate v. micellar casein at rest and after resistance exercise in elderly men. British Journal of Nutrition. 2012;**108**:958-962.

[106] Mitchell CJ, Della Gatta PA, Petersen AC, Cameron-Smith D. Soy protein ingestion results in less prolonged p70S6 kinase phosphorylation compared to whey protein after resistance exercise in older men. Journal of the International Society of Sports Nutrition 2015; **12**:6. DOI: 10.1186/s12970-015-0070-2.

[107] Di Girolamo FG, Situlin R, Mazzucco S. Omega-3 fatty acids and protein metabolism: Enhancement of anabolic interventions for sarcopenia. Nutrition in Clinical Practice. 2013;**28(6)**:684-690. DOI: 10.1177/0884533613507607.

[108] Stehle J, Reuss S, Riemann R, Seidel A, Vollrath L. The role of arginine-vasopressin for pineal melatonin synthesis in the rat: Involvement of vasopressinergic receptors. Neuroscience Letters 1991;**123**:131-134.

[109] Dawson D, Encel N. Melatonin and sleep in humans. Journal of Pineal Research 1993;**15**:1-12.

[110] Pechanova O, Paulis L, Simko F. Peripheral and central effects of melatonin on blood pressure regulation. International Journal of Molecular Sciences 2014, 15, 17920-17937.

[111] Erkanl N K, Kayalar N, Ercan F, Sener G, KNrali K. Melatonin protects against ischemia/reperfusion injury in skeletal muscle. Journal of Pineal Research. 2005;**39**:238-242

[112] Lee JY, Kim JH, Lee DC. Urine melatonin levels are inversely associated with sarcopenia in postmenopausal women. Menopause. 2014; **21(1)**:39-44. DOI: 10.1097/GME.0b013e318291f6c8.

[113] Ramis MR, Esteban S, Miralles A, Tan DX, Reiter R. Protective effects of melatonin and mitochondria-targeted antioxidants against oxidative stress: A review. Current Medicinal Chemistry 2015;**22**:2690-2711

[114] Kim CH, Kim KH, Yoo YM. Melatonin-induced autophagy is associated with degradation of MyoD protein in C2C12 myoblast cells. Journal of Pineal Research 2012;53:289-297

[115] Borges LS, Dermargos A, da Silva J EP, Weimann E, Lambertucci RH, Hatanaka E. Melatonin decreases muscular oxidative stress and inflammation induced by strenuous exercise and stimulates growth factor synthesis. Journal of Pineal Research. 2015;**58**:166-172.

[116] Ochoa JJ, Díaz-Castro J, Kajarabille N, García C, Guisado IM, de Teresa C, Guisado R. Melatonin supplementation ameliorates oxidative stress and inflammatory signaling induced by strenuous exercise in adult human males. Journal of Pineal Research 2011;**51**:373-380.

[117] Coto-Montes A, Boga JA, Reite RJ. Melatonin as a potential agent in the treatment of sarcopenia. International Journal of Molecular Sciences 2016;**17(10)**:177. DOI: 10.3390/ijms17101771

[118] Aaron RK, Ciombor DM, Simon BJ. Treatment of nonunions with electric and electromagnetic fields. Clinical Orthopaedics 2004;**419**:21-29.

[119] Pesce M, Patruno A, Speranza L, and Reale M. Extremely low frequency electromagnetic field and wound healing: Implication of cytokines as biological mediators. European Cytokine Network 2013;**24**:1-10

[120] Rasouli J, Lekhraj R, White NM, Flamm ES, Pilla AA, Strauch B, Casper D. Attenuation of interleukin-1beta by pulsed electromagnetic fields after traumatic brain injury. Neuroscience Letters 2012;**519**:4-8.

[121] Nelson FR, Zvirbulis R, and Pilla AA. Non-invasive electromagnetic field therapy produces rapid and substantial pain reduction in early knee osteoarthritis: A randomized double-blind pilot study. Rheumatology International 2013;**33**:2169-2173.

[122] Pesce M, Patruno A, Speranza L, and Reale M. Extremely low frequency electromagnetic field and wound healing: Implication of cytokines as biological mediators. European Cytokine Network 2013;**24**:1-10.

[123] Heden, P and Pilla AA. Effects of pulsed electromagnetic fields on postoperative pain: A double-blind randomized pilot study in breast augmentation patients. Aesthetic Plastic Surgery 2008; 32, 660-666

[124] Saggini R, Bellomo RG, Saggini A, Iodice P, Toniato E. Rehabilitative treatment for low back pain with external pulsed electromagnetic fields. International Journal of Immunopathology and Pharmacology. 2009;**22(3 suppl)**:25-28

[125] Saggini R, Scarcello L, Carmignano SM, Khodor H, Visciano C, Giuliani L. Complex Rehabilitation Project in Leigh syndrome. Journal of Clinical Trials. 2014;**4**:196

[126] Lappin MS, Lawrie FW, Richards TL, Kramer ED. Effects of a pulsed electromagnetic therapy on multiple sclerosis fatigue and quality of life: A double-blind, placebo controlled trial. Alternative Therapies in Health and Medicine. 2003;**9(4)**:38-48

[127] Di Bonaventura G, Saggini R, Giuliani L, Bellomo RG et al. Exposure to extremely low frequencies electromagnetic field aspects biofilm formation by cystic fibrosis pathogens. Future Microbiology 2014;**10**.

[128] Gerardi G, De Ninno A, Prosdocimi M, Ferrari V, Barbaro F, et al. Effects of electromagnetic fields of low frequency and low intensity on rat metabolism. BioMagnetic Research and Technology 2008;**6**:3.

[129] Hernandez A, Cheng A, Westerblad H. Antioxidants and skeletal muscle performance: "common knowledge" vs. experimental evidence. Frontiers in Physiology. 2012;**3**:46. DOI: 10.3389/fphys.2012.00046

[130] Hurley BF, Hanson ED, Sheaff AK. Strength training as a countermeasure to aging muscle and chronic disease. Sports Medicine 2011;**41**:289.

[131] Binder E, Schechtman K, Ehsani A, Steger-May KMA, Brown M, Sinacore DR, et al. Effects of exercise training on frailty in community-dwelling elderly adults: Results of a randomized, controlled trial. Journal of the American Geriatrics Society. 2002;**50(12)**:1921-1928

[132] Schulte JN, Yarasheski KE. Effects of resistance training on the rate of muscle protein synthesis in frail elderly people. International Journal of Sport Nutrition and Exercise Metabolism 2001;**11**:S111-S118.

[133] Candow DG, Chilibeck PD, Abeysekara S, Zello GA J. Short-term heavy resistance training eliminates age-related deficits in muscle mass and strength in healthy older males. Journal of Strength and Conditioning Research. 2011;**25(2)**:326-333.

[134] Liu CJ, Latham NK. Progressive resistance strength training for improving physical function in older adults. Cochrane Database of Systematic Reviews. 2009;**8(3)**:CD002759.

[135] Reid KF, Callahan DM, Carabello RJ, Phillips EM, Frontera WR, Fielding RA. Lower extremity power training in elderly subjects with mobility limitations: A randomized controlled trial. Aging Clinical and Experimental Research. 2008;**20(4)**:337-343.

[136] American Geriatrics Society, British Geriatrics Society, and American Academy of Orthopaedic Surgeons Panel on Falls Prevention. Guideline for the prevention of falls in older persons. Journal of the American Geriatrics Society. 2001;**49(5)**:664-672

[137] Bellomo RG, Iodice P, Maffulli N, Maghradze T, Coco V, Saggini R. Muscle strength and balance training in sarcopenic elderly: A pilot study with randomized controlled trial. European Journal of Inflammation. 2013;**11**:193-201

[138] Bellomo RG, Khodor H, Barassi G, Carmignano SM, Di Stefano A, Di Pancrazio L, Saggini R. Global bioprogressive rehabilitation program and postural instability in Parkinson's disease. European Scientific Journal. 2014;**2**:310-321

[139] Saggini R, Di Pancrazio L, Pisciella V, Iodice P, Marri A, Bellomo RG. Postural anti-gravitational reprogramming in the elderly with flexed posture. European Journal of Physical and Rehabilitation Medicine. 2010;**46** - suppl.1 - No.2. ISSN: 1973-9087.

[140] Saggini R, Di Stefano A, Capogrosso F, Carmignano SM, D'Ettole S, Iodice P et al.Task-oriented physical exercise using postural re-alignment with body weight support in chronic stroke. European Journal of Inflammation. 2013;**11(3)**:739-749

[141] Bellomo RG, Pisciella V, Di Pancrazio L, Saggini R. The virtual images into physical rehabilitation. In: book abstract SIMFER the Italian Society of Physical and Rehabilitation Medicine 37th National Congress. Campobasso, Italy; 20-23 September 2009; 189.

[142] Devereux K, Robertson D, Briffa NK. Effects of a water-based training on women 65 years and over: A randomised controlled trial. The Australian Journal of Physiotherapy 2005;**51**:102-108

[143] Montero-Fernández N, Serra-Rexach JA. Role of exercise on sarcopenia in the elderly. European Journal of Physical and Rehabilitation Medicine. 2013;**49(1)**:131-143

[144] Phu S, Boersma D, Duque G. Exercise and sarcopenia. Journal of Clinical Densitometry. 2015;**18(4)**:488-492

10

Frailty and Cardiovascular Disease

Vinod Chainani, Russell Riehl, Geeta Chainani,
Abir Abdo, Mauricio G. Cohen, Carlos Alfonso,
Pedro Martinez-Clark, Carl J. Lavie, John P. Reilly and
Nidal Abi-Rafeh

Abstract

Cardiovascular disease (CVD) comprises a vast spectrum of disease states ranging from hypertension (HTN) to valvular heart disease (VHD). CVD is known to be the leading cause of morbidity, mortality, and health-care expenditure throughout the world. According to the World Health Organization, coronary artery disease (CAD) and stroke, both subsets of CVD, are the world's biggest killers, accounting for a combined 15 million deaths in 2015. These diseases have remained the leading causes of death globally in the last 15 years. In 2010, CAD alone was projected to cost the U.S. $108.9 billion including the cost of health-care services, medications, and lost productivity. The presence of frailty significantly worsens outcomes for patients suffering from CAD. With just this one example of how frailty affects CVD, it is clear that understanding the impact of frailty upon patients afflicted with the spectrum of cardiovascular disease is integral for the care of this very significant patient population.

Keywords: frailty, cardiovascular disease, valvular heart disease, outcomes in cardiovascular disease, hypertension, coronary artery disease, peripheral vascular disease, lipid dysregulation

1. Introduction

Cardiovascular disease (CVD) comprises a vast spectrum of disease states ranging from hypertension (HTN) to valvular heart disease (VHD) and is known to be the leading cause of morbidity, mortality, and health-care expenditure throughout the world. According to the World Health Organization, coronary heart disease (CHD) and stroke, both subsets of CVD, are the world's most impactful causes of mortality, accounting for a combined 15 million deaths in

2015. These diseases have remained the leading causes of death globally in the last 15 years. In 2010, CHD alone was projected to cost the United States (US) $108.9 billion including the cost of health-care services, medications, and lost productivity. The presence of frailty significantly worsens outcomes for patients suffering from CHD [1]. With just this one example of how frailty affects CVD, it is clear that understanding the impact of frailty upon patients afflicted with the spectrum of CVD is integral for the care of this very significant patient population.

While frailty as an entity is manifested by the interplay of multiple factors, there are some that are pertinent to the relationship between CVD and frailty. Endocrine dysregulation and higher levels of inflammatory markers have been found in frail compared with non-frail persons, and these derangements have been appreciated in patients with CHD. Elevations in some markers of frailty are also risk factors for the development of progressive vascular and CHD [2]. So while it can be inferred that CVD and frailty share common links, the effect of frailty upon the outcomes of CVD is still an area of interest and continued study [3].

We now know that CVD can worsen sarcopenia and lead to frailty, while frailty worsens morbidity and mortality in CVD [4, 5]. Maximal aerobic power (MAP), a measure of frailty, decreases with age due to a decrease in cardiac output. And though CVD is not the primary cause of decline of MAP, CVD clearly exacerbates the said decline [5]. Recently, in a meta-analysis of 54,250 elderly individuals with a mean follow-up of 6.2 years, the presence of atherosclerotic CVD was associated with the coexistence of frailty syndrome (FS) with an odds ratio (OR) of 2.7–4.1 [6]. Also, in patients who did not begin the study with FS, CVD was associated with the onset of FS during follow-up of these patients. There have been several studies that highlight the relationship between CVD and frailty, as described in **Tables 1** and **2**.

Study	Study type/number of patients	Objective	Outcome
Chin et al. [7]	Population-based cohort study/545 men	Assess association between classic cardiovascular risk factors and subsequent functional disability and mental well-being in elderly men.	Combined classic cardiovascular risk factors are predictive of functional disability.
Newman et al. [8]	Observational cohort/4375 patients	Assess the relationship between subclinical cardiovascular disease and frailty.	Cardiovascular disease was associated with an increased likelihood of frail health.
Chaves et al. [9]	Prospective population based cohort/670 patients	Examined the cross-sectional relationship between hemoglobin (Hb) and a recently-validated measure of frailty in community-dwelling older women, and whether this relationship was modified by cardiovascular disease (CVD) status.	Mildly low and low-normal Hb levels were independently associated with increased frailty risk. This risk was synergistically modified by the presence of CVD.
Woods et al. [10]	Prospective study, the Women's Health Initiative Observational Study/40.657 women	Identified risk factors for frailty as targets for prevention. Investigated the predictive validity of this frailty classification for death, hospitalization, hip fracture, and activity of daily living (ADL) disability.	Community-dwelling older women with CVD and cardiovascular risk factors were at higher risk of developing incident frailty.

Table 1. Effect of cardiovascular disease on frailty.

Study	Study type/ number of patients	Objective	Outcome
Klein et al. [11]	Prospective cohort/2962 patients	Association of measures of frailty to disease outcomes and survival in a population-based study of Midwestern adults.	Greater frailty was significantly associated with cardiovascular disease and hypertension.
Cacciatore et al. [12]	Prospective cohort/1259 patients	This study aimed to examine the predictive role of frailty on long-term mortality in elderly subjects with CHF.	Frailty represents a new independent variable for predicting long-term mortality in elderly subjects with CHF.
Purser et al. [13]	Observational cohort/309 patients	To characterize physiological variation in hospitalized older adults with severe coronary artery disease (CAD) and evaluate the prevalence of frailty in this sample, to determine whether single-item performance measures are good indicators of multidimensional frailty, and to estimate the association between frailty and 6-month mortality.	Gait speed frailty was the strongest predictor of mortality in a population with CAD and may add to traditional risk assessments when predicting outcomes in this population.
Boxer et al. [14]	Prospective cohort/60 patients	To assess the distance on the 6-min walk test (6MWT) as a measure of frailty in 60 older HF patients (ejection fraction <or= 40%) compared with frailty phenotype (FP).	The 6MWT may be useful to identify frailty and those in transition to frailty.
Dumurgier et al. [15]	Prospective cohort study/3208 men and women	Study the relation between low walking speed and the risk of death in older people, both overall and with regard to the main causes of death.	Slow gait speed was associated with a threefold increase in cardiovascular mortality over 5 years but no difference in death due to cancer or death due to other causes, implying a specific effect of frailty on CVD.
Ekerstad et al. [5]	Prospective cohort/307 patients	To analyze how frailty predicts short-term outcomes for elderly non-ST-segment elevation myocardial infarction patients.	Frailty is strongly and independently associated with in-hospital mortality, 1-month mortality, prolonged hospital care, and the study's primary composite outcome which included endpoints like all-cause mortality, reinfarction, revascularization, and even dialysis in older patients after non-ST elevation myocardial infarction (NSTEMI).

Table 2. Effect of frailty on cardiovascular disease.

A scoring system easily used on an inpatient basis highlights the interplay of CVD and frailty [16]. Sanchis et al. described seven independent predictors of frailty: age ≥75 years, female sex, prior CHD, admission for heart failure (HF), hemoglobin ≤12.5 g/dL, vitamin D ≤9 ng/mL, and cystatin-C ≥1.2 mg, which could be measured on an inpatient basis. Defining frailty as positive when there were ≥3 had a good correlation with the Fried score of frailty.

In this chapter, we delve into a basic understanding of the underlying pathophysiology of CVD in relation to frailty and how it is worsened by the latter, inflammatory markers that have proven significant in CVD and frailty, and how frailty affects a vast spectrum of CVD, ranging from lipid dysregulation to outcomes in VHD.

2. Pathophysiology

The pathophysiology of CVD and frailty relates to a baseline chronic inflammatory state [17–20]. This phenomenon is caused by a metabolic imbalance in the body, hereby systemic demand is not met by metabolic supply, and consequently the body becomes primarily catabolic, oxidative stress increases, and ultimately a low-level inflammatory phenotype is established [18, 21–28].

Multiple diseases place systemic stress demands on the body [1] that in turn leads to the inability of the body to keep pace with the demands of daily living, such as thermoregulation, aerobic respiration, glycolysis, and oxidative phosphorylation [17, 22, 29]. As a consequence of this baseline mismatch between the body's demand and its ability to supply, the body enters a pro-catabolic state and begins to metabolize itself for nutrient utilization [17, 25]. During this state, more inefficient systems are used to produce energy, and weakness and weight loss occur [30]. A pro-catabolic state is frequently seen in both CHD and frailty and leads to, as we already know exists in frailty, a pro-inflammatory state [18, 24].

The aforementioned pro-inflammatory state is highlighted by the presence of elevated inflammatory markers. There are markers specific to frailty and others that are common between CVD and frailty. Interleukin (IL)-6 is the most consistently seen inflammatory marker in patients with frailty, and is thought to be central to the pathogenesis of the phenotype [18, 21, 24, 26–28]. Studies have reported seeing elevated plasma uric acid, D-dimer, white blood cells (WBCs), erythrocyte sedimentation rate (ESR), triglycerides, homocysteine, glucose, hemoglobin A1C (HbA1c), creatinine, cystatin C, insulin-like growth factor (IGF)-1, fibrinogen, von Willebrand factor, factors VIII and IX, oxidized proteins, protein carbonylation, as well as decreased vitamin D and testosterone in patients with frailty [31]. In order to highlight the common role inflammation plays in both CVD and frailty, we can appreciate that elevations of C-reactive protein (CRP), factor VIII, and D-dimer are commonly seen even after correction of CVD [32]. Particularly, D-dimer, CRP, IL-6, and tumor necrosis factor (TNF)-alpha will be discussed where pertinent.

3. Frailty and hypertension (HTN)

Though not all frail patients are hypertensive, there is some evidence to suggest that HTN is independently associated with frailty [33]. The mechanism behind this finding is further elucidated by the fact that frail patients have a decreased ability to use adenosine triphosphate (ATP) [23, 29, 34]. This leads to a decreased ability of smooth muscle to use ATP to pump calcium back into the sarcoplasmic reticulum, which is marked by a slower rate of decay of the calcium transit. In practical terms, this means the blood vessels of frail patients have decreased compliance and difficulty relaxing, which leads to HTN.

The renin-angiotensin-aldosterone system (RAAS) is one of the primary systems used by the body to regulate blood pressure (BP) (**Figure 1**) [35, 36]. Chronic inflammation directly stimulates RAAS, which causes HTN [37]. Since frail patients have persistently increased inflammation, stimulating RAAS, they are more likely to develop HTN. Thus, there is a direct link between the chronic inflammation phenotype and HTN in frail patients.

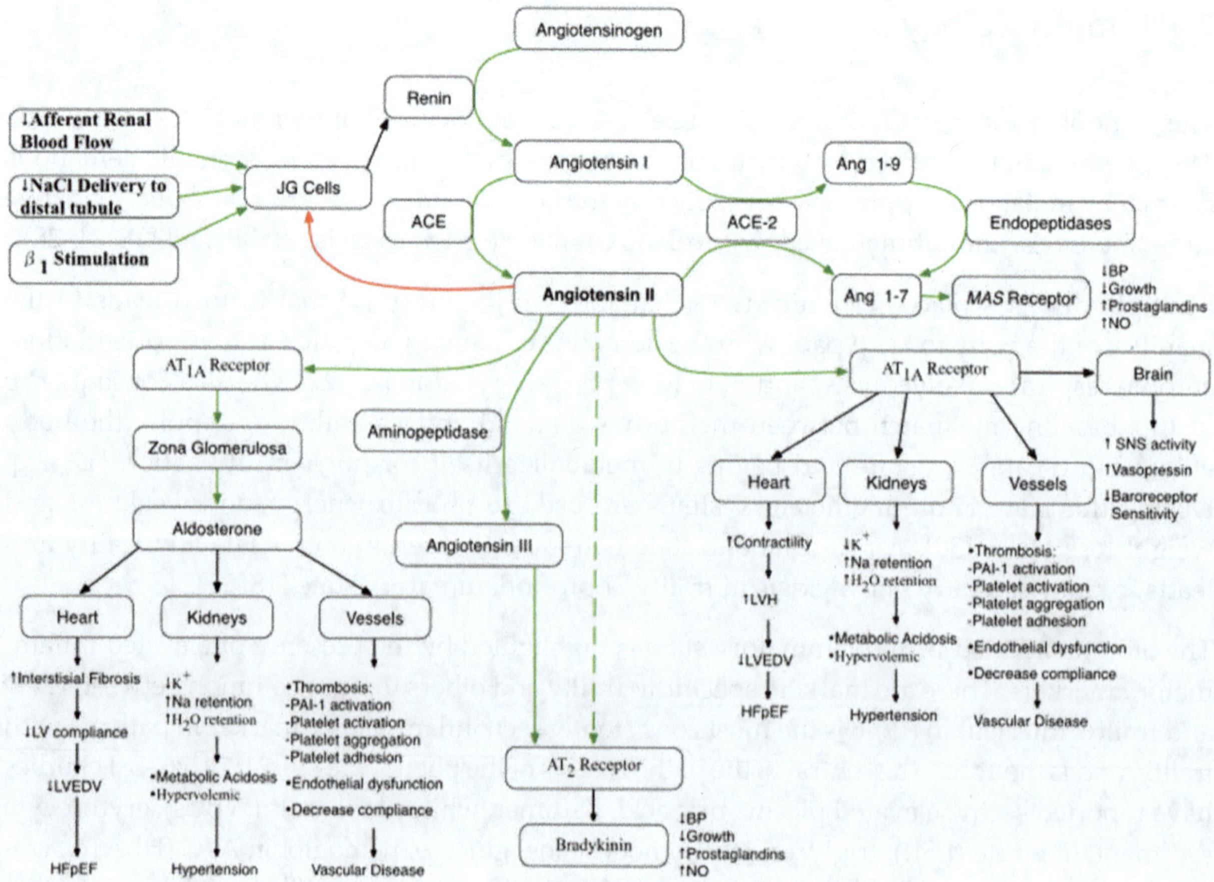

Figure 1. Renin-angiotensin-aldosterone system. ACE I, angiotensin-converting enzyme inhibitor; ACE-2, angiotensin-converting enzyme-2; Ang, angiotensin; BK, bradykinin; BP, blood pressure; HFpEF, heart failure with preserved ejection fraction; JG, juxtaglomerular; LV, left ventricle; LVEDV, left ventricular end diastolic volume; LVH, left ventricular hypertrophy; NO, nitric oxide; PAI-1, plasminogen activator inhibitor-1; SNS, sympathetic nervous system.

Evidence from randomized controlled trials over the past decade indicates there is benefit to treating hypertension in older patients [38, 39]. This is inconsistent with earlier observational and subgroup analyses of previous randomized control trials which were inconclusive [40, 41]. The HYVET trial in 2008 specifically focused the treatment of hypertension in elderly patients and found that antihypertensive treatment in patients older than 80 was beneficial [39]. In 2015, the Systolic Blood Pressure Intervention Trial (SPRINT) was undertaken. This trial should not be confused with the Sarcopenia and Physical Frailty in Older People: Multicomponent Treatment Strategies (SPRINTT) trial, which aims to provide a clear operational definition of physical frailty and assess the impact a multi-component intervention has on its progression [42]. The SPRINT trial showed that among patients >50 years old, lowering BP to <120 mmHg, particularly in the elderly, was associated with a significant decrease in mortality compared to a target of less than 140 mmHg at 5 years (5.2% vs. 6.8%; hazard ratio (HR): 0.75; 95% confidence interval (CI): 0.64–0.89, $p < 0.001$) [38]. Of note, patients who were >75 years old tended to fare better than younger patients. Taken together, this suggests that all elderly patients benefit from antihypertensive treatments, but there is an important caveat to both of these studies: enrolled patients tended to be relatively healthy patients and specifically excluded patients with heart failure, stroke, and end-stage renal disease [35, 38].

The exclusion criteria for HYVET and SPRINT raise concern that their findings may not be generalizable to frail patients [43]. A subgroup analysis of patients enrolled in HYVET addressed this concern [44]. Participants in both the control and treatment groups were given a frailty index according to 60 different variables. The impact of the frailty index on subsequent risk of stroke, mortality, and cardiac events was found to be non-significant, suggesting that benefits associated with BP lowering were conserved in frail patients. A frailty index was calculated for SPRINT participants using a similar set of 36 variables [45]. The frailty index distribution among the participants was comparable to general population cohorts. This suggests the heterogeneity of frailty among participants is similar to the general population.

Another 2015 report as a part of the Zwolle Outpatient Diabetes Project Integrating Available Care-34 (ZODIAC-34) cohort study, this time including all-comers, confirmed what observational studies had shown: for all-cause mortality (especially frail patients), there was an inverse relationship between blood pressure and all-cause mortality with a hazard ratio for systolic blood pressure of 0.92 (95% CI: 0.87–0.98) and 0.83 for diastolic blood pressure (95% CI: 0.73–0.93) [46]. This suggested that among all patients >75 years of age, this time including those with less than 1 year life expectancy and DM, lower BP was associated with an increase in mortality. Contiguously, intensive lowering of BP in patients with low gate speed (a commonly used proxy for frailty) did not reduce mortality and the rate of CVD events ($p = 0.05$, 0.28, respectively) [47].

4. Frailty and lipids

The metabolism of lipids has been shown to affect aging, such that having a high-density lipoprotein (HDL) level above 70 mg/dL is referred to as longevity syndrome. The Invecchiamento e Longevità nel Sirente (ilSERENTE) study showed that the HDL levels of the patients in their study who died during follow-up were significantly lower than the levels of the survivors. This finding contributed to the understanding of the effect of HDL on lifespan, highlighting the role of lipid metabolism in decreasing mortality in the frail, elderly patient [48]. Another study of the same group of patients showed that, among frail patients, those with the highest HDL levels had the best functional states [49]. To further support this idea, another study done in 2015 supported frailty as an independent risk factor for various diseases along the CVD spectrum. A low HDL level was one of the parameters [50]. As a part of the Longitudinal Aging Study Amsterdam, it was described that a lower total cholesterol was related to a higher rate of decline on information-processing speed indicating, ultimately, that lower total cholesterol may be considered to be a marker of frailty and predictive of lower cognitive function in the elderly [51]. As described earlier, there has been significant study regarding the relationship between frailty, HDL status, and its effect on mortality. Conversely, the relation between low-density lipoprotein (LDL) levels and frailty has yet to be established. Also, whereas the effect of lipids in the frail patient has been studied, the effect of frailty on the patient with a lipid disorder has yet to be established.

There has been speculation upon the metabolism of lipids in the frail patient. As there is a pro-inflammatory milieu in the frail patient, this inflammation may affect lipid metabolism and, hence, lipid profiles in those who are frail. There may also be some correlation between dysfunctional lipid metabolism due to endocrine dysregulation evidenced by lower IGF-1 and growth hormone levels in frail patients, lower HDL levels, and resultant poorer outcomes in CHD [52, 53]. A study on metabolic syndrome and disability showed a correlation between high triglycerides and a limitation in mobility and activities of daily living [54]. Overall, the effect of frailty, its pro-inflammatory state, and the collective effect on lipids seems to be contiguous with an elevation in triglycerides (TGs) and a decrease in HDL likely contributing to the elevated CVD risk in the frail population.

5. Frailty and atrial fibrillation (AF)

The up-regulation of the RAAS system in frail patients, as mentioned earlier, mediates an up-regulation of endothelin-1, which in turn mediates an increase in cardiac fibrosis [55]. Cardiac fibrosis, in turn, increases the likelihood of AF by disrupting the cardiac neuroconduction pathways [23]. Additionally, frailty may be an independent risk factor for AF [46] due to a decreased ability to modulate heart rate, resulting in an increased likelihood of a patient developing AF [56, 57]. Additionally, an increased calcium influx, as discussed earlier, causes changes in the trans-cellular membrane potential, which in turn makes a patient more likely to develop AF [23].

Frail patients have a 4.4 times higher chance (95% CI: 2.104–9.080, $p < 0.001$) of having AF compared to the general population [57]. Additionally, Polidoro et al. found that even after adjusting for age, sex, CVD, and CVD risk factors, AF was associated with a fourfold increase in frailtyhighlighting the relation between frailty and AF [58]. Additional evidence supporting the link between frailty and AF is the impairment of autonomic control vis-à-vis decreased heart rate variability which often precedes episodes of paroxysmal AF [57]. Similarly, there is decreased heart rate variability in frail patients.

AF has a significant impact on outcomes, including mortality, in frail patients [59]. Nguyen et al. found that in patients with AF, there was a 2.69 times higher risk of death in frail patients over a 6-month period after hospitalization (HR: 2.69, 95% CI: 1.53–4.74). This relationship held even after correction for potential co-founders (HR: 2.33; 95% CI: 1.31–4.14). It may be plausible to infer that AF also causes significant risk for cognitive decline to these patients seeing as they are already at an increased risk for microbleeds as discussed subsequently in the section on cerebrovascular disease. Furthermore, the strong risk of stroke and TIA outlined in the subsequent text is indubitably linked with AF [60].

Despite the increased risk of death with AF, frail patients have an eightfold less likelihood of being discharged home on an oral anticoagulant after hospitalization [57]. In fact, frailty is the third most cited reason for not prescribing an oral anticoagulant. This makes the report by Granzera et al. more pertinent as the population ages [61]. In this study, he provides an approach to deciding if oral anticoagulation is appropriate in elderly frail patients (**Figure 2**).

Granziera et al. also discussed what factors should go into making the decision of whether to use warfarin or novel oral anticoagulants (NOACs) in frail patients [61]. Severe renal impairment, severe liver impairment, and poor adherence favored the use of warfarin. The exceptions

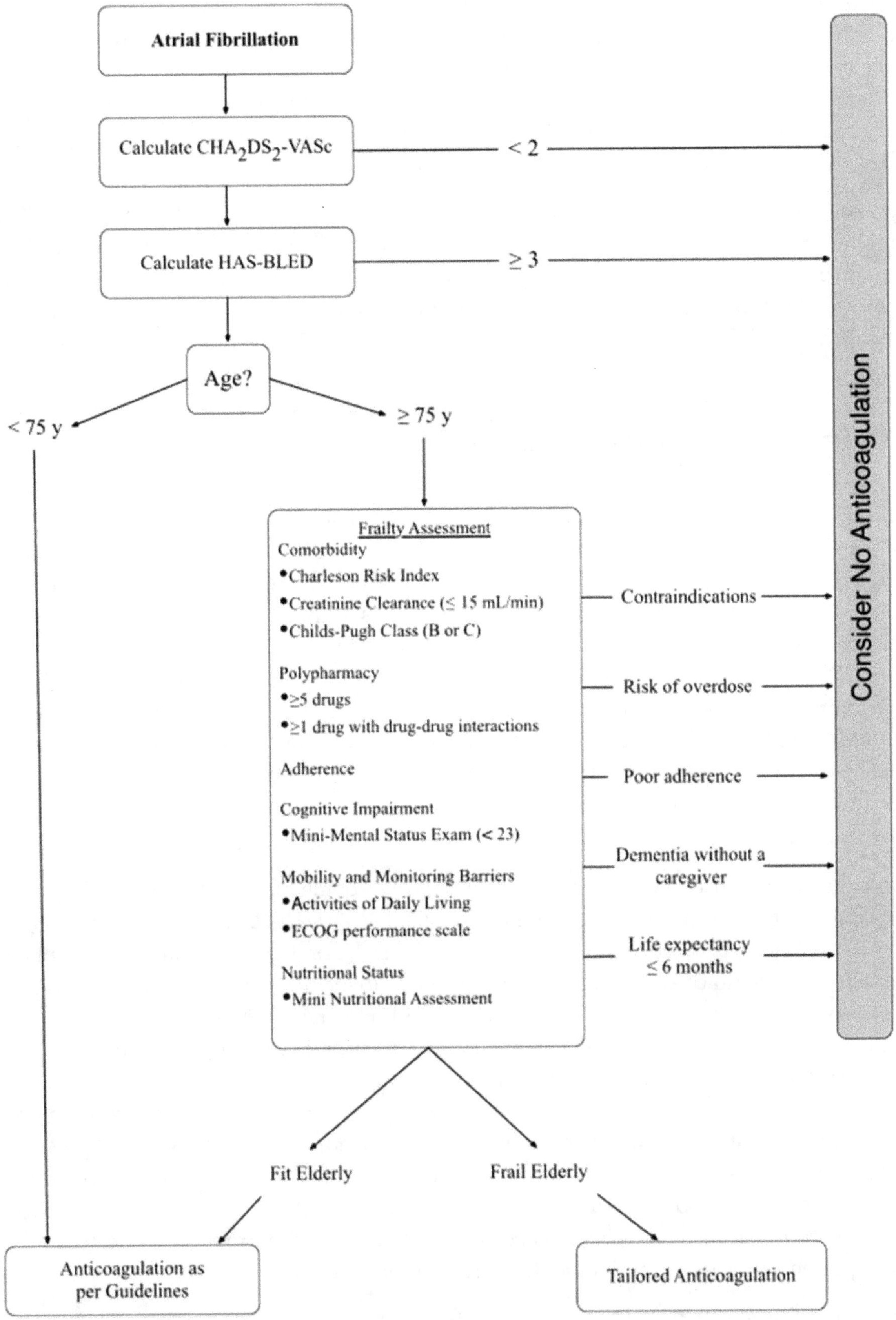

Figure 2. Decision algorithm for use of oral anticoagulants in elderly frail patients (<75 vs. ≥75 years). Adapted from Granziera et al. [61].

to favoring warfarin in renal impairment are apixaban and edoxaban, both of which may be prescribed in patients with compromised renal function. Decreased renal and hepatic clearances have minimal effect on warfarin. In patients at risk for poor compliance, their risk for stroke will not revert to baseline if a dose is missed. For patients with decreased mobility, they are less likely to comply with nutritional changes for warfarin and have polypharmacy; NOACs are the better choice for improved compliance.

Frail patients may have less of a benefit from device therapy than healthy patients [57]. In a combined analysis of four clinical trials, the benefits of implantable cardioverter defibrillators were inversely proportional to the number of comorbidities. This line of thought was further supported by a retrospective study of 83,792 undergoing ICD implantation in which frail patients had a 22% risk of mortality at 1 year compared to 12% overall.

6. Frailty and cerebrovascular disease

Several studies have indicated that frailty is associated with low cognitive performance. This is attributed to multiple causes including increased rates of Alzheimer's disease (AD), mild cognitive impairment, and a distinct subtype of frailty—cognitive frailty [62, 63]. Cognitive frailty is a clinical syndrome found in elderly patients without AD or other dementias, and occurs concurrently with physical frailty [63]. The key feature differentiating this syndrome from AD and other dementias is its potential for reversibility. The proposed mechanism for cognitive frailty is similar to physical frailty—a decrease in physiological reserves for responding to systemic stressors that manifests as an erosion of homeostatic mechanisms. The erosion of homeostatic mechanisms seen in cognitive frailty is manifested as β-amyloid accumulation. These changes are independent other causes of dementia such as vascular and Alzheimer's dementia.

Frail patients were also more likely to have any form of dementia (HR 1.85; 95% CI: 1.01–3.40) and vascular dementia in particular (HF 2.68; 95% CI: 1.16–7.17) [62]. Frail patients are 3.38 times (95% CI: 2.37–4.81, $p < 0.001$) more likely to have a stroke or TIA than non-frail patients [60]. This association with cerebrovascular disease extends to include pre-frail patients, who have a 1.98 times greater risk of having a stroke versus non-frail patients (95% CI: 1.53–2.57, $p < 0.001$). Another manifestation of cerebrovascular disease, cerebromicrobleeds, is one of the primary lesions responsible for vascular dementia. When the number of lesions is low (only one or two), there is usually no clinical evidence of microbleed, but when there is a larger lesion burden, patients present with stroke or dementia [64]. Even when adjusted for age, sex, and presence of vascular risk factors (CHD, chronic kidney disease, and global cognitive impairment), the lesion number was positively correlated with the severity of physical frailty. Chung et al. also found that the severity of physical frailty was positively correlated with proportion of cerebromicrobleeds present in the deep and infratentorial regions of the brain.

Furthermore, a study performed on patients undergoing carotid endarterectomy (CEA) using the American College of Surgeons National Surgical Quality Improvement Program (NSQIP) database from 2005 to 2011 showed that frailty is a predictor of increased stroke, mortality, myocardial infarction, and length of stay after CEA, further supporting the idea that CVD and frailty are strongly interlinked with frail patients suffering poorer outcomes postintervention [65].

6.1. Inflammatory markers in CHD

The relationship between frailty and CHD is one that has been extensively studied as well. Chronic inflammation is a shared mechanism between atherosclerosis and frailty [18, 66, 67]. In Libby et al.'s strong and well-cited review article, they show that, in addition to plaque characteristics, acute coronary syndromes are also caused by a chronic inflammatory state [59]. This link is most strongly seen by four markers of inflammation shared by both frailty and coronary vascular disease: IL-6, CRP, fibrinogen, and D-dimer [26, 27].

Hunter et al. made the strong case that IL-6 is a keystone mediator of systemic inflammation in multiple disease processes, especially CVD [28]. There have been numerous other studies linking IL-6 and CHD [18, 66, 67]. This suggests that IL-6 is central to the immunogenic dysregulation that accounts for the disease burden suffered by patients with both CVD and frailty [28]. Another significant marker of chronic inflammation shared between both CHD and frailty is CRP [26, 27]. Like IL-6, this marker is elevated in frailty even when CHD is accounted for [32].

Fibrinogen is an acute-phase reactant shown to be elevated with chronic inflammation and is strongly correlated with both frailty and atherosclerosis [26, 66]. Elevated fibrinogen is an independent risk factor for CVD events [66]. The mechanism is thought to be caused by fibrinogen affecting the plaque phenotype, causing it to be more permeable, able to accumulate oxidized LDL, increase platelet reactivity, and aggregation. A direct association between frailty and fibrinogen has been observed independent of chronic disease states [26].

Similar to fibrinogen, D-dimer fragments are an independent risk factor for CHD to the point where they are considered a biomarker for atherothrombosis [66]. Moreover, elevated D-dimers are also independently associated with frailty [32].

7. Frailty and CHD

A meta-analysis of 54,250 elderly individuals with a mean follow-up of 6.2 years showed that the presence of atherosclerotic CVD was associated with the coexistence of frailty syndrome with an odds ratio of 2.7–4.1 [6]. The relationship between CVD and frailty is significantly bidirectional [6, 60]. This is highlighted by the twofold increase in mortality among frail CHD patients compared to non-frail patients even when adjusted for age and comorbidities [68]. In the Women's Health Initiative Study, women with CHD were more likely to become frail over the subsequent 6 years; likewise, the Health, Aging, and Body Composition Study showed that older adults with frailty were more likely to develop CHD. This same study showed that the presence of frailty, assessed by gait speed, was associated with an increased risk of incident CVD. After adjustment for potential confounding factors, a slower gait was associated with an increased incidence of CVD events and all-cause mortality compared with individuals having higher walking speed [69]. Furthering the complexity of this disease interplay is the fact that patients with both frailty and CHD have a higher frequency of multivessel disease and left main disease (74%) than non-frail patients (60%) and moderately frail (68%) patients ($p = 0.019$) [70]. These differences persisted even after correcting for age and gender ($p = 0.005$). The wealth of evidence clearly defines the effect of frailty upon CHD.

Interestingly, atherogenesis is also affected by sarcopenia. This effect is partially due to the replacement of muscle with adipose tissue, and partially to the neurohumoral dysregulation and decreased mobility brought on by sarcopenia [71–73]. Atherogenesis is worsened by the presence of sarcopenia and frailty in humans as evidenced by the association between carotid atherosclerosis, arterial stiffness, and sarcopenia [6]. It, therefore, seems natural that frail patients fare worse after an acute CHD event compared to non-frail patients. This notion was validated by Dodson et al., who found that at 1 year after an acute CHD event, older adults with slow gait speed (<0.8 m/s measured 1 month after the event) were more likely to die or be re-admitted to the hospital than those with faster speeds (35.4% vs. 18.5%; $p = 0.006$) [74]. However, it is important to note that the majority of these events were re-admissions—not death.

Regarding interventions, there has been an extensive amount of investigation into whether coronary artery bypass grafting (CABG) is better than percutaneous coronary intervention (PCI) in frail patients. Fifty-six percent of frail patients who underwent CABG had postoperative complications compared to seventeen percent of those who were non-frail ($p < 0.001$) [75]. Frailty was also an independent predictor of in-hospital mortality after CABG (OR 1.8; 92% CI: 1.1–3.0). Similarly, PCI also carried significant risks. Frailty was associated with a longer hospital stay (HR 4.8, 95% CI: 1.4–16.3; $p = 0.013$), higher 30-day mortality (HR 4.8, 95% CI: 1.4–16.3; $p = 0.01$), and higher 1-year mortality (HR 5.9, 95% CI: 2.5–13.8; $p < 0.001$) [76, 77]. Importantly, there is evidence that there is no significant difference in change in frailty at 30 months between CABG and PCI ($p = 0.090$) [78]. In patients ≥75 years old treated with either PCI or CABG, there was a significantly different trajectory in their frailty score at 30 months (0.188 vs. 247, respectively) and at baseline (0.164 vs. 0.189, respectively; $p = 0.041$). Including frailty as part of the three-tiered criterion in the assessment of a patient undergoing PCI improved the discriminatory ability of the Mayo Clinic risk score [79]. Of great importance is the decision as to which modality of intervention is most effective in the frail population with obstructive coronary artery disease (CAD). Although we suspect that being less invasive in frail patients may be preferable, a prospective, randomized trial in the frail population addressing this quandary, as well as whether revascularization impacts frailty, would be beneficial.

8. Frailty and peripheral arterial disease (PAD)

Clearly, PAD is a pandemic condition that could potentially lead to the literal loss of life and limb. It manifests as tissue hypoperfusion caused by acute insult upon a limb with preexisting underlying atherosclerosis. This disease process is a significant cause of morbidity and mortality in both the frail and non-frail populations [80, 81].

Frailty has been shown to be associated with and worsen outcomes in patients with PAD. A study of the participants >50 years of age in the National Health and Nutritional Examination Survey (NHANES) showed that, in multivariable multinomial logistic regression models, ankle brachial index (ABI) <0.9 predicted frailty and pre-frailty. A higher prevalence of frailty was seen in participants with ABI ≥1.4. Frailty predicted general and CVD mortality in participants with ABI <0.9. Hence, this study suggested that frailty mediates increased morbidity and mortality in PAD [82]. A cross-sectional study was carried out in a geriatric population of ≥65-year-old residents of Taichung, Taiwan, in June 2009 to assess the association between frailty and subclinical PAD. It reported findings suggesting that frail individuals had a significantly increased risk for subclinical PAD with an odds ratio of 3.168 [83]. In a study assessing gait in patients with PAD versus non-PAD both with and without frailty, the pre-frail group defined by the Fried Frailty Index had a diminished difference between study groups. This indicated that pre-frail patients have a poor functional status overall, which may overshadow the level of dysfunction imposed upon them by PAD alone [84].

Another study assessing the effect of frailty on outcomes after vascular surgery showed that frailty, assessed by the modified Frailty Index (mFI), predicted mortality in patients undergoing open procedures and Clavien-Dindo class IV (life-threatening) complications for both open and endovascular abdominal aortic aneurysm repairs [85]. Affecting disposition and, hence, patient wellness and health-care expenditure, frailty also increases the propensity of home-dwelling patients classified as frail to be discharged to a facility other than their home after elective vascular interventions [86]. There is also evidence to support the idea that frail females are potentially at the highest risk of death after vascular surgery, suggesting that female gender may be an additive risk factor [87].

9. Frailty and heart failure

The pathogenesis of HF has significant overlap with the processes leading to the frailty phenotype [17, 88]. With HF, much like frailty, the metabolic demands of the body outstrip physiologic reserves. The findings of Lavie et al. likewise show that a loss of fat (reserves) signals a worsening prognosis in HF [30].

Frail patients and patients with HF consistently have a similar biochemical profile of elevated CRP and interleukin-6, which in turn promote mitochondrial dysfunction [18, 22, 31]. Mitochondrial dysfunction produces excessive reactive oxygen species producing a pro-apoptotic intracellular environment. In the case of HF, apoptosis of cardiomyocytes fosters a local pro-inflammatory atmosphere, leading to cardiac fibrosis and ultimately decreased contractility. Likewise, when applied to skeletal muscle, this process causes sarcopenia, one of the hallmarks and precursors of frailty.

The likelihood of a frail patient to manifest HF is 8.76 times higher than that of a non-frail patient and, compared to any other element of CVD, HF is the most strongly linked with frailty [60, 89]. However, it should be noted that frailty is not limited to geriatric heart failure patient, and been observed in up to one-third of younger patients with HF [68]. The prevalence of frailty among heart failure patients is important because frailty is an even stronger predictor of mortality than is HF per se [88]. Cacciatore et al. assessed the role frailty had on mortality in HF patients ($n = 1139$) over a 12-year period compared to patients without CHF ($n = 120$) and found that frailty was independently associated with mortality in HF (HR 1.48, 95% CI: 1.04–2.11; $p = 0.0032$) and control group patients (HR 1.36, 95% CI: 1.17–1.57; $p < 0.001$), proving that it indeed was a more important predictor of mortality than HF itself [12]. Lupon et al. found that among 622 outpatient HF patients, frailty was an independent predictor of mortality even after adjustment for HF (HR 2.09, 95% CI: 1.11–3.92; $p = 0.022$) [90].

Discerning which patients are frail versus non-frail also has an impact on clinic resources. Frail patients versus non-frail patients in one study had a 92% increase in Emergency Department (ED) visits (HR 1.92, 1.60; 95% CI: 1.30–2.83) and 65% increased risk for hospitalizations (HR 1.65; 95% CI: 1.17–2.35) [91]. Of note, there was no significant association between outpatient visits in HF patients and frailty. This raises the question as to whether or not more intensive outpatient management of frail HF patients would decrease ED and hospital utilization.

One possible intervention to decrease the amount of hospital utilization in frail patients and, moreover, improve their morbidity and mortality is specifically resistance exercise [92]. As noted by Lavie et al., there is compelling evidence that muscle mass and muscle strength are protective in HF patients [93]. Moreover, a lack of muscular fitness overall is a strong determinant of cardiac cachexia which, as mentioned earlier, may be seen as a classification of frailty. There is evidence to suggest that maximal aerobic power, a measure of frailty, decreases with age, due to a decrease in cardiac output, and is exacerbated by CVD. Importantly, this is a measure of frailty which could be addressed with an increase in muscle mass and anaerobic exercise [94]. It is important to note that resistance training is the most well-validated countermeasure to slow the decline of muscle mass and muscle strength, even in frail patients [92]. By slowing the decline in muscle strength, the decline into frailty is consequently retarded. Taken together, this evidence points to muscle bulk, or the lack thereof, as being a significant marker of disease progression in HF and element of CVD.

The choice of pursuing advanced therapeutic options in the frail population with HF is a difficult one. As Joyce points out, HF itself and its ensuing sequelae can simulate the frailty phenotype [95]. Discerning between frailty caused specifically by HF and frailty attributable to non-CVD causes has significant implications in this selection of patients for destination therapy with left ventricular assist devices (LVADs). In patients with HF as the primary driver of his or her frailty, implantation of an LVAD led to restoration of aberrant cardiac output and metabolism. Flint et al. sorted out frail patients receiving an LVAD into three groups: LVAD-responsive, LVAD-independent, and LVAD-intermediate. In the LVAD-responsive group, whose frailty was primarily due to HF, implantation of LVAD caused a significant decrease in post-LVAD frailty as measured by hand-grip strength compared to both the LVAD-intermediate and LVAD-independent patients. These LVAD-responsive patients may be more accurate representatives of cardiac cachexia versus frailty.

Frailty in the heart-transplant (HT) population has more significant and far-reaching importance. Frail patients who underwent HT in one study had a 1-year survival rate of 52 ± 23% versus 100% in the non-frail control arm. This has significant implications in the way HT therapy is allocated. This is a realm that requires more study, though studies will be sparse given the requirements for HT approval, including appropriate performance on pre-HT cardiopulmonary testing, in which frail and pre-frail patient would likely have suboptimal results.

10. Frailty and valvular heart disease (VHD)

In industrialized countries, the prevalence of VHD is estimated at 2.5%. Degenerative calcification seems to augment the prevalence of VHD markedly after the age of 65 years, particularly regarding aortic stenosis (AS) and mitral regurgitation (MR). These two disease entities account for three in four cases of VHD. Also contributing to the incidence of VHD is infective endocarditis, the incidence of which is approximately 30 cases per million individuals per year worldwide. Finally, rheumatic heart disease (RHD) is another very significant contributor to the incidence of VHD and still represents a significant health burden with over 15 million cases of RHD worldwide, 282,000 new cases, and 233,000 deaths annually [96]. Health-care expenditure for these disease entities is substantial. In fact, US expenditure estimates close to $2 billion annually for symptomatic and asymptomatic aortic VHD, and $2.6 billion for symptomatic and asymptomatic mitral VHD [97, 98].

Patients who meet indications for VHD surgery are frequently not offered surgery due to prohibitive risk features. As an example in the mitral VHD population, among patients who meet the current indications for surgical treatment of MR, almost 50% are not offered therapy due to several factors, including high surgical risk from comorbidities and frailty associated with advanced age [99, 100]. Importantly, though some patients may tolerate a surgical procedure, meaningful functional recovery is not achieved if they demonstrate marked frailty prior to the intervention [101]. Unfortunately, such patients are left with few clinical options, resulting in frequent referrals to palliative care and hospice programs. Fortunately, as we now know, patients earlier deemed inoperable or high risk for conventional VHD surgery have minimally invasive options to address their comorbid state. These include transcatheter aortic valve replacement (TAVR), transcatheter mitral valve replacement (TMVR), and Mitraclip. These procedures may be the ones most suitable for the frail population as they are part of the aforementioned patient populations that would otherwise be left without options. Currently, of the interventions for VHD that are performed, the three mentioned earlier are the ones that have the most impact on the frail population.

In a study aimed at studying inflammatory markers in patients undergoing TAVR in an attempt to estimate preoperative risk, two inflammatory markers were studied. Neopterin, a pteridine synthesized by activated macrophages, and immune activation-mediated tryptophan and its subsequent degradation had both been shown prior to be associated with frailty and chronic disease. Ultimately, increased immune activation and associated tryptophan degradation underscored the prognostic role of baseline inflammation for outcome in patients with severe AS undergoing TAVR [102]. The aforementioned inflammatory markers like IL-6, TNF-alpha, D-dimer, and CRP have not yet been studied in the frail population in regard to outcomes in VHD but may prove to be valuable area of further research.

Frailty is well known in the VHD population to be associated with poorer outcomes when compared to non-frail patients. Patients with a moderate to severe degree of frailty (defined as requiring assistance to ambulate or attend to their own bodily needs, or a modified Rankin score 4) are generally considered high risk for valvular surgery [103]. In a study conducted by Sepeheri et al., frailty had a strong positive relationship with the risk of major adverse cardiovascular and cerebrovascular events (MACCE) (odds ratio, 4.89; 95% confidence interval, 1.64–14.60) [104]. Relationships were stronger in older patients undergoing TAVR than younger patients undergoing CABG and VHD surgery (hazard ratio for frailty in TAVR, 3.31–4.89 vs. hazard ratio for non-TAVR, 1.10–3.16). One single-center experience of all cardiac operations demonstrated frailty to be an independent predictor of in-hospital mortality, institutional discharge, and reduced midterm survival [105]. In a study assessing the effect of frailty on mortality, length of stay (LOS), and discharge destination in patients post-TAVR, Chauhan et al. showed that frailty portended an increase in LOS and mortality [106]. Additionally, a study assessing preoperative computed tomography (CT) scans that are done as part of the workup for transcatheter therapeutic interventions for VHD shows that these CTs have proven useful in measuring the patient's skeletal mass index (SMI) and, thus, preoperative sarcopenia. This correlated directly to length of stay more strongly than the frailty index [107].

Many of the frail patients afflicted with MR, however, tolerate MitraClip and are able to recover from the femoral venotomy and general anesthesia required for this procedure. In one study assessing effectiveness of transcutaneous mitral valve repair with Mitraclip in 564 patients, frailty was noted in 57% of patients. The procedural success rate, nonetheless, was 91% defined as MR less than or equal to grade 2 and surviving the hospital stay. A majority of patients were discharged home with moderate or less MR than prior [108]. Patients with severe frailty who are bedridden and/or require constant nursing care may be too disabled to achieve meaningful benefit from MitraClip and may also be considered prohibitive for TAVR [101]. This, though, has yet to be assessed prospectively.

The interesting aspect of frailty in VHD is that the novel interventions in this field are generally aimed to treat non-operable or high, prohibitive risk individuals. Frail patients comprise a significant portion of this population indicating that understanding how best to treat these patients is of significant import for the field in its gestalt. As this field continues to develop more prolifically, addressing the frail patient will prove to be an area of in-depth study. Many practitioners share the belief that current interventions prove to reverse certain aspects of frailty but this has yet to be studied in a prospective trial.

11. Conclusions

Frailty is a significant disease entity affecting a myriad of clinical situations. How it affects the spectrum of CVD has been an area of interest and study for a number of years. With the advent of novel procedures in the realm of VHD and the expansion of patient populations now being considered as candidates for interventions, the topic of frailty, its interplay with CVD, and how it affects outcomes in patients with CVD are of the utmost import. As discussed earlier, current risk scores for patients undergoing cardiovascular surgery (STS and euroSCORE) have yet to include frailty as official criteria in their scoring systems, yet many practitioners still note frailty to be a condition predisposing patients to unfavorable outcomes and, thus, precluding them from interventions.

That frail patient suffers poorer outcomes is significant. From postintervention mortality to disposition postdischarge, frail patients perform suboptimally when compared to their non-frail counterparts. The generalized debility to which frail patients are predisposed may make them less tolerant of therapeutic postintervention treatments that would otherwise improve their outcomes, such as physical therapy and progressive exercise training. Their subclinical inflammatory state may further prevent wound healing and resolution. Also, their comorbid conditions may prevent complete healing and recovery as well. These hypotheses have not yet been studied and warrant further investigation for the purpose of elucidating ways to counteract the aforementioned poorer outcomes experienced by frail patients.

Frailty can be treated, potentially, with specific modalities, such as exercise, protein-calorie supplementation, vitamin D, and reduction of polypharmacy [109]. This shows that, although frailty is incredibly significant and has undeniable impacts on morbidity and mortality, it is something that is potentially reversible. With further study and therapeutic interventions tailored specifically to the frail patient, we may be able to expand our indications and improve the quality of life for a patient population known to suffer with a disease process different from any other.

Author details

Vinod Chainani[1*], Russell Riehl[1], Geeta Chainani[5], Abir Abdo[2], Mauricio G. Cohen[3], Carlos Alfonso[3], Pedro Martinez-Clark[3], Carl J. Lavie[1], John P. Reilly[1] and Nidal Abi-Rafeh[4]

*Address all correspondence to: vinod.chainani@gmail.com

1 Ochsner Health System, John Ochsner Heart and Vascular Institute, Jefferson, Louisiana, USA

2 Louisiana State University Health Sciences Center, New Orleans, Louisiana, USA

3 University of Miami Miller School of Medicine, Miami, Florida, USA

4 Tulane University School of Medicine, New Orleans, Louisiana, USA

5 Windsor University School of Medicine, Saint kitts, Carribean

References

[1] Go AS, Mozaffarian D, Roger VL, et al. Heart disease and stroke statistics—2013 update: A report from the American Heart Association. Circulation. 2013;**127**(1):e6-e245

[2] Tracy RP. Emerging relationships of inflammation, cardiovascular disease and chronic diseases of aging. International Journal of Obesity and Related Metabolic Disorders. 2003;**27**(Suppl 3):S29-S34

[3] Singh M, Alexander K, Roger VL, et al. Frailty and its potential relevance to cardiovascular care. Mayo Clinic Proceedings. 2008;**83**(10):1146-1153

[4] Bouillon K, Batty GD, Hamer M, et al. Cardiovascular disease risk scores in identifying future frailty: The Whitehall II prospective cohort study. Heart. 2013;**99**(10):737-742

[5] Ekerstad N, Swahn E, Janzon M, et al. Frailty is independently associated with short-term outcomes for elderly patients with non-ST-segment elevation myocardial infarction. Circulation. 2011;**124**(22):2397-2404

[6] Afilalo J, Karunananthan S, Eisenberg MJ, Alexander KP, Bergman H. Role of frailty in patients with cardiovascular disease. American Journal of Cardiology. 2009;**103**(11): 1616-1621

[7] Chin A Paw MJ, Dekker JM, Feskens EJ, Schouten EG, Kromhout D. How to select a frail elderly population? A comparison of three working definitions. Journal of Clinical Epidemiology. 1999;**52**(11):1015-1021

[8] Newman AB, Gottdiener JS, Mcburnie MA, et al. Associations of subclinical cardiovascular disease with frailty. Journal of Gerontology: Series A Biological Sciences and Medical Sciences. 2001;**56**(3):M158-M166

[9] Chaves PH, Semba RD, Leng SX, et al. Impact of anemia and cardiovascular disease on frailty status of community-dwelling older women: The Women's Health and Aging Studies I and II. Journal of Gerontology: Series A Biological Sciences and Medical Sciences. 2005;**60**(6):729-735

[10] Woods NF, LaCroix AZ, Gray SL, et al. Frailty: Emergence and consequences in women aged 65 and older in the Women's Health Initiative Observational Study. Journal of American Geriatrics Society. 2005;**53**(8):1321-1330

[11] Klein BE, Klein R, Knudtson MD, Lee KE. Frailty, morbidity and survival. Archives of Gerontology and Geriatrics. 2005;**41**(2):141-149

[12] Cacciatore F, Abete P, Mazzella F, et al. Frailty predicts long-term mortality in elderly subjects with chronic heart failure. European Journal of Clinical Investigation. 2005;**35**(12):723-730

[13] Purser JL, Kuchibhatla MN, Fillenbaum GG, Harding T, Peterson ED, Alexander KP. Identifying frailty in hospitalized older adults with significant coronary artery disease. Journal of American Geriatrics Society. 2006;**54**(11):1674-1681

[14] Boxer RS, Wang Z, Walsh SJ, Hager D, Kenny AM. The utility of the 6-minute walk test as a measure of frailty in older adults with heart failure. The American Journal of Geriatric Cardiology. 2008;**17**(1):7-12

[15] Dumurgier J, Elbaz A, Ducimetière P, Tavernier B, Alpérovitch A, Tzourio C. Slow walking speed and cardiovascular death in well functioning older adults: Prospective cohort study. British Medical Journal. 2009;**339**:b4460

[16] Sanchis J, Núñez E, Ruiz V, et al. Usefulness of clinical data and biomarkers for the identification of frailty after acute coronary syndromes. Canadian Journal of Cardiology. 2015;**31**(12):1462-1468

[17] Fried LP, Tangen CM, Walston J, et al. Frailty in older adults: Evidence for a phenotype. The Journal of Gerontology: Series A Biological Sciences and Medical Sciences. 2001;**56**(3):M146-M156

[18] Fedarko NS. The biology of aging and frailty. Clinics in Geriatric Medicine. 2011;**27**(1):27-37

[19] Wang Z, Nakayama T. Inflammation, a link between obesity and cardiovascular disease. Mediators of Inflammation. 2010;**2010**:535918

[20] Zakynthinos E, Pappa N. Inflammatory biomarkers in coronary artery disease. Journal of Cardiology. 2009;**53**(3):317-333

[21] Yao X, Li H, Leng SX. Inflammation and immune system alterations in frailty. Clinics in Geriatric Medicine. 2011;**27**(1):79-87

[22] Biala AK, Dhingra R, Kirshenbaum LA. Mitochondrial dynamics: Orchestrating the journey to advanced age. Journal of Molecular and Cellular Cardiology. 2015;**83**:37-43

[23] Keller KM, Howlett SE. Sex differences in the biology and pathology of the aging heart. Canadian Journal of Cardiology. 2016;**32**(9):1065-1073

[24] Liu CK, Lyass A, Larson MG, et al. Biomarkers of oxidative stress are associated with frailty: The Framingham Offspring Study. Age (Dordr). 2016;**38**(1):1

[25] Morley JE, Malmstrom TK. Frailty, sarcopenia, and hormones. Endocrinology & Metabolism Clinics of North America. 2013;**42**(2):391-405

[26] Soysal P, Stubbs B, Lucato P, et al. Inflammation and frailty in the elderly: A systematic review and meta-analysis. Ageing Research Reviews. 2016;**31**:1-8

[27] Michaud M, Balardy L, Moulis G, et al. Proinflammatory cytokines, aging, and age-related diseases. Journal of the American Medical Directors Association. 2013;**14**(12):877-882

[28] Hunter CA, Jones SA. IL-6 as a keystone cytokine in health and disease. Nature Immunology. 2015;**16**(5):448-457

[29] Akki A, Yang H, Gupta A, et al. Skeletal muscle ATP kinetics are impaired in frail mice. Age (Dordr). 2014;**36**(1):21-30

[30] Lavie CJ, De Schutter A, Alpert MA, Mehra MR, Milani RV, Ventura HO. Obesity paradox, cachexia, frailty, and heart failure. Heart Failure Clinics. 2014;**10**(2):319-326

[31] Niedernhofer LJ, Kirkland JL, Ladiges W. Molecular pathology endpoints useful for aging studies. Ageing Research Reviews. 2016;**35**:241-249

[32] Lang PO, Mitchell WA, Lapenna A, Pitts D, Aspinall R. Immunological pathogenesis of main age-related diseases and frailty: Role of Immunosenescence. European Geriatric Medicine. 2010;**1**:112-121

[33] Khan H, Kalogeropoulos AP, Georgiopoulou VV, et al. Frailty and risk for heart failure in older adults: The health, aging, and body composition study. American Heart Journal. 2013;**166**(5):887-894

[34] Feridooni HA, Dibb KM, Howlett SE. How cardiomyocyte excitation, calcium release and contraction become altered with age. Journal of Molecular and Cellular Cardiology. 2015;**83**:62-72

[35] Kalidindi SR, Tang WH, Francis GS. Drug insight: Aldosterone-receptor antagonists in heart failure--the journey continues. Nature Clinical Practice Cardiovascular Medicine. 2007;**4**(7):368-378

[36] Singh A, Williams GH. Textbook of Nephro-Endocrinology. 1st ed. Amsterdam, Boston: Elsevier/Academic Press; 2009

[37] Muñoz-Durango N, Fuentes CA, Castillo AE, et al. Role of the renin-angiotensin-aldosterone system beyond blood pressure regulation: Molecular and cellular mechanisms involved in end-organ damage during arterial hypertension. International Journal of Molecular Science. 2016;**17**(7):797

[38] Wright JT, Williamson JD, Whelton PK, et al. A randomized trial of intensive versus standard blood-pressure control. New England Journal of Medicine. 2015;**373**(22):2103-2116

[39] Beckett NS, Peters R, Fletcher AE, et al. Treatment of hypertension in patients 80 years of age or older. New England Journal of Medicine. 2008;**358**(18):1887-1898

[40] Langer RD, Criqui MH, Barrett-Connor EL, Klauber MR, Ganiats TG. Blood pressure change and survival after age 75. Hypertension. 1993;**22**(4):551-559

[41] Gueyffier F, Bulpitt C, Boissel JP, et al. Antihypertensive drugs in very old people: A subgroup meta-analysis of randomised controlled trials. INDANA Group. Lancet. 1999;**353**(9155):793-796

[42] Landi F, Cesari M, Calvani R, et al. The "Sarcopenia and Physical fRailty IN older people: Multi-componenT Treatment strategies" (SPRINTT) randomized controlled trial: Design and methods. Aging Clinical and Experimental Research. 2017;**29**(1):89-100

[43] Materson BJ, Garcia-Estrada M, Preston RA. Hypertension in the frail elderly. Journal of the American Society of Hypertension. 2016;**10**(6):536-541

[44] Warwick J, Falaschetti E, Rockwood K, et al. No evidence that frailty modifies the positive impact of antihypertensive treatment in very elderly people: An investigation of the impact of frailty upon treatment effect in the HYpertension in the Very Elderly Trial (HYVET) study, a double-blind, placebo-controlled study of antihypertensives in people with hypertension aged 80 and over. Boston Medical Center Medicine. 2015;**13**:78

[45] Pajewski NM, Williamson JD, Applegate WB, et al. Characterizing Frailty Status in the Systolic Blood Pressure Intervention Trial. The Journal of Gerontology Series A Biological Sciences and Medical Sciences. 2016;**71**(5):649-655

[46] van Hateren KJ, Hendriks SH, Groenier KH, et al. Frailty and the relationship between blood pressure and mortality in elderly patients with type 2 diabetes (Zwolle Outpatient Diabetes project Integrating Available Care-34). Journal of Hypertension. 2015;**33**(6):1162-1166

[47] Won CW, Kim S. Use of frailty in deciding clinical treatment goals for chronic disease in elderly patients in the community. Journal of the American Medical Directors Association. 2016;**17**(11):967-969

[48] Landi F, Russo A, Pahor M, et al. Serum high-density lipoprotein cholesterol levels and mortality in frail, community-living elderly. Gerontology. 2008;**54**(2):71-78

[49] Landi F, Russo A, Cesari M, Pahor M, Bernabei R, Onder G. HDL-cholesterol and physical performance: Results from the ageing and longevity study in the sirente geographic area (ilSIRENTE Study). Age Ageing. 2007;**36**(5):514-520

[50] Ramsay SE, Arianayagam DS, Whincup PH, et al. Cardiovascular risk profile and frailty in a population-based study of older British men. Heart. 2015;**101**(8):616-622

[51] van den Kommer TN, Dik MG, Comijs HC, Fassbender K, Lütjohann D, Jonker C. Total cholesterol and oxysterols: Early markers for cognitive decline in elderly? Neurobiology of Aging. 2009;**30**(4):534-545

[52] Roubenoff R, Parise H, Payette HA, et al. Cytokines, insulin-like growth factor 1, sarcopenia, and mortality in very old community-dwelling men and women: The Framingham Heart Study. American Journal of Medicine. 2003;**115**(6):429-435

[53] Hwang AC, Liu LK, Lee WJ, et al. Association of frailty and cardiometabolic risk among community-dwelling middle-aged and older people: Results from the I-Lan Longitudinal Aging Study. Rejuvenation Research. 2015;**18**(6):564-572

[54] Carriere I, Pérès K, Ancelin ML, et al. Metabolic syndrome and disability: Findings from the prospective three-city study. The Journal of Gerontology Series A Biological Sciences and Medical Sciences. 2014;**69**(1):79-86

[55] Wang X, Guo Z, Ding Z, et al. Endothelin-1 upregulation mediates aging-related cardiac fibrosis. Journal of Molecular and Cellular Cardiology. 2015;**80**:101-109

[56] Pulignano G, Del Sindaco D, Tinti MD, et al. Atrial fibrillation, cognitive impairment, frailty and disability in older heart failure patients. Journal of Cardiovascular Medicine (Hagerstown). 2016;**17**(8):616-623

[57] Bibas L, Levi M, Touchette J, et al. Implications of frailty in elderly patients with electrophysiological conditions. JACC: Clinical Electrophysiology. 2016;**2**(3):288-294

[58] Polidoro A, Stefanelli F, Ciacciarelli M, Pacelli A, Di Sanzo D, Alessandri C. Frailty in patients affected by atrial fibrillation. Archives of Gerontology and Geriatrics. 2013;**57**(3):325-327

[59] Nguyen TN, Cumming RG, Hilmer SN. The impact of frailty on mortality, length of stay and re-hospitalisation in older patients with atrial fibrillation. Heart, Lung and Circulation. 2016;**25**(6):551-557

[60] Veronese N, Cereda E, Stubbs B, et al. Risk of cardiovascular disease morbidity and mortality in frail and pre-frail older adults: Results from a meta-analysis and exploratory meta-regression analysis. Ageing Research Reviews. 2017;**35**:63-73

[61] Granziera S, Cohen AT, Nante G, Manzato E, Sergi G. Thromboembolic prevention in frail elderly patients with atrial fibrillation: A practical algorithm. Journal of the American Medical Directors Association. 2015;**16**(5):358-364

[62] Solfrizzi V, Scafato E, Frisardi V, et al. Frailty syndrome and the risk of vascular dementia: The Italian Longitudinal Study on Aging. Alzheimer's & Dementia. 2013;**9**(2):113-122

[63] Ruan Q, Yu Z, Chen M, Bao Z, Li J, He W. Cognitive frailty, a novel target for the prevention of elderly dependency. Ageing Research Review. 2015;**20**:1-10

[64] Chung CP, Chou KH, Chen WT, et al. Cerebral microbleeds are associated with physical frailty: A community-based study. Neurobiology of Aging. 2016;**44**:143-150

[65] Melin AA, Schmid KK, Lynch TG, et al. Preoperative frailty Risk Analysis Index to stratify patients undergoing carotid endarterectomy. Journal of Vascular Surgery. 2015;**61**(3):683-689

[66] Borissoff JI, Spronk HM, ten Cate H. The hemostatic system as a modulator of atherosclerosis. New England Journal of Medicine. 2011;**364**(18):1746-1760

[67] Libby P. Mechanisms of acute coronary syndromes and their implications for therapy. New England Journal of Medicine. 2013;**368**(21):2004-2013

[68] Afilalo J, Alexander KP, Mack MJ, et al. Frailty assessment in the cardiovascular care of older adults. Journal of American College of Cardiology. 2014;**63**(8):747-762

[69] Newman AB, Simonsick EM, Naydeck BL, et al. Association of long-distance corridor walk performance with mortality, cardiovascular disease, mobility limitation, and disability. Journal of American Medical Association. 2006;**295**(17):2018-2026

[70] Gharacholou SM, Roger VL, Lennon RJ, et al. Comparison of frail patients versus nonfrail patients ≥65 years of age undergoing percutaneous coronary intervention. American Journal of Cardiology. 2012;**109**(11):1569-1575

[71] Goodpaster BH, Carlson CL, Visser M, et al. Attenuation of skeletal muscle and strength in the elderly: The Health ABC Study. Journal of Applied Physiology (1985). 2001;**90**(6):2157-2165

[72] Srinivas-Shankar U, Roberts SA, Connolly MJ, et al. Effects of testosterone on muscle strength, physical function, body composition, and quality of life in intermediate-frail and frail elderly men: A randomized, double-blind, placebo-controlled study. Journal of Clinical Endocrinology and Metabolism. 2010;**95**(2):639-650

[73] Waters DL, Qualls CR, Dorin RI, Veldhuis JD, Baumgartner RN. Altered growth hormone, cortisol, and leptin secretion in healthy elderly persons with sarcopenia and mixed body composition phenotypes. The Journal of Gerontology Series A Biological Sciences and Medical Sciences. 2008;**63**(5):536-541

[74] Dodson JA, Arnold SV, Gosch KL, et al. Slow gait speed and risk of mortality or hospital readmission after myocardial infarction in the translational research investigating underlying disparities in recovery from acute myocardial infarction: Patients' Health Status Registry. Journal of American Geriatric Society. 2016;**64**(3):596-601

[75] O'Neill DE, Knudtson ML, Kieser TM, Graham MM. Considerations in cardiac revascularization for the elderly patient: age isn't everything. Canadian Journal of Cardiology. 2016;**32**(9):1132-1139

[76] Kang L, Zhang SY, Zhu WL, et al. Is frailty associated with short-term outcomes for elderly patients with acute coronary syndrome? Journal of Geriatric Cardiology. 2015;**12**(6):662-667

[77] Murali-Krishnan R, Iqbal J, Rowe R, et al. Impact of frailty on outcomes after percutaneous coronary intervention: A prospective cohort study. Open Heart. 2015;**2**(1):e000294

[78] Freiheit EA, Hogan DB, Patten SB, et al. Frailty trajectories after treatment for coronary artery disease in older patients. Circulation: Cardiovascular Quality and Outcomes. 2016;**9**(3):230-238

[79] Singh M, Rihal CS, Lennon RJ, Spertus JA, Nair KS, Roger VL. Influence of frailty and health status on outcomes in patients with coronary disease undergoing percutaneous revascularization. Circulation: Cardiovascular Quality and Outcomes. 2011;**4**(5):496-502

[80] Thukkani AK, Kinlay S. Endovascular intervention for peripheral artery disease. Circulation Research. 2015;**116**(9):1599-1613

[81] Suzuki J, Shimamura M, Suda H, et al. Current therapies and investigational drugs for peripheral arterial disease. Hypertension Research. 2016;**39**(4):183-191

[82] Ochi M, Kohara K, Tabara Y, et al. Arterial stiffness is associated with low thigh muscle mass in middle-aged to elderly men. Atherosclerosis. 2010;**212**(1):327-332

[83] Lin CH, Chou CY, Liu CS, Huang CY, Li TC, Lin CC. Association between frailty and subclinical peripheral vascular disease in a community-dwelling geriatric population: Taichung Community Health Study for Elders. Geriatrics & Gerontology International. 2015;**15**(3):261-267

[84] Toosizadeh N, Stocker H, Thiede R, Mohler J, Mills JL, Najafi B. Alterations in gait parameters with peripheral artery disease: The importance of pre-frailty as a confounding variable. Vascular Medicine. 2016;**21**(6):520-527

[85] Ehlert BA, Najafian A, Orion KC, Malas MB, Black JH, Abularrage CJ. Validation of a modified Frailty Index to predict mortality in vascular surgery patients. Journal of Vascular Surgery. 2016;**63**(6):1595-1601.e1592

[86] Arya S, Long CA, Brahmbhatt R, et al. Preoperative frailty increases risk of nonhome discharge after elective vascular surgery in home-dwelling patients. Annals in Vascular Surgery. 2016;**35**:19-29

[87] Brahmbhatt R, Brewster LP, Shafii S, et al. Gender and frailty predict poor outcomes in infrainguinal vascular surgery. Journal of Surgical Research. 2016;**201**(1):156-165

[88] Jha SR, Ha HS, Hickman LD, et al. Frailty in advanced heart failure: A systematic review. Heart Failure Reviews. 2015;**20**(5):553-560

[89] Nadruz W, Kitzman D, Windham BG, et al. Cardiovascular dysfunction and frailty among older adults in the community: The ARIC study. The Journal of Gerontology Series A Biological Sciences and Medical Sciences. 2016;**72**:958-964

[90] Lupón J, González B, Santaeugenia S, et al. Prognostic implication of frailty and depressive symptoms in an outpatient population with heart failure. Revista Española de Cardiología. 2008;**61**(8):835-842

[91] McNallan SM, Singh M, Chamberlain AM, et al. Frailty and healthcare utilization among patients with heart failure in the community. JACC Heart Failure. 2013;**1**(2):135-141

[92] Rolland Y, Dupuy C, Abellan van Kan G, Gillette S, Vellas B. Treatment strategies for sarcopenia and frailty. Medical Clinics of North America. 2011;**95**(3):427-438, ix

[93] Lavie CJ, Forman DE, Arena R. Bulking up skeletal muscle to improve heart failure prognosis. JACC Heart Failure. 2016;**4**(4):274-276

[94] Pendergast DR, Fisher NM, Calkins E. Cardiovascular, neuromuscular, and metabolic alterations with age leading to frailty. Journal of Gerontology. 1993;**48** Spec No:61-67

[95] Joyce E. Frailty in advanced heart failure. Heart Failure Clinics. 2016;**12**(3):363-374

[96] Carapetis JR, Steer AC, Mulholland EK, Weber M. The global burden of group A streptococcal diseases. The Lancet Infectious Diseases. 2005;**5**(11):685-694

[97] Kern DM, DeVore S, Kim J, et al. Abstract 53: Health care utilization and cost among type 2 diabetes mellitus (T2DM) patients with cardiovascular disease (CVD) or cardiovascular disease risk factors. Circulation: Cardiovascular Quality and Outcomes. 2015;**6**(Suppl 1):A53

[98] Chen J, Mallow PJ, Moore M, Rizzo JA. Abstract 257: The direct healthcare expenditures of aortic valve disease: Evidence from US National Survey Data. Circulation: Cardiovascular Quality and Outcomes. 2016;**9**(Suppl 2):A257

[99] Mirabel M, Iung B, Baron G, et al. What are the characteristics of patients with severe, symptomatic, mitral regurgitation who are denied surgery? European Heart Journal. 2007;**28**(11):1358-1365

[100] Bach DS, Awais M, Gurm HS, Kohnstamm S. Failure of guideline adherence for intervention in patients with severe mitral regurgitation. Journal of American College of Cardiology. 2009;**54**(9):860-865

[101] Vesely MR, Benitez RM, Robinson SW, Collins JA, Dawood MY, Gammie JS. Surgical and transcatheter mitral valve repair for severe chronic mitral regurgitation: A review of clinical indications and patient assessment. Journal of the American Heart Association. 2015;**4**(12):e002424

[102] Csordas A, Fuchs D, Frangieh AH, et al. Immunological markers of frailty predict outcomes beyond current risk scores in aortic stenosis following transcatheter aortic valve replacement: Role of neopterin and tryptophan. IJC Metabolic & Endocrine. 2016;**10**:7-15

[103] Nishimura RA, Otto CM, Bonow RO, et al. 2014 AHA/ACC guideline for the management of patients with valvular heart disease: a report of the American College of Cardiology/American Heart Association Task Force on Practice Guidelines. Journal of Thoracic and Cardiovascular Surgery. 2014;**148**(1):e1-e132

[104] Sepehri A, Beggs T, Hassan A, et al. The impact of frailty on outcomes after cardiac surgery: A systematic review. Journal of Thoracic and Cardiovascular Surgery. 2014;**148**(6):3110-3117

[105] Lee DH, Buth KJ, Martin BJ, Yip AM, Hirsch GM. Frail patients are at increased risk for mortality and prolonged institutional care after cardiac surgery. Circulation. 2010;**121**(8):973-978

[106] Chauhan D, Haik N, Merlo A, et al. Quantitative increase in frailty is associated with diminished survival after transcatheter aortic valve replacement. American Heart Journal. 2016;**182**:146-154

[107] Dahya V, Xiao J, Prado CM, et al. Computed tomography-derived skeletal muscle index: A novel predictor of frailty and hospital length of stay after transcatheter aortic valve replacement. American Heart Journal. 2016;**182**:21-27

[108] Sorajja P, Mack M, Vemulapalli S, et al. Initial experience with commercial transcatheter mitral valve repair in the United States. Journal of American College of Cardiology. 2016;**67**(10):1129-1140

[109] Morley JE, Vellas B, van Kan GA, et al. Frailty consensus: A call to action. Journal of American Medical Directors Association. 2013;**14**(6):392-397

11

Allogeneic Mesenchymal Stem Cells as a Treatment for Aging Frailty

Bryon A. Tompkins, Ana Marie Landin,
Victoria Florea, Makoto Natsumeda,
Angela C. Rieger, Wayne Balkan,
Ivonne Hernandez Schulman and Joshua M. Hare

Abstract

As life expectancy is projected to increase in the ensuing decades, individuals of older age continue to exceed the previous generation's lifespan. Advancing age is associated with a reduction in physical and mental functional capacity, and chronic inflammation is a major factor contributing to this decline. A heightened inflammatory state can lead to exhaustion, weakness, weight loss, slow gate speed, and an overall decrease in activity level. These phenotypes define the onset of the disease process known as frailty. Frailty is a growing epidemic, which severely undermines a person's ability to deal with outside stressors, and increases their rate of hospitalization, institutionalization, and mortality. Current interventions focus on preventative care by improving exercise capacity, strength, nutritional supplementation, diet, and mobility. However, a biological cure has heretofore remained elusive. Here, we introduce the novel therapeutic principle that mesenchymal stem cell (MSC) therapy may represent a safe, practical, and efficacious both the treatment and prevention of frailty in individuals of advancing age. To date, a phase I safety trial reveals an excellent safety profile and suggests that mesenchymal stem cells can ameliorate signs and symptoms of frailty. These early studies lay the groundwork for future large-scale clinical trials of this exciting and novel therapeutic concept that has the potential to expand health span in the aging population.

Keywords: mesenchymal stem cells, immunomodulation, frailty, tumor necrosis factor-alpha, regenerative medicine

1. Introduction

Projected life expectancy continues to grow worldwide owing to the advancement of new treatments and technologies for leading causes of death such as cardiovascular disease and cancer [1]. Meanwhile, frailty is gaining relevance as a significant clinical syndrome that is associated with increased risk of falls, depression, and disability, leading to higher mortality [2]. Frailty is defined by an age-related decline in reserve and function leading to a reduced ability to cope with acute or external stressors [3] and is characterized by easy tiring, decreased libido, mood disturbance, accelerated osteoporosis, diminished muscle strength, and susceptibility to disease. However, the pathophysiology underlying this syndrome is complex and not clearly understood [4].

Inflammation is a pathophysiologic change that is closely linked with frailty [5]. Aging is associated with immunosenescence or the dysregulation of the innate immune system, resulting in an increase of pro-inflammatory cytokines such as tumor necrosis factor (TNF)-α, interleukin (IL)-6, and IL-1β, further leading to a chronic low-grade inflammatory state [6]. Chronic inflammatory response inhibits the repair, turnover, and adaptation of many tissues, including skeletal muscle [6]. Regeneration of skeletal muscle involves the cross-talk of muscle cells with immune cells, where the pro-inflammatory phenotype of immune cells promotes migration of satellite cells to the injured area, activates satellite cells, and matures newly formed muscle fibers [7]. Muscular degeneration caused by the altered pro-inflammatory state in frail patients is referred to as sarcopenia, another critical physiologic component of frailty.

Aging also produces physiologic changes in the brain, contributing to the development of frailty. Neurons with high metabolic demands, such as the hippocampal pyramidal neurons, are an important mediator in the pathophysiology of cognitive decline and are a key component of the stress response [3]. Concomitant with changes in the immune system, microglial cells, which are the resident immune cells of the central nervous system, are also structurally and functionally altered with aging and undergo senescence, likely causing damage and neuronal death [8]. Accumulating evidence supports an association between frailty, cognitive impairment, and dementia [9, 10].

The brain and endocrine system are intrinsically linked through the hypothalamo-pituitary axis, controlling metabolism via a series of homeostatic hormones. Four major circulating hormones are affected by aging: first, the decrease of insulin-like growth factor 1 (IGF-1) is associated with lower strength and decreased mobility [11]. Second, decreased sex hormone (estradiol and testosterone) increases the release of luteinizing hormone and follicle-stimulating hormone [12]. Third, decreased activity of the adrenocortical cells produces the major sex steroid precursor dehydroepiandrosterone sulfate (DHEA-S), which is associated with a gradual rise in cortisol. DHEA-S directly maintains muscle mass and indirectly prevents the inflammatory pathways that contribute to muscle decline [13, 14]. Finally, the reduced level of 25(OH) vitamin D is associated with the development of osteoporosis [15].

Due to the complexity of multiple inter-related physiological systems that contribute to frailty, there is no gold standard for diagnosing the syndrome. There are currently two models for evaluating frailty: the phenotype model and the cumulative deficit model that forms the basis

Frailty phenotypes	MSC response	Postulated mechanism of action
Weight loss	Maintains total caloric expenditure	↓ Inflammation which suppresses the onset of sarcopenia
Exhaustion	↑ Pulmonary function, ↓ chronic inflammation	↑ Endothelial function, ↓ markers of inflammation
Weakness	↑ Physical performance	↑ Mitochondrial transfer, ↑endogenous stem cell function
Slow gate speed	↑ 6-minute walk distance	↑ Endothelial function, ↑ cardiac performance, ↑skeletal muscle performance
Decreased activity level	↓ Chronic inflammation, ↑ quality of life	↓ TNF-α, ↓ IL-1β, ↑ IL-10

Notes: MSCs home to sites of injury and to enhance repair of damaged tissue (heart, joints, muscle, and blood vessels) and exert their regenerative effects via paracrine signaling, mitochondrial transfer, direct cellular contact, and exosome excretion.

Table 1. The effect of MSCs on the phenotypes of frailty.

of the Canadian Study of Health and Aging (CSHA) frailty index [16]. The phenotype model defines frailty as meeting three or more of five criteria: weight loss (>5% of body weight in the previous year), exhaustion (positive response to questions regarding effort required for activity), weakness (decreased grip strength), slow gait speed (>6–7 seconds for walking 15 feet), decreased physical activity, or low energy expenditure (kcal spent per week: males expending <383 kcal, females expending <270 kcal) (**Table 1**) [17]. This model is simple and easy to use; however, it fails to include factors such as cognitive impairment and highly prevalent conditions associated with functional decline and disability [3].

The cumulative deficit model is based on the accumulation of illnesses, functional and cognitive declines, and social situations that are added together to calculate frailty [16]. This model utilizes 20 or more medically and functionally related questions and 92 baseline variables. The deficit model fashioned the origin of the CSHA frailty index [3]. The frailty index measures a number of age-associated health deficits (signs, symptoms, and laboratory values) [18], which is calculated by dividing each 'deficit' by the total number tested [3]. The higher the number of deficits, the higher the score, with '1' being the maximum index, which indicates a poorer prognosis. Specifically, Rockwood and Mitnitski noted that an index >0.7 indicates a high risk of mortality [19]. In an effort to simplify this index, the same authors proposed the CSHA clinical frailty score, a 7-point rapid screening tool that was highly correlated with the frailty index; with 7 being the maximum score, indicating "severe frailty" [20]. The clinical frailty score is currently widely used in clinical practice [21].

2. Epidemiology

Universal characteristics that are associated with an increased prevalence of frailty include: chronological age, female sex, racial, and ethnic minority, those in supportive residential settings, and lower income [22]. The prevalence among community-dwelling people over 65 years of age ranges from 4 to 17% in studies with varying geographic features [23, 24]. There are similar trends in Japan, the country with the highest life expectancy in the world. The reason for longevity in Japan is multifactorial. The universal health insurance system, the high population density with close access to hospitals, fish-based diets, awareness of healthy aging in the general public, and lower prevalence of lung cancer despite a higher population of smokers are some contributors [25]. Interestingly, a meta-analyses of frail Japanese patients using the phenotype model demonstrated that the age-stratified-weighted prevalence of frailty was lower in younger age groups (1.9% in 65–69 years, 3.8% in 70–74 years), the same in the 75–79-year age groups (10.0%), but higher in older age groups (20.4% in 80–84 years, 35.1% in ≥85 years) when compared to Western countries [25]. One explanation is that non-Japanese frail older individuals die younger, while Japanese frail older individuals survive longer, leading to a higher prevalence of frailty in their 80s.

3. Intervention and preventive care

While there is no cure for frailty, exercise is considered the most effective intervention to improve quality of life and functionality in frail adults. Improvements in muscle strength and mobility [26, 27] are among the most successful changes reported. Several studies have demonstrated an improvement in muscle strength in older persons with resistance exercise [28–30]. A longitudinal study of aging showed that physical activity is associated with a slower progression in functional limitations in older adults over a follow-up period of 6 months [31]. A randomized, placebo-controlled trial compared resistance exercise training, multinutrient supplementation, both interventions, and neither intervention (control group) in frail adults over a period of 10 weeks. The study suggested that high-intensity resistance exercise training improved muscle strength, gait velocity, and stair-climbing power. However, nutritional supplementation did not reduce muscle weakness or physical frailty [28]. Similarly, the LIFE-P (lifestyle interventions and independence for Elders pilot) exploratory study demonstrated that regular physical activity reduces frailty prevalence at a 12-month follow-up time point [32].

Another approach to delay frailty is the use of nutritional supplements, which increase protein and caloric daily intake. Administration of leucine-enriched essential amino acids can increase muscle synthesis through stimulation of the mechanistic target of rapamycin (mTOR) signaling pathway [33]. The PROT-AGE study [34] reviewed the dietary protein intake in older healthy people (>65 years). They found that the optimal protein intake in older persons with sarcopenia is 1.0–1.2 g/kg body weight per day, and higher protein intake >1.2 g/kg body weight per day for those who are exercising. The PROVIDE trial [35] assessed protein supplements enriched in leucine and vitamin D in sarcopenic older adults at high risk for disability. The study demonstrated that the group receiving high quantity protein supplements gained significantly more muscle mass and improved their chair stand ability relative to the control group.

The randomized Controlled Trial of Community-based Nutritional, Physical and Cognitive Training Intervention Programmes for At Risk Frail Elderly (FIT) compared the effects of 6-month interventions with either nutritional supplementation, cognitive training, physical activity, the combination treatments, or no intervention (control) in prefrail and frail adults [36]. Frailty score and status were measured at 3, 6 and 12 months. While these parameters were reduced in all groups, including the controls, the other four groups were significantly improved compared to the controls, at all three time points. However, none of the interventions improved the secondary endpoints, which included: hospitalizations, falls, and performance of activities of daily living [36]. Recent studies suggest that vitamin D plays a role in the pathogenesis and management of frailty [37, 38]. One such study demonstrated that daily doses of ≥800 IU of vitamin D has beneficial effects on balance and muscle strength [39]; while another reported an improvement in balance with a single large dose of vitamin D [40]. While an analysis of 53 trials showed that vitamin D supplementation alone does not prevent fractures in older adults [41], supplementation of vitamin D in combination with calcium can prevent disabling hip fractures among others [41].

While diet and exercise have been thoroughly evaluated, hormone therapy has also been tested. Testosterone undecanoate plus a high-calorie supplement (2108–2416 kJ/day) was compared with a control group (placebo plus a low-calorie supplement (142–191 kJ/day)) in a randomized controlled trial. The results showed that there were no significant differences in frailty scores at either 6- or 12-month follow-up between the groups [42]. While testosterone treatment improves muscle strength, it also increases incidence of adverse cardiovascular events [43]. Estrogen in combination with progestin therapy in postmenopausal women increases the risk of incident breast cancer after 5.6- or 7.1-years of follow-up [44, 45]. Likewise, the benefits of dehydroepiandrosterone sulfate (DHEA-S) supplementation in frail patients have not been demonstrated. Older subjects who received DHEA for 2 years exhibited no beneficial effects on body composition, physical performance, or quality of life [46]. Similarly, 1 year of treatment with insulin-like growth factor 1 (IGF-1) did not alter bone mineral density, fat mass, muscle strength, blood lipid parameters, and measures of postprandial glucose disposal in postmenopausal women [47].

Frailty is increasingly recognized as a clinical state of vulnerability with increased risk of adverse health outcomes. The pathogenesis that underlies this syndrome is multifactorial and elusive, and there is not yet a gold standard for diagnosis or treatment. Exercise and nutritional supplementations are currently the key interventions for frailty. Although helpful, none of them have been proven to treat the disease process. Therefore, an alternative approach to treating frail adults needs to be investigated. Here, we focus on a novel intervention, allogeneic mesenchymal stem cells (allo-MSCs) as a potential therapy for the treatment of frailty. While the mechanism is as yet unclear, we propose that the beneficial effects of MSCs for frailty are due, in large part, to a combination of their immunomodulatory, antifibrotic, and pro-regenerative effects.

4. Regenerative medicine

Frailty is a multifactorial condition triggered by genetic and environmental factors. As previously described, there is a direct association between frailty and the loss of proliferative homeostasis, neurodegeneration, DNA/mitochondrial mutations, free radical accumulation, a rise in pro-inflammatory markers, and increased immunosenescence. Stem cell depletion is a key mechanism postulated to contribute to frailty and its epigenetic dysregulation [48–50]. Thus, the repletion of stem cells is an appealing approach to treat this multifactorial dysregulation and MSCs are a particularly attractive candidate. MSCs are a multipotent, self-renewing somatic progenitor cell type that exhibits immunoprivileged properties [51–53] and are relatively easy to collect (bone marrow harvest), isolate, and expand [54, 55].

MSCs home to sites of injury, upregulate endogenous stem cells, and reduce inflammation and organ dysfunction [56–61]. With respect to age-related diseases, MSCs have demonstrated improvements in ischemic and nonischemic cardiomyopathies [62–64], stroke [65], systemic inflammation [66], and Parkinson's, among others [67]. Although not completely understood, the beneficial effects of stem cells are likely due primarily to paracrine signaling [68, 69] including microvesicle/exosome release [70, 71] and secondarily to direct cellular contact including gap junction formation [72] and mitochondrial exchange via tunneling nanotubes [73, 60].

MSC effects at the molecular level are secondary to the secretion of growth factors, chemokines, and metalloproteinases, including vascular endothelial growth factor (VEGF), angiopoetin-1, fibroblast growth factor, placental growth factor, stem cell-derived factor (SDF), plasminogen activator [74], hepatocyte growth factor/scatter factor (HGF/SF) [75], secreted frizzled-related protein 2 (Sfrp2), hypoxic-induced Akt-regulated stem cell factor (HASF) and IGF-1 and -2 [76]. These molecules stimulate the Akt pathway [77], promote vasculogenesis [56], and protect native cells under hypoxic conditions [68]. In the heart, injection of MSCs produces antifibrotic, anti-inflammatory, and proangiogenic [57–59] effects and upregulates the proliferation of endogenous cardiac stem cells [60, 61], while improving the preservation of function of the cells surrounding the sites of injection.

MSCs mediate metabolic changes and stimulate resident cell activation after injury. *In vitro* studies have shown that MSC-conditioned culture media stimulates resident cardiac stem cells to proliferate, differentiate, and migrate [53, 78] via IGF-1. HASF and Sfrp2 prevent cardiomyocyte apoptosis, promote cardiac stem cell differentiation, and reduce fibrosis after myocardial infarction (MI) [79–81].

The absence of major histocompatibility complex (MHC) class II antigens underlies the lack of allo-MSCs to stimulate a major immune response [82] and has generated an interest in their systemic and local application without the need for immunosuppression [62]. In the clinical setting, multiple trials have evaluated and proven the safety and efficacy of MSC therapy [63, 64, 83–85]. Several disease processes have been studied in humans: autoimmune diseases, organ transplantation, and as a therapeutic agent after solid organ injury.

5. Immune biomarkers in aging and frailty

Aging and frailty are associated with a dramatic impairment of the ability of the immune system to provide protection from new pathogens. Older frail individual has serious complications that cause adverse health outcomes including acute illness, heightened inflammatory state, and immune dysregulation, which cause a severe impairment in both innate and adaptive immunity and greater susceptibility to infectious diseases, comorbidities, and increased mortality [86, 87]. The accumulation of reactive oxygen species (ROS) in the aging process leads, in part, to chronic activation of Toll-like receptors (TLRs), which in turn leads to an increase in the inflammatory process [88–90]. In frailty, the immune phenotype is dysregulated due to incrementing chronic inflammation known as inflammaging and includes increased IL-6, C-reactive peptide (CRP), and TNF-α [87]. Inflammaging plays an important role in the suppression of the immune system and the remodeling of the immune phenotype (**Figure 1**). The remodeling of the immune phenotype in aging is known as immunosenescence and is marked by several immune biomarkers described below.

The immune risk phenotype (IRP), which is the ratio of CD4+ to CD8+ T cells, decreases to <1 in aging and frailty, has been linked to increased risk of mortality [91, 92]. The decreased IRP associated with aging and frailty is due to an expansion of the CD8+ compartment in comparison to the CD4+ compartment. In spite of the expansion of the CD8+ T-cell compartment, the effector T cells in frail individuals have diminished function mostly due to antigen experienced CD8+ T cells re-expressing the naïve marker CD45RA, also known as TEMRA T cells [87]. This expansion of the TEMRA T cell population is exacerbated by factors such as chronic activation due to Cytomegalovirus (CMV) exposure known to be present in >60% of the US population [93]. Finally, the ability to produce protective antibodies upon new antigenic exposure is also severely impaired in aging and frailty due to a remodeling of the B cell compartment. In addition, there is an intrinsic defect in B cells in aging, which causes a decrease in the enzyme, activation-induced cytidine deaminase (AID) leading to diminished ability to switch antibody isotype, which has been correlated to increased TNF-α [94]. The inflammaging process depletes the B cell compartment of switched memory B cells, which are a predictive biomarker for protective vaccine response. In addition, the refractory/exhausted B cell compartment is expanded filling up the B cell niche with unresponsive cells [86, 94, 95].

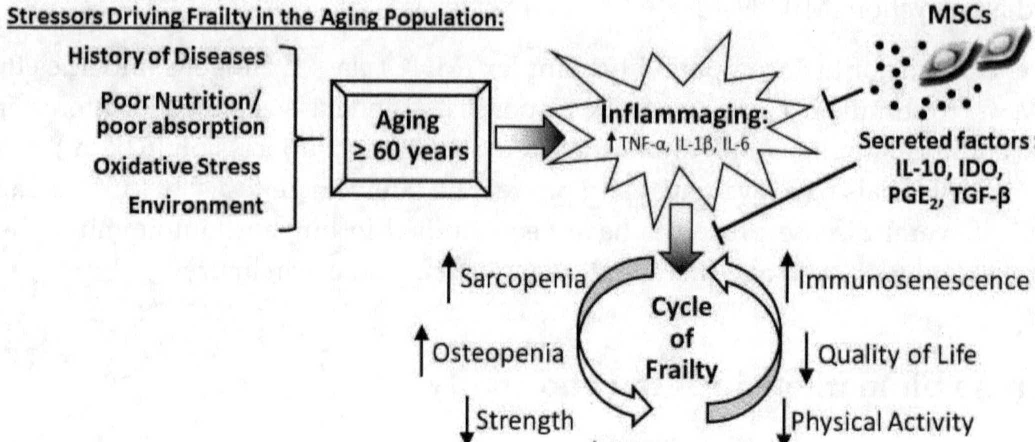

Figure 1. The role of stressors, aging, and inflammation in frailty and the effects of mesenchymal stem cells. As individuals grow older, several stressors (poor nutrition, diseases, oxidative stress, and environmental factors) increase the inflammaging process leading to frailty. Mesenchymal stem cells (MSCs) secrete several factors that block or reverse the inflammaging process and ultimately reverses the effects of frailty.

6. The role of MSCs in inflammaging and immune modulation

Human bone marrow-derived MSCs downregulate the expression of pro-inflammatory cytokines TNF-α, IL-1β, IL-6, and monocyte chemoattractant protein-1 (**Figure 2**) [96, 32]. Other immunomodulatory properties include the inhibition of dendritic cells, natural killer cells [97–99], and T/B cell proliferation via the downregulation of the molecules programmed death-1 (PD-1) transforming growth factor-β, HGF, nitric oxide, indoleamine 2,3-dioxygenase, and prostaglandin-E2 release [52, 68]. Interestingly, MSCs are able to transform pro-inflammatory macrophages (M1) into anti-inflammatory macrophages (M2) by upregulating IGF-1 and IL-10 [100], thereby promoting angiogenesis and cardiomyocyte recovery [101, 102]. Most importantly, MSCs suppress T cell activation, which is crucial due to the high incidence of CMV virus among the US population, causing chronic activation of T cells leading to an exhausted immune phenotype [103].

Ground-breaking immune-modulatory results in the Randomized Comparison of Allogeneic Versus Autologous Mesenchymal Stem Cells for Nonischemic Dilated Cardiomyopathy: POSEIDON-DCM study demonstrated that 6 months post-TESI, allogeneic human mesenchymal stem cells (hMSCs) were more efficient than auto-hMSCs in reducing serum levels of TNF-α, increased switched memory B cells, decreased exhausted B cells concomitant with a decrease in the percentage of B cells expressing TNF-α, decreased T cell activation and decreased TEMRA T cells [62]. This reversal on the effects of chronic inflammation on these immune biomarkers opens up the feasibility of using allo-hMSC as a treatment to reverse the process of inflammaging and immunosenescence.

Together, these findings are indicative of the safety of MSC therapy in a variety of disease processes. Furthermore, given that MSCs are known to elicit immunomodulatory, neoangiogenic,

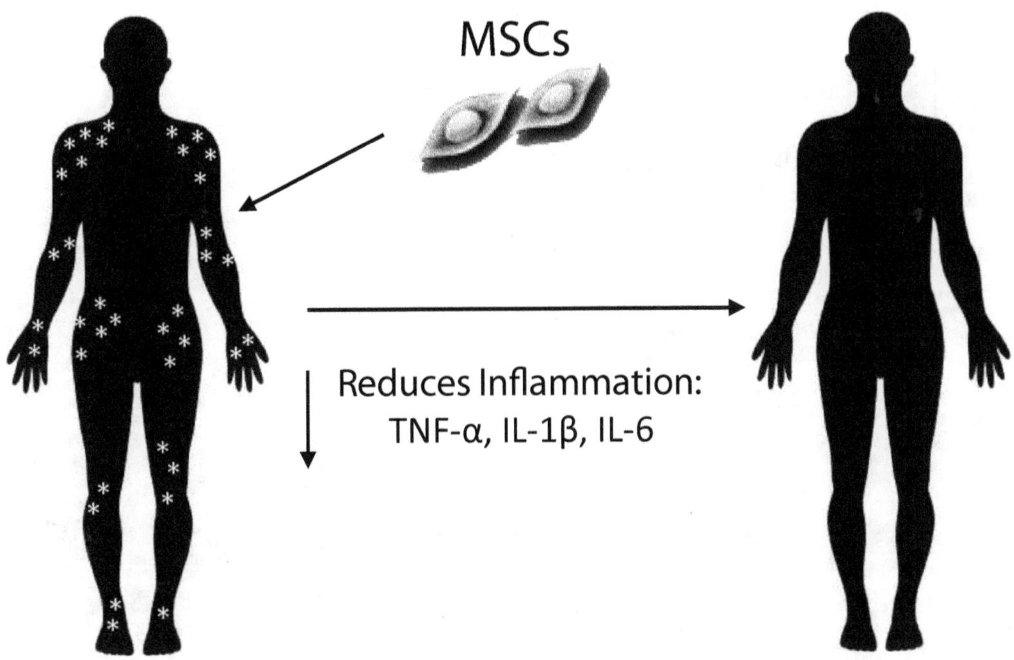

Figure 2. MSCs serve as an anti-inflammatory treatment. (A) Depiction of systemic inflammation (white asterisks'). (B). The anti-inflammatory effects of MSCs. Reproduced from Golpanian et al., with permission from the publisher.

endogenous cellular proliferative, and antifibrotic effects post-MI in both animal models and clinical trials alike, we anticipate that MSC therapy will act in a similar manner and prove beneficial in older individuals with frailty.

7. CRATUS phase I and II

The therapeutic interventions available to frail older individuals focus on improving the functionality of a precipitously declining quality of life. With the understanding that deteriorating endogenous stem cell function is a key mechanism behind this disease process, the allogeneic human mesenchymal stem cells (allo-hMSC) in patients with aging FRAilTy via intravenous delivery (CRATUS) trial (**Figure 3**) was established to reverse the untoward effects of frailty. Conducted at the University of Miami Miller School of Medicine, the pilot phase was designed to establish an optimal dose, and tested the hypothesis that allo-hMSCs were safe, well tolerated, and reduced the signs and symptoms of the disease [104]. The study was conducted in a nonrandomized, nonblinded, escalating dosage via peripheral intravenous infusion in 15 frail subjects [104]. Donors were healthy males and females between the ages of 20 and 45 [104]. Three groups of five patients each received either 20 million (M)-, 100M-, or 200M-cells [104]. Patients were followed out to 1-year postinfusion. The pilot phase revealed the two most salient doses (100M- and 200M-cells) [55] and was followed by

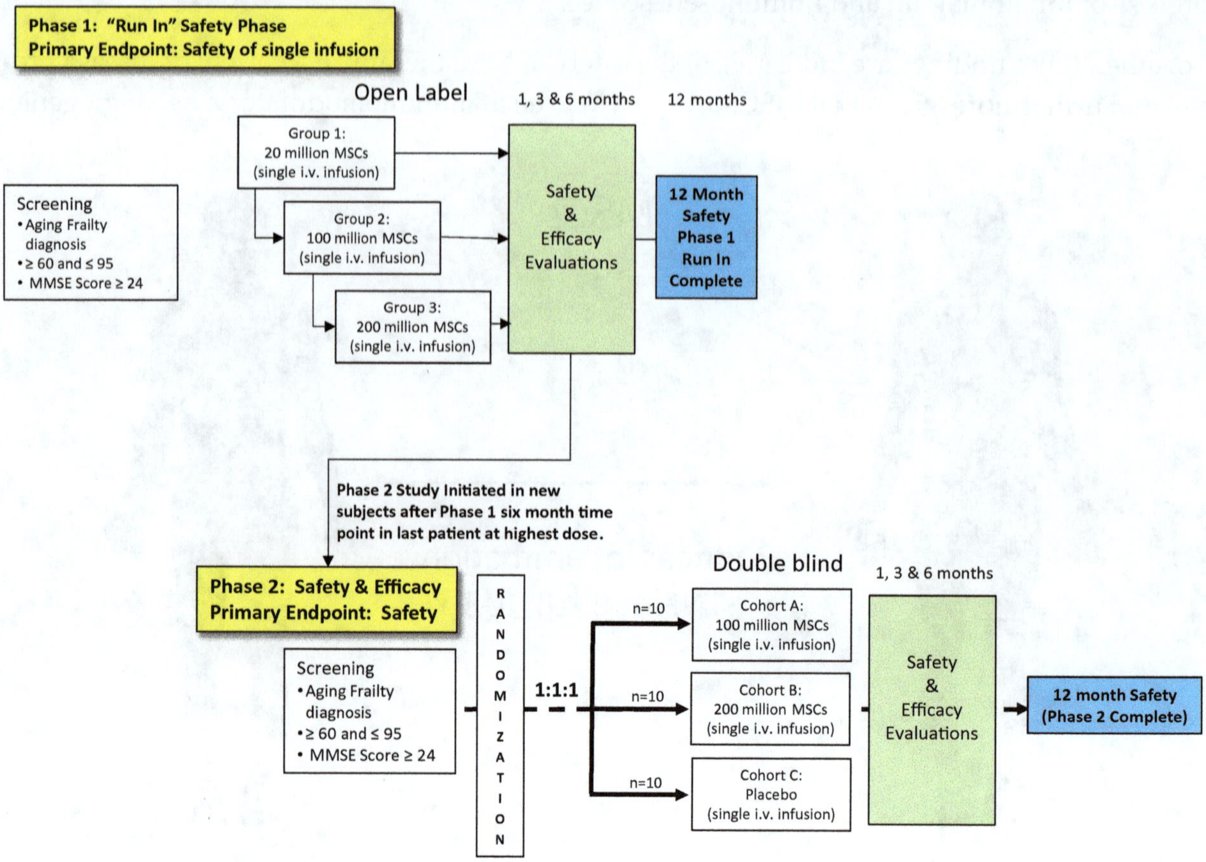

Figure 3. Schematic of the CRATUS pilot and randomized phases.

phase II, a randomized, double-blinded, placebo-controlled trial that further tested the safety and efficacy of allo-hMSCs in frail older individuals.

7.1. Results of the phase I study

The 15 subjects in the pilot phase had an average age of 78.4 ± 4.7 years [55]. Eight patients were categorized as vulnerable to frailty with a CSHA score of 4 and the others were mild, with a score of 6 (n = 6) and moderate with a score of 7 (n = 1) [55]. Most importantly, the primary endpoint, treatment-emergent serious adverse events (TE-SAE) at 1-month postinfusion, was met with no adverse reactions in any group [55].

Efficacy outcomes were measured out to 6 months postinfusion as a secondary endpoint. The 6-minute walk distance (6-MWD) test is a measure of functional exercise capacity [105], which can reflect a frail subject's ability to perform basic activities of daily living. The test has been specifically used to assess subjects with diseases of the musculoskeletal, pulmonary, and cardiovascular systems [106–108]; and as such, the subjects experienced a significant improvement in all treatment groups at 3 and 6 months postinfusion with the greatest improvement in the 100M cell-dose group in the phase I [55]. Pulmonary function was measured via FEV1, and improved in the 200M cell-dose group [55]. In regard to physical and quality of life improvement, the SF-36 questionnaire, which has a physical and mental component, yielded an improvement in the 100M-group in the pilot phase. Immunomodulation was also reported with a significant reduction in the pro-inflammatory biomarker serum TNF-α in the 100M and 200M cell-dose groups at 6 months postinfusion [55].

7.2. Update on the phase II study

The 30 subjects in phase II had a mean age of 75.5 ± 7.3 and a mean frailty score of 4 based on the CSHA Clinical Frailty Scale, and were equally randomized to receive 100M-, 200M-cells, or placebo [109]. Safety was the primary endpoint of the study and was measured via the occurrence of TE-SAE at 1-month postinfusion. The trial has completed enrollment, however, as reported in phase 1, preliminary findings show that the treatment is safe and produces significant improvements in the treated subjects in both quality of life and functional status [109].

8. Conclusion

Frailty has increasingly been recognized as a constellation of waning physical and mental qualities secondary to outside stressors, which relate to aging, and confer a vulnerability to adverse health outcomes [110]. Biologically, inflammation and stem cell depletion are at the forefront of this disease process. Early intervention is warranted at the onset of recognized symptoms to reduce the burden of disease progression, hospitalizations, and associated healthcare costs [111, 112]. To date, several important multimodal interventions are available to manage frailty; however, a disease-specific treatment has yet to emerge [112, 113]. Given the positive results of numerous studies utilizing MSCs in a variety of disease processes common to frailty as defined by the physical phenotype model, we believe stem cell therapy will be a treatment of choice for this disease process.

Future indications applicable to frailty	Response to MSCs	Proposed mechanisms of action
Osteoporosis	Improved bone mineral content and reduced rate of fractures	Reduction in ROS and increased AMPK
Heart disease	Improved function	Increased endothelial function, decreased inflammation, reduced cardiac fibrosis, and increased cardiomyogenesis
Delayed healing in Injury	Increased wound healing	Decrease inflammation (TNF-α and IL-1β), Increased IL-10
Autoimmunity	Delayed onset/prevention	Suppress TH17, induce T regs, and promote TH2 response

Table 2. MSCs and future indications.

Future implications of stem cell administration in frail or prefrail older individuals may be useful in settings where undo stress may cause rapid physical deterioration. There are a number of medical procedures (breast/colorectal cancer treatment, cardiac surgery, non-cardiac elective surgery, etc.) that are taxing to a young healthy individual let alone older individuals [114–116]. A preemptive or perioperative administration of MSCs may dampen the immune response, aid in the healing process, and keep at-risk older individuals from declining in functional status (**Table 2**) [56, 117–120]. Given the results from the CRATUS, pilot dose finding [55] and randomized placebo controlled study [109] and the number of medical procedures older individuals undergo, large, randomized, double-blinded clinical trials are warranted to elucidate the efficacy of stem cell therapy in regard to the disease process in itself and its ability to suppress the progression of frailty after strenuous medical interventions.

In summary, allogeneic MSCs are immunotolerant in frail older individuals providing clinically meaningful improvements in functional capacity, inflammatory biomarkers, and quality of life patient-reported outcomes. Frailty, the multimodal biologically mediated decline in physiologic reserve, may now have an optimistic therapeutic option.

Author details

Bryon A. Tompkins[1,2], Ana Marie Landin[1], Victoria Florea[1], Makoto Natsumeda[1], Angela C. Rieger[1], Wayne Balkan[1,3], Ivonne Hernandez Schulman[1,3] and Joshua M. Hare[1,3]*

*Address all correspondence to: jhare@med.miami.edu

1 The Interdisciplinary Stem Cell Institute, University of Miami Miller School of Medicine, Miami, USA

2 The Department of Surgery, University of Miami Miller School of Medicine, Miami, USA

3 The Department of Medicine, University of Miami Miller School of Medicine, Miami, USA

References

[1] Writing Group M, Mozaffarian D, Benjamin EJ, Go AS, Arnett DK, Blaha MJ, Cushman M, Das SR, de Ferranti S, Despres JP, Fullerton HJ, Howard VJ, Huffman MD, Isasi CR, Jimenez MC, Judd SE, Kissela BM, Lichtman JH, Lisabeth LD, Liu S, Mackey RH, Magid DJ, McGuire DK, Mohler ER, 3rd, Moy CS, Muntner P, Mussolino ME, Nasir K, Neumar RW, Nichol G, Palaniappan L, Pandey DK, Reeves MJ, Rodriguez CJ, Rosamond W, Sorlie PD, Stein J, Towfighi A, Turan TN, Virani SS, Woo D, Yeh RW, Turner MB, American Heart Association Statistics C, Stroke Statistics S. Heart disease and stroke statistics-2016 update: A report from the american heart association. Circulation. 2016;133(4):e38-360. DOI: 10.1161/CIR.0000000000000350

[2] Soysal P, Stubbs B, Lucato P, Luchini C, Solmi M, Peluso R, Sergi G, Isik AT, Manzato E, Maggi S, Maggio M, Prina AM, Cosco TD, Wu YT, Veronese N. Inflammation and frailty in the elderly: A systematic review and meta-analysis. Ageing Research Reviews. 2016;**31**:1-8. DOI: 10.1016/j.arr.2016.08.006

[3] Clegg A, Young J, Iliffe S, Rikkert MO, Rockwood K. Frailty in elderly people. Lancet. 2013;**381**(9868):752-762. DOI: 10.1016/S0140-6736(12)62167-9

[4] Gomes MJ, Martinez PF, Pagan LU, Damatto RL, Cezar MD, Lima AR, Okoshi K, Okoshi MP. Skeletal muscle aging: Influence of oxidative stress and physical exercise. Oncotarget. 2017;**8**(12):20428-20440. DOI: 10.18632/oncotarget.14670

[5] Chen X, Mao G, Leng SX. Frailty syndrome: An overview. Clinical Interventions in Aging. 2014;**9**:433-441. DOI: 10.2147/CIA.S45300

[6] Franceschi C, Campisi J. Chronic inflammation (inflammaging) and its potential contribution to age-associated diseases. The Journals of Gerontology. Series A, Biological Sciences and Medical Sciences. 2014;**69**(Suppl 1):S4-9. DOI: 10.1093/gerona/glu057

[7] Tidball JG, Villalta SA Regulatory interactions between muscle and the immune system during muscle regeneration. The American Journal of Physiology. 2010;**298**(5):R1173-1187. DOI: 10.1152/ajpregu.00735.2009

[8] Luo XG, Ding JQ, Chen SD. Microglia in the aging brain: Relevance to neurodegeneration. Molecular Neurodegeneration. 2010;**5**:12. DOI: 10.1186/1750-1326-5-12

[9] Boyle PA, Buchman AS, Wilson RS, Leurgans SE, Bennett DA. Physical frailty is associated with incident mild cognitive impairment in community-based older persons. Journal of the American Geriatrics Society. 2010;**58**(2):248-255. DOI: 10.1111/j.1532-5415.2009.02671.x

[10] Song X, Mitnitski A, Rockwood K. Nontraditional risk factors combine to predict Alzheimer disease and dementia. Neurology. 2011;**77**(3):227-234. DOI: 10.1212/WNL.0b013e318225c6bc

[11] Cappola AR, Xue QL, Ferrucci L, Guralnik JM, Volpato S, Fried LP. Insulin-like growth factor I and interleukin-6 contribute synergistically to disability and mortality in older women. The Journal of Clinical Endocrinology & Metabolism. 2003;**88**(5):2019-2025. DOI: 10.1210/jc.2002-021694

[12] Travison TG, Nguyen AH, Naganathan V, Stanaway FF, Blyth FM, Cumming RG, Le Couteur DG, Sambrook PN, Handelsman DJ. Changes in reproductive hormone concentrations predict the prevalence and progression of the frailty syndrome in older men: The concord health and ageing in men project. The Journal of Clinical Endocrinology & Metabolism. 2011;**96**(8):2464-2474. DOI: 10.1210/jc.2011-0143

[13] Leng SX, Cappola AR, Andersen RE, Blackman MR, Koenig K, Blair M, Walston JD. Serum levels of insulin-like growth factor-I (IGF-I) and dehydroepiandrosterone sulfate (DHEA-S), and their relationships with serum interleukin-6, in the geriatric syndrome of frailty. Aging Clinical and Experimental Research. 2004;**16**(2):153-157

[14] Lamberts SW. The endocrinology of aging and the brain. Archives of Neurology. 2002; **59**(11):1709-1711

[15] Puts MT, Visser M, Twisk JW, Deeg DJ, Lips P. Endocrine and inflammatory markers as predictors of frailty. Clin Endocrinology (Oxf). 2005;**63**(4):403-411. DOI: 10.1111/j.1365-2265.2005.02355.x

[16] Rockwood K, Mitnitski A. Frailty in relation to the accumulation of deficits. The Journals of Gerontology. Series A, Biological Sciences and Medical Sciences. 2007;**62**(7):722-727

[17] Fried LP, Tangen CM, Walston J, Newman AB, Hirsch C, Gottdiener J, Seeman T, Tracy R, Kop WJ, Burke G, McBurnie MA, Cardiovascular Health Study Collaborative Research G. Frailty in older adults: Evidence for a phenotype. The Journals of Gerontology. Series A, Biological Sciences and Medical Sciences. 2001;**56**(3):M146-156

[18] Rockwood K, Blodgett JM, Theou O, Sun MH, Feridooni HA, Mitnitski A, Rose RA, Godin J, Gregson E, Howlett SE. A frailty index based on deficit accumulation quantifies mortality risk in humans and in mice. Scientific Reports. 2017;**7**:43068. DOI: 10.1038/srep43068

[19] Rockwood K, Mitnitski A. Limits to deficit accumulation in elderly people. Mechanisms of Ageing and Development. 2006;**127**(5):494-496. DOI: 10.1016/j.mad.2006.01.002

[20] Rockwood K, Song X, MacKnight C, Bergman H, Hogan DB, McDowell I, Mitnitski A. A global clinical measure of fitness and frailty in elderly people. Canadian Medical Association Journal. 2005;**173**(5):489-495. DOI: 10.1503/cmaj.050051

[21] Ritt M, Ritt JI, Sieber CC, Gassmann KG. Comparing the predictive accuracy of frailty, comorbidity, and disability for mortality: A 1-year follow-up in patients hospitalized in geriatric wards. Clinical Interventions in Aging. 2017;**12**:293-304. DOI: 10.2147/CIA.S124342

[22] Bandeen-Roche K, Seplaki CL, Huang J, Buta B, Kalyani RR, Varadhan R, Xue QL, Walston JD, Kasper JD. Frailty in older adults: A nationally representative profile in the United States. The Journals of Gerontology. Series A, Biological Sciences and Medical Sciences. 2015;**70**(11):1427-1434. DOI: 10.1093/gerona/glv133

[23] Collard RM, Boter H, Schoevers RA, Oude Voshaar RC. Prevalence of frailty in community-dwelling older persons: A systematic review. Journal of the American Geriatrics Society. 2012;**60**(8):1487-1492. DOI: 10.1111/j.1532-5415.2012.04054.x

[24] Santos-Eggimann B, Cuenoud P, Spagnoli J, Junod J Prevalence of frailty in middle-aged and older community-dwelling Europeans living in 10 countries. The Journals of Gerontology. Series A, Biological Sciences and Medical Sciences. 2009;**64**(6):675-681. DOI: 10.1093/gerona/glp012

[25] Kojima G, Iliffe S, Taniguchi Y, Shimada H, Rakugi H, Walters K. Prevalence of frailty in Japan: A systematic review and meta-analysis. Journal of Epidemiology. 2016; pii:S0917-5040(16):30083-1. DOI: 10.1016/j.je.2016.09.008

[26] Clegg AP, Barber SE, Young JB, Forster A, Iliffe SJ. Do home-based exercise interventions improve outcomes for frail older people? Findings from a systematic review. Reviews in Clinical Gerontology. 2012;**22**(1):68-78. DOI: 10.1017/S0959259811000165

[27] Theou O, Stathokostas L, Roland KP, Jakobi JM, Patterson C, Vandervoort AA, Jones GR. The effectiveness of exercise interventions for the management of frailty: A systematic review. Journal of Aging Research. 2011;**2011**:569194. DOI: 10.4061/2011/569194

[28] Fiatarone MA, O'Neill EF, Ryan ND, Clements KM, Solares GR, Nelson ME, Roberts SB, Kehayias JJ, Lipsitz LA, Evans WJ. Exercise training and nutritional supplementation for physical frailty in very elderly people. New England Journal of Medicine. 1994;**330**(25):1769-1775. DOI: 10.1056/NEJM199406233302501

[29] Tieland M, Dirks ML, van der Zwaluw N, Verdijk LB, van de Rest O, de Groot LC, van Loon LJ. Protein supplementation increases muscle mass gain during prolonged resistance-type exercise training in frail elderly people: A randomized, double-blind, placebo-controlled trial. Journal of the American Medical Directors Association. 2012;**13**(8):713-719. DOI: 10.1016/j.jamda.2012.05.020

[30] Churchward-Venne TA, Tieland M, Verdijk LB, Leenders M, Dirks ML, de Groot LC, van Loon LJ. There are no nonresponders to resistance-type exercise training in older men and women. Journal of the American Medical Directors Association. 2015;**16**(5):400-411. DOI: 10.1016/j.jamda.2015.01.071

[31] Miller ME, Rejeski WJ, Reboussin BA, Ten Have TR, Ettinger WH. Physical activity, functional limitations, and disability in older adults. Journal of the American Geriatrics Society. 2000;**48**(10):1264-1272

[32] Cesari M, Vellas B, Hsu FC, Newman AB, Doss H, King AC, Manini TM, Church T, Gill TM, Miller ME, Pahor M, Group LS. A physical activity intervention to treat the frailty syndrome in older persons-results from the LIFE-P study. The Journals of Gerontology. Series A, Biological Sciences and Medical Sciences. 2015;**70**(2):216-222. DOI: 10.1093/gerona/glu099

[33] Malafarina V, Uriz-Otano F, Iniesta R, Gil-Guerrero L. Effectiveness of nutritional supplementation on muscle mass in treatment of sarcopenia in old age: A systematic review. Journal of the American Medical Directors Association. 2013;**14**(1):10-17. DOI: 10.1016/j.jamda.2012.08.001

[34] Bauer J, Biolo G, Cederholm T, Cesari M, Cruz-Jentoft AJ, Morley JE, Phillips S, Sieber C, Stehle P, Teta D, Visvanathan R, Volpi E, Boirie Y. Evidence-based recommendations

for optimal dietary protein intake in older people: A position paper from the PROT-AGE Study Group. Journal of the American Medical Directors Association. 2013;**14**(8):542-559. DOI: 10.1016/j.jamda.2013.05.021

[35] Bauer JM, Verlaan S, Bautmans I, Brandt K, Donini LM, Maggio M, McMurdo ME, Mets T, Seal C, Wijers SL, Ceda GP, De Vito G, Donders G, Drey M, Greig C, Holmback U, Narici M, McPhee J, Poggiogalle E, Power D, Scafoglieri A, Schultz R, Sieber CC, Cederholm T. Effects of a vitamin D and leucine-enriched whey protein nutritional supplement on measures of sarcopenia in older adults, the PROVIDE study: A randomized, double-blind, placebo-controlled trial. Journal of the American Medical Directors Association. 2015;**16**(9):740-747. DOI: 10.1016/j.jamda.2015.05.021

[36] Ng TP, Feng L, Nyunt MS, Feng L, Niti M, Tan BY, Chan G, Khoo SA, Chan SM, Yap P, Yap KB. Nutritional, physical, cognitive, and combination interventions and frailty reversal among older adults: A randomized controlled trial. The American Journal of Medicine. 2015;**128**(11):1225-1236 e1221. DOI: 10.1016/j.amjmed.2015.06.017

[37] Wong YY, Flicker L. Hypovitaminosis D and frailty: Epiphenomenon or causal? Maturitas. 2015;**82**(4):328-335. DOI: 10.1016/j.maturitas.2015.07.027

[38] Artaza-Artabe I, Saez-Lopez P, Sanchez-Hernandez N, Fernandez-Gutierrez N, Malafarina V. The relationship between nutrition and frailty: Effects of protein intake, nutritional supplementation, vitamin D and exercise on muscle metabolism in the elderly. A systematic review. Maturitas. 2016;**93**:89-99. DOI: 10.1016/j.maturitas.2016.04.009

[39] Muir SW, Montero-Odasso M. Effect of vitamin D supplementation on muscle strength, gait and balance in older adults: A systematic review and meta-analysis. Journal of the American Geriatrics Society. 2011;**59**(12):2291-2300. DOI: 10.1111/j.1532-5415.2011.03733.x

[40] Dhesi JK, Jackson SH, Bearne LM, Moniz C, Hurley MV, Swift CG, Allain TJ. Vitamin D supplementation improves neuromuscular function in older people who fall. Age and Ageing. 2004;**33**(6):589-595. DOI: 10.1093/ageing/afh209

[41] Avenell A, Mak JC, O'Connell D. Vitamin D and vitamin D analogues for preventing fractures in post-menopausal women and older men. The Cochrane Database of Systematic Reviews. 2014;(4):CD000227. DOI: 10.1002/14651858.CD000227.pub4

[42] Theou O, Chapman I, Wijeyaratne L, Piantadosi C, Lange K, Naganathan V, Hunter P, Cameron ID, Rockwood K, Visvanathan R. Can an intervention with testosterone and nutritional supplement improve the frailty level of under-nourished older people? The Journal of Frailty & Aging. 2016;**5**(4):247-252. DOI: 10.14283/jfa.2016.108

[43] Basaria S, Coviello AD, Travison TG, Storer TW, Farwell WR, Jette AM, Eder R, Tennstedt S, Ulloor J, Zhang A, Choong K, Lakshman KM, Mazer NA, Miciek R, Krasnoff J, Elmi A, Knapp PE, Brooks B, Appleman E, Aggarwal S, Bhasin G, Hede-Brierley L, Bhatia A, Collins L, LeBrasseur N, Fiore LD, Bhasin S. Adverse events associated with testosterone administration. The New England Journal of Medicine. 2010;**363**(2):109-122. DOI: 10.1056/NEJMoa1000485

[44] Rossouw JE, Anderson GL, Prentice RL, LaCroix AZ, Kooperberg C, Stefanick ML, Jackson RD, Beresford SA, Howard BV, Johnson KC, Kotchen JM, Ockene J, Writing Group for the Women's Health Initiative I. Risks and benefits of estrogen plus progestin in healthy postmenopausal women: Principal results from the women's health initiative randomized controlled trial. Journal of the American Medical Association. 2002;**288**(3):321-333

[45] Prentice RL, Manson JE, Langer RD, Anderson GL, Pettinger M, Jackson RD, Johnson KC, Kuller LH, Lane DS, Wactawski-Wende J, Brzyski R, Allison M, Ockene J, Sarto G, Rossouw JE. Benefits and risks of postmenopausal hormone therapy when it is initiated soon after menopause. American Journal of Epidemiology. 2009;**170**(1):12-23. DOI: 10.1093/aje/kwp115

[46] Nair KS, Rizza RA, O'Brien P, Dhatariya K, Short KR, Nehra A, Vittone JL, Klee GG, Basu A, Basu R, Cobelli C, Toffolo G, Dalla Man C, Tindall DJ, Melton 3rd LJ, Smith GE, Khosla S, Jensen MD. DHEA in elderly women and DHEA or testosterone in elderly men. The New England Journal of Medicine. 2006;**355**(16):1647-1659. DOI: 10.1056/NEJMoa054629

[47] Friedlander AL, Butterfield GE, Moynihan S, Grillo J, Pollack M, Holloway L, Friedman L, Yesavage J, Matthias D, Lee S, Marcus R, Hoffman AR. One year of insulin-like growth factor I treatment does not affect bone density, body composition, or psychological measures in postmenopausal women. The Journal of Clinical Endocrinology and Metabolism. 2001;**86**(4):1496-1503. DOI: 10.1210/jcem.86.4.7377

[48] Peffers MJ, Collins J, Loughlin J, Proctor C, Clegg PD.. A proteomic analysis of chondrogenic, osteogenic and tenogenic constructs from ageing mesenchymal stem cells. Stem Cell Research & Therapy. 2016;**7**(1):133. DOI: 10.1186/s13287-016-0384-2

[49] Sethe S, Scutt A, Stolzing A2006. Aging of mesenchymal stem cells. Ageing Research Reviews. 2006;**5**(1):91-116. DOI: 10.1016/j.arr.2005.10.001

[50] Stolzing A, Jones E, McGonagle D, Scutt A. Age-related changes in human bone marrow-derived mesenchymal stem cells: Consequences for cell therapies. Mechanisms of Ageing and Development. 2008;129(3):163-173. DOI: 10.1016/j.mad.2007.12.002

[51] Chapel A, Bertho JM, Bensidhoum M, Fouillard L, Young RG, Frick J, Demarquay C, Cuvelier F, Mathieu E, Trompier F, Dudoignon N, Germain C, Mazurier C, Aigueperse J, Borneman J, Gorin NC, Gourmelon P, Thierry D. Mesenchymal stem cells home to injured tissues when co-infused with hematopoietic cells to treat a radiation-induced multi-organ failure syndrome. The Journal of Gene Medicine 2003;**5**(12):1028-1038. DOI: 10.1002/jgm.452

[52] Augello A, Tasso R, Negrini SM, Amateis A, Indiveri F, Cancedda R, Pennesi G. Bone marrow mesenchymal progenitor cells inhibit lymphocyte proliferation by activation of the programmed death 1 pathway. European Journal of Immunology. 2005;35(5):1482-1490. DOI: 10.1002/eji.200425405

[53] Mourkioti F, Rosenthal N. IGF-1, inflammation and stem cells: Interactions during muscle regeneration. Trends in Immunology. 2005;**26**(10):535-542. DOI: 10.1016/j.it.2005.08.002

[54] Sanina C, Hare JM. Mesenchymal stem cells as a biological drug for heart disease: Where are we with cardiac cell-Based Therapy? Circulation Research. 2005;**117**(3):229-233. DOI: 10.1161/CIRCRESAHA.117.306306

[55] Golpanian S, DiFede DL, Khan A, et al. Allogeneic Human Mesenchymal Stem Cell Infusions for Aging Frailty. J Gerontol A Biol Sci Med Sci. DOI: 10.1093/gerona/glx056.

[56] Golpanian S, Wolf A, Hatzistergos KE, Hare JM. Rebuilding the damaged heart: Mesenchymal stem cells, cell-based therapy, and engineered heart tissue. Physiological Reviews. 2016;**96**(3):1127-1168. DOI: 10.1152/physrev.00019.2015

[57] Cao Y, Gomes S, Rangel EB, Paulino EC, Fonseca TL, Li J, Telxelra MB, Gouvela CH, Bianco AC, Kapiloff MS, Balkan W, Hare JM. S-nitrosoglutathione reductase–dependent PPARγ denitrosylation participates in adipogenesis and osteogenesis. The Journal of Clinical Investigation. 2015;**125**(4):1679-91. DOI: 10.1172/JCI73780

[58] Karantalis V, Hare JM. Use of mesenchymal stem cells for therapy of cardiac disease. Circulation Research. 2015;**116**(8):1413-1430. DOI: 10.1161/CIRCRESAHA.116.303614

[59] Karantalis V, DiFede DL, Gerstenblith G, Pham S, Symes J, Zambrano JP, Fishman J, Pattany P, McNiece I, Conte J, Schulman S, Wu K, Shah A, Breton E, Davis-Sproul J, Schwarz R, Feigenbaum G, Mushtaq M, Suncion VY, Lardo AC, Borrello I, Mendizabal A, Karas TZ, Byrnes J, Lowery M, Heldman AW, Hare JM. Autologous mesenchymal stem cells produce concordant improvements in regional function, tissue perfusion, and fibrotic burden when administered to patients undergoing coronary artery bypass grafting: The prospective randomized study of mesenchymal stem cell therapy in patients undergoing Cardiac Surgery (PROMETHEUS) trial. Circulation Research. 2014;**114**(8):1302-1310. DOI: 10.1161/CIRCRESAHA.114.303180

[60] Hatzistergos KE, Quevedo H, Oskouei BN, Hu Q, Feigenbaum GS, Margitich IS, Mazhari R, Boyle AJ, Zambrano JP, Rodriguez JE, Dulce R, Pattany PM, Valdes D, Revilla C, Heldman AW, McNiece I, Hare JM . Bone marrow mesenchymal stem cells stimulate cardiac stem cell proliferation and differentiation. Circulation Research. 2010;**107**(7):913-922. DOI: 10.1161/CIRCRESAHA.110.222703

[61] Premer C, Blum A, Bellio MA, Schulman IH, Hurwitz BE, Parker M, Dermarkarian CR, DiFede DL, Balkan W, Khan A, Hare JM. Allogeneic mesenchymal stem cells restore endothelial function in heart failure by stimulating endothelial progenitor cells. EBioMedicine. 2015;**2**(5):467-475. DOI: 10.1016/j.ebiom.2015.03.020

[62] Hare JM, DiFede DL, Castellanos AM, Florea V, Landin AM, El-Khorazaty J, Khan A, Mushtaq M, Lowery MH, Byrnes JJ, Hendel RC, Cohen MG, Alfonso CE, Valasaki K, Pujol MV, Golpanian S, Ghersin E, Fishman JE, Pattany P, Gomes SA, Delgado C, Miki R, Abuzeid F, Vidro-Casiano M, Premer C, Medina A, Porras V, Hatzistergos KE, Anderson E, Mendizabal A, Mitrani R, Heldman AW. Randomized comparison of allogeneic

vs. autologous mesenchymal stem cells for non-Ischemic dilated cardiomyopathy: POSEIDON-DCM trial. Journal of the American College of Cardiology. 2016; pii: S0735-1097(16)36906-6. DOI:10.1016/j.jacc.2016.11.009

[63] Hare JM, Traverse JH, Henry TD, Dib N, Strumpf RK, Schulman SP, Gerstenblith G, DeMaria AN, Denktas AE, Gammon RS, Hermiller JB, Jr., Reisman MA, Schaer GL, Sherman W. A randomized, double-blind, placebo-controlled, dose-escalation study of intravenous adult human mesenchymal stem cells (prochymal) after acute myocardial infarction. Journal of the American College of Cardiology. 2009;**54**(24):2277-2286. DOI: 10.1016/j.jacc.2009.06.055

[64] Hare JM, Fishman JE, Gerstenblith G, DiFede Velazquez DL, Zambrano JP, Suncion VY, Tracy M, Ghersin E, Johnston PV, Brinker JA, Breton E, Davis-Sproul J, Schulman IH, Byrnes J, Mendizabal AM, Lowery MH, Rouy D, Altman P, Wong Po Foo C, Ruiz P, Amador A, Da Silva J, McNiece IK, Heldman AW, George R, Lardo A. Comparison of allogeneic vs autologous bone marrow-derived mesenchymal stem cells delivered by transendocardial injection in patients with ischemic cardiomyopathy: The POSEIDON randomized trial. Journal of the American Medical Association. 2012;**308**(22):2369-2379. DOI: 10.1001/jama.2012.25321

[65] Gutierrez-Fernandez M, Rodriguez-Frutos B, Otero-Ortega L, Ramos-Cejudo J, Fuentes B, Diez-Tejedor E. Adipose tissue-derived stem cells in stroke treatment: From bench to bedside. Discovery Medicine. 2013;**16**(86):37-43

[66] Weiss DJ, Casaburi R, Flannery R, LeRoux-Williams M, Tashkin DP. A placebo-controlled, randomized trial of mesenchymal stem cells in COPD. Chest. 2013;**143**(6):1590-1598. DOI: 10.1378/chest.12-2094

[67] Trounson A, McDonald C. Stem cell therapies in clinical trials: Progress and challenges. Cell Stem Cell. 2015;**17**(1):11-22. DOI: http://dx. DOI.org/10.1016/j.stem.2015.06.007

[68] Hodgkinson CP, Bareja A, Gomez JA, Dzau VJ. Emerging concepts in paracrine mechanisms in regenerative cardiovascular medicine and biology. Circulation Research. 2016;**118**(1):95-107. DOI: 10.1161/CIRCRESAHA.115.305373

[69] Ranganath SH, Levy O, Inamdar MS, Karp JM. Harnessing the mesenchymal stem cell secretome for the treatment of cardiovascular disease. Cell Stem Cell. 2012;**10**(3):244-258. DOI: 10.1016/j.stem.2012.02.005

[70] Figeac F, Lesault PF, Le Coz O, Damy T, Souktani R, Trebeau C, Schmitt A, Ribot J, Mounier R, Guguin A, Manier C, Surenaud M, Hittinger L, Dubois-Rande JL, Rodriguez AM.. Nanotubular crosstalk with distressed cardiomyocytes stimulates the paracrine repair function of mesenchymal stem cells. Stem Cells. 2014;**32**(1):216-230. DOI: 10.1002/stem.1560

[71] Akyurekli C, Le Y, Richardson RB, Fergusson D, Tay J, Allan DS. A systematic review of preclinical studies on the therapeutic potential of mesenchymal stromal cell-derived microvesicles. Stem Cell Reviews. 2014;**11**(1):150-60. DOI: 0.1007/s12015-014-9545-9

[72] Hahn JY, Cho HJ, Kang HJ, Kim TS, Kim MH, Chung JH, Bae JW, Oh BH, Park YB, Kim HS. Pre-treatment of mesenchymal stem cells with a combination of growth factors enhances gap junction formation, cytoprotective effect on cardiomyocytes, and therapeutic efficacy for myocardial infarction. Journal of the American College of Cardiology. 2008;**51**(9):933-943. DOI: 10.1016/j.jacc.2007.11.040

[73] Mazhari R, Hare JM. Mechanisms of action of mesenchymal stem cells in cardiac repair: Potential influences on the cardiac stem cell niche. Nature Clinical Practice Cardiovascular Medicine. 2007;**4**(Suppl 1):S21-26. DOI: 10.1038/ncpcardio0770

[74] Kinnaird T, Stabile E, Burnett MS, Lee CW, Barr S, Fuchs S, Epstein SE. Marrow-derived stromal cells express genes encoding a broad spectrum of arteriogenic cytokines and promote in vitro and in vivo arteriogenesis through paracrine mechanisms. Circulation Research. 2004;**94**(5):678-685. DOI: 10.1161/01.RES.0000118601.37875.AC 01.RES.0000118601.37875.AC [pii]

[75] Weimar IS, Miranda N, Muller EJ, Hekman A, Kerst JM, de Gast GC, Gerritsen WR. Hepatocyte growth factor/scatter factor (HGF/SF) is produced by human bone marrow stromal cells and promotes proliferation, adhesion and survival of human hematopoietic progenitor cells (CD34+). Experimental Hematology. 1998;**26**(9):885-894

[76] Cheng SL, Zhang SF, Mohan S, Lecanda F, Fausto A, Hunt AH, Canalis E, Avioli LV. Regulation of insulin-like growth factors I and II and their binding proteins in human bone marrow stromal cells by dexamethasone. The Journal of Cellular Biochemistry. 1998;**71**(3):449-458

[77] Gnecchi M, He H, Liang OD, Melo LG, Morello F, Mu H, Noiseux N, Zhang L, Pratt RE, Ingwall JS, Dzau VJ. Paracrine action accounts for marked protection of ischemic heart by Akt-modified mesenchymal stem cells. Nature Medicine. 2005;**11**(4):367-368

[78] Engels MC, Rajarajan K, Feistritzer R, Sharma A, Nielsen UB, Schalij MJ, de Vries AA, Pijnappels DA, Wu SM. Insulin-like growth factor promotes cardiac lineage induction in vitro by selective expansion of early mesoderm. Stem Cells. 2014;**32**(6):1493-1502. DOI: 10.1002/stem.1660

[79] Schmeckpeper J, Verma A, Yin L, Beigi F, Zhang L, Payne A, Zhang Z, Pratt RE, Dzau VJ, Mirotsou M. Inhibition of Wnt6 by Sfrp2 regulates adult cardiac progenitor cell differentiation by differential modulation of Wnt pathways. Journal of Molecular and Cellular Cardiology. 2015;**85**:215-225. DOI: 10.1016/j.yjmcc.2015.06.003

[80] Kobayashi K, Luo M, Zhang Y, Wilkes DC, Ge G, Grieskamp T, Yamada C, Liu TC, Huang G, Basson CT, Kispert A, Greenspan DS, Sato TN. Secreted frizzled-related protein 2 is a procollagen C proteinase enhancer with a role in fibrosis associated with myocardial infarction. Nature Cell Biology. 2009;**11**(1):46-55. DOI: 10.1038/ncb1811

[81] Mastri M, Shah Z, Hsieh K, Wang X, Wooldridge B, Martin S, Suzuki G, Lee T. Secreted frizzled-related protein 2 as a target in antifibrotic therapeutic intervention. American Journal of Physiology Cell physiology. 2014;**306**(6):C531-539. DOI: 10.1152/ajpcell.00238.2013

[82] Karantalis V, Schulman IH, Balkan W, Hare JM. Allogeneic cell therapy: A new paradigm in therapeutics. Circulation Research. 2015;**116**(1):12-15. DOI: 10.1161/CIRCRESAHA.114.305495

[83] Hare JM, DiFede DL, Rieger AC, Florea V, Landin AM, El-Khorazaty J, Khan A, Mushtaq M, Lowery MH, Byrnes JJ, Hendel RC, Cohen MG, Alfonso CE, Valasaki K, Pujol MV, Golpanian S, Ghersin E, Fishman JE, Pattany P, Gomes SA, Delgado C, Miki R, Abuzeid F, Vidro-Casiano M, Premer C, Medina A, Porras V, Hatzistergos KE, Anderson E, Mendizabal A, Mitrani R, Heldman AW. Randomized comparison of allogeneic versus autologous mesenchymal stem cells for nonischemic dilated cardiomyopathy: POSEIDON-DCM trial. Journal of the American College of Cardiology. 2017;**69**(5):526-537. DOI: 10.1016/j.jacc.2016.11.009

[84] Chen SL, Fang WW, Ye F, Liu YH, Qian J, Shan SJ, Zhang JJ, Chunhua RZ, Liao LM, Lin S, Sun JP. Effect on left ventricular function of intracoronary transplantation of autologous bone marrow mesenchymal stem cell in patients with acute myocardial infarction. The American Journal of Cardiology. 2004;**94**(1):92-95. DOI: 10.1016/j.amjcard.2004.03.034

[85] Chullikana A, Majumdar AS, Gottipamula S, Krishnamurthy S, Kumar AS, Prakash VS, Gupta PK. Randomized, double-blind, phase I/II study of intravenous allogeneic mesenchymal stromal cells in acute myocardial infarction. Cytotherapy. 2015;**17**(3):250-261. DOI: 10.1016/j.jcyt.2014.10.009

[86] Frasca D, Blomberg BB . Inflammaging decreases adaptive and innate immune responses in mice and humans. Biogerontology. 2016;**17**(1):7-19. DOI: 10.1007/s10522-015-9578-8

[87] Mitnitski A, Collerton J, Martin-Ruiz C, Jagger C, von Zglinicki T, Rockwood K, Kirkwood TB. Age-related frailty and its association with biological markers of ageing. BMC Medicine. 2015;**13**:161. DOI: 10.1186/s12916-015-0400-x

[88] Cannizzo ES, Clement CC, Sahu R, Follo C, Santambrogio L. Oxidative stress, inflammaging and immunosenescence. Journal of Proteomics. 2011;**74**(11):2313-2323. DOI: 10.1016/j.jprot.2011.06.005

[89] Albert C. Shaw SJ, Hannah Greenwood, Alexander Panda, and Janet M. Lord. Aging of the Innate Immune System. Current Opinion in Immunology. 2010;**22**(4):507-513. DOI: 10.1016/j.coi.2010.05.003

[90] Dewan SK, Zheng SB, Xia SJ, Bill K . Senescent remodeling of the immune system and its contribution to the predisposition of the elderly to infections. Chinese Medical Journal(Engl)). 2012;**125**(18):3325-3331

[91] Wikby A, Ferguson F, Forsey R, Thompson J, Strindhall J, Lofgren S, Nilsson BO, Ernerudh J, Pawelec G, Johansson B. An immune risk phenotype, cognitive impairment, and survival in very late life: Impact of allostatic load in Swedish octogenarian and nonagenarian humans. Journals of Gerontology Series A Biological Sciences and Medical Sciences. 2005;**60**(5):556-565

[92] Pawelec G. Immunity and ageing in man. Experimental Gerontology. 2006;**41**(12):1239-1242. DOI: 10.1016/j.exger.2006.09.005

[93] Zhang LJ, Hanff P, Rutherford C, Churchill WH, Crumpacker CS. Detection of human cytomegalovirus DNA, RNA, and antibody in normal donor blood. Journal of Infectious Diseases. 1995;**171**(4):1002-1006

[94] Frasca D, Diaz A, Romero M, Landin AM, Phillips M, Lechner SC, Ryan JG, Blomberg BB. Intrinsic defects in B cell response to seasonal influenza vaccination in elderly humans. Vaccine. 2010;**28**(51):8077-8084

[95] Frasca D, Diaz A, Romero M, Phillips M, Mendez NV, Landin AM, Blomberg BB. Unique biomarkers for B-cell function predict the serum response to pandemic H1N1 influenza vaccine. International Immunology. 2012;**24**(3):175-182. DOI: 10.1093/intimm/dxr123

[96] Ortiz LA, Dutreil M, Fattman C, Pandey AC, Torres G, Go K, Phinney DG. Interleukin 1 receptor antagonist mediates the antiinflammatory and antifibrotic effect of mesenchymal stem cells during lung injury. Proceedings of the National Academy of Sciences of the United States of America . 2007;**104**(26):11002-11007. DOI: 10.1073/pnas.0704421104

[97] Djouad F, Charbonnier LM, Bouffi C, Louis-Plence P, Bony C, Apparailly F, Cantos C, Jorgensen C, Noel D. Mesenchymal stem cells inhibit the differentiation of dendritic cells through an interleukin-6-dependent mechanism. Stem Cells. 2007;**25**(8):2025-2032. DOI: 10.1634/stemcells.2006-0548

[98] Spaggiari GM, Abdelrazik H, Becchetti F, Moretta L. MSCs inhibit monocyte-derived DC maturation and function by selectively interfering with the generation of immature DCs: Central role of MSC-derived prostaglandin E2. Blood. 2009;**113**(26):6576-6583. DOI: 10.1182/blood-2009-02-203943

[99] Spaggiari GM, Capobianco A, Abdelrazik H, Becchetti F, Mingari MC, Moretta L. Mesenchymal stem cells inhibit natural killer-cell proliferation, cytotoxicity, and cytokine production: Role of indoleamine 2,3-dioxygenase and prostaglandin E2. Blood. 2008;**111**(3):1327-1333. DOI: 10.1182/blood-2007-02-074997

[100] Burchfield JS, Iwasaki M, Koyanagi M, Urbich C, Rosenthal N, Zeiher AM, Dimmeler S. Interleukin-10 from transplanted bone marrow mononuclear cells contributes to cardiac protection after myocardial infarction. Circulation Research. 2008;**103**(2):203-211. DOI: 10.1161/circresaha.108.178475

[101] Yano T, Miura T, Whittaker P, Miki T, Sakamoto J, Nakamura Y, Ichikawa Y, Ikeda Y, Kobayashi H, Ohori K, Shimamoto K. Macrophage colony-stimulating factor treatment after myocardial infarction attenuates left ventricular dysfunction by accelerating infarct repair. Journal of the American College of Cardiology. 2006;**47**(3):626-634. DOI: 10.1016/j.jacc.2005.09.037

[102] Troidl C, Mollmann H, Nef H, Masseli F, Voss S, Szardien S, Willmer M, Rolf A, Rixe J, Troidl K, Kostin S, Hamm C, Elsasser A. Classically and alternatively activated macrophages

contribute to tissue remodelling after myocardial infarction. Journal of Cellular and Molecular Medicine. 2009;**13**(9b):3485-3496. DOI: 10.1111/j.1582-4934.2009.00707.x

[103] van der Heiden M, van Zelm MC, Bartol SJ, de Rond LG, Berbers GA, Boots AM, Buisman A-M. Differential effects of Cytomegalovirus carriage on the immune phenotype of middle-aged males and females. Scientific Reports. 2016;**6**:26892

[104] Golpanian S, DiFede DL, Pujol MV, Lowery MH, Levis-Dusseau S, Goldstein BJ, Schulman IH, Longsomboon B, Wolf A, Khan A, Heldman AW, Goldschmidt-Clermont PJ, Hare JM. Rationale and design of the allogeneiC human mesenchymal stem cells (hMSC) in patients with aging fRAilTy via intravenoUS delivery (CRATUS) study: A phase I/II, randomized, blinded and placebo controlled trial to evaluate the safety and potential efficacy of allogeneic human mesenchymal stem cell infusion in patients with aging frailty. Oncotarget. 2016;**7**(11):11899-11912. DOI: 10.18632/oncotarget.7727

[105] Guyatt GH, Sullivan MJ, Thompson PJ, Fallen EL, Pugsley SO, Taylor DW, Berman LB.. The 6-minute walk: A new measure of exercise capacity in patients with chronic heart failure. Canadian Medical Association Journal. 1985;**132**(8):919-923

[106] Castillo-Moreno JA, Garcia-Escribano IA, Martinez-Pascual-de-Riquelme M, Jaulent-Huertas L, Dau-Villarreal DF, Rubio-Paton R, Giner-Caro JA, Bonaque-Gonzalez JC, Consuegra-Sanchez L. Prognostic usefulness of the 6-minute walk test in patients with severe aortic stenosis. American Journal of Cardiology. 2016;**118**(8):1239-1243. DOI: 10.1016/j.amjcard.2016.07.042

[107] Albarrati AM, Gale NS, Enright S, Munnery MM, Cockcroft JR, Shale DJ. A simple and rapid test of physical performance inchronic obstructive pulmonary disease. International Journal of Chronic Obstructive Pulmonary Disease. 2016;**11**:1785-1791. DOI: 10.2147/COPD.S106151

[108] Bello L, Campadello P, Barp A, Fanin M, Semplicini C, Soraru G, Caumo L, Calore C, Angelini C, Pegoraro E. Functional changes in Becker muscular dystrophy: Implications for clinical trials in dystrophinopathies. Scientific Reports. 2016;**6**:32439. DOI: 10.1038/srep32439

[109] Hare JM, Difede DL, Khan A, Landin AM, Tompkins B, Goldschmidt PJ, Mendizabal A. Allogeneic mesenchymal stem cells to treat aging frailty: A randomized, placebo-controlled intervention study. The Gerontologist. 2016;**56**(Suppl 3):50-51

[110] Walston J, Hadley EC, Ferrucci L, Guralnik JM, Newman AB, Studenski SA, Ershler WB, Harris T, Fried LP. Research agenda for frailty in older adults: Toward a better understanding of physiology and etiology: Summary from the American Geriatrics Society/National Institute on Aging Research Conference on Frailty in Older Adults. Journal of the American Geriatrics Society. 2006;**54**(6):991-1001. DOI: 10.1111/j.1532-5415.2006.00745.x

[111] Cerreta F, Eichler HG, Rasi G. Drug policy for an aging population--the European Medicines Agency's geriatric medicines strategy. The New England Journal of Medicine. 2012;**367**(21):1972-1974. DOI: 10.1056/NEJMp1209034

[112] Morley JE, Vellas B, van Kan GA, Anker SD, Bauer JM, Bernabei R, Cesari M, Chumlea WC, Doehner W, Evans J, Fried LP, Guralnik JM, Katz PR, Malmstrom TK, McCarter RJ, Gutierrez Robledo LM, Rockwood K, von Haehling S, Vandewoude MF, Walston J. Frailty consensus: A call to action. Journal of the American Medical Directors Association 2013;**14**(6):392-397. DOI: 10.1016/j.jamda.2013.03.022

[113] Xue QL. The frailty syndrome: Definition and natural history. Clinics in Geriatric Medicine 2011;**27**(1):1-15. DOI: 10.1016/j.cger.2010.08.009

[114] van Abbema D, van Vuuren A, van den Berkmortel F, van den Akker M, Deckx L, Buntinx F, van Kampen R, Lambooij E, de Boer M, de Vos-Geelen J, Tjan-Heijnen VC. Functional status decline in older patients with breast and colorectal cancer after cancer treatment: A prospective cohort study. Journal of Geriatric Oncology. 2017; pii: S1879-4068(17)30023-1. DOI:10.1016/j.jgo.2017.01.003

[115] Kim DH, Kim CA, Placide S, Lipsitz LA, Marcantonio ER. Preoperative frailty assessment and outcomes at 6 months or later in older adults undergoing cardiac surgical procedures: A systematic review. Annals of Internal Medicine. 2016;**165**(9):650-660. DOI: 10.7326/M16-0652

[116] CA Polanczyk, E Marcantonio, L Goldman, LEP Rohde, J Orav, CM Mangione, TH Lee. Impact of Age on Perioperative Complications and Length of Stay in Patients Undergoing Noncardiac Surgery. **Annals of Internal Medicine** 2001;**134**:637-643

[117] Sharaf-Eldin WE, Abu-Shahba N, Mahmoud M, El-Badri N. The modulatory effects of mesenchymal stem cells on osteoclastogenesis. Stem Cells International. 2016;2016:1908365. DOI: 10.1155/2016/1908365

[118] Takano T, Li YJ, Kukita A, Yamaza T, Ayukawa Y, Moriyama K, Uehara N, Nomiyama H, Koyano K, Kukita T. Mesenchymal stem cells markedly suppress inflammatory bone destruction in rats with adjuvant-induced arthritis. Laboratory Investigation. 2014;**94**(3):286-296. DOI: 10.1038/labinvest.2013.152

[119] Wei X, Yang X, Han ZP, Qu FF, Shao L, Shi YF. Mesenchymal stem cells: A new trend for cell therapy. Acta Pharmacologica Sinica. 2013;**34**(6):747-754. DOI: 10.1038/aps.2013.50

[120] Rastegar F, Shenaq D, Huang J, Zhang W, Zhang BQ, He BC, Chen L, Zuo GW, Luo Q, Shi Q, Wagner ER, Huang E, Gao Y, Gao JL, Kim SH, Zhou JZ, Bi Y, Su Y, Zhu G, Luo J, Luo X, Qin J, Reid RR, Luu HH, Haydon RC, Deng ZL, He TC. Mesenchymal stem cells: Molecular characteristics and clinical applications. World Journal of Stem Cells. 2010;**2**(4):67-80. DOI: 10.4252/wjsc.v2.i4.67

Permissions

All chapters in this book were first published in FSODCC, by InTech Open; hereby published with permission under the Creative Commons Attribution License or equivalent. Every chapter published in this book has been scrutinized by our experts. Their significance has been extensively debated. The topics covered herein carry significant findings which will fuel the growth of the discipline. They may even be implemented as practical applications or may be referred to as a beginning point for another development.

The contributors of this book come from diverse backgrounds, making this book a truly international effort. This book will bring forth new frontiers with its revolutionizing research information and detailed analysis of the nascent developments around the world.

We would like to thank all the contributing authors for lending their expertise to make the book truly unique. They have played a crucial role in the development of this book. Without their invaluable contributions this book wouldn't have been possible. They have made vital efforts to compile up to date information on the varied aspects of this subject to make this book a valuable addition to the collection of many professionals and students.

This book was conceptualized with the vision of imparting up-to-date information and advanced data in this field. To ensure the same, a matchless editorial board was set up. Every individual on the board went through rigorous rounds of assessment to prove their worth. After which they invested a large part of their time researching and compiling the most relevant data for our readers.

The editorial board has been involved in producing this book since its inception. They have spent rigorous hours researching and exploring the diverse topics which have resulted in the successful publishing of this book. They have passed on their knowledge of decades through this book. To expedite this challenging task, the publisher supported the team at every step. A small team of assistant editors was also appointed to further simplify the editing procedure and attain best results for the readers.

Apart from the editorial board, the designing team has also invested a significant amount of their time in understanding the subject and creating the most relevant covers. They scrutinized every image to scout for the most suitable representation of the subject and create an appropriate cover for the book.

The publishing team has been an ardent support to the editorial, designing and production team. Their endless efforts to recruit the best for this project, has resulted in the accomplishment of this book. They are a veteran in the field of academics and their pool of knowledge is as vast as their experience in printing. Their expertise and guidance has proved useful at every step. Their uncompromising quality standards have made this book an exceptional effort. Their encouragement from time to time has been an inspiration for everyone.

The publisher and the editorial board hope that this book will prove to be a valuable piece of knowledge for researchers, students, practitioners and scholars across the globe.

List of Contributors

Harnish P Patel
Academic Geriatric Medicine, University Hospital Southampton, UK
Department of Medicine for Older People, University Hospital Southampton, UK
NIHR Biomedical Research Centre, Southampton, UK
MRC Lifecourse Epidemiology Unit, University of Southampton, Southampton, UK

Esther Clift and Lucy Lewis
Health Education England, Wessex, UK

Cyrus Cooper
MRC Lifecourse Epidemiology Unit, University of Southampton, Southampton, UK
University of Oxford, Oxford, UK

Rosaly Correa-de-Araujo
Division of Geriatrics and Clinical Gerontology, National Institute on Aging, National Institutes of Health, U.S. Department of Health and Human Services, Bethesda, MD, USA

Zhuowei Yu and Qingwei Ruan
Shanghai Institute of Geriatrics and Gerontology, Shanghai Key Laboratory of Clinical Geriatrics, Huadong Hospital, Shanghai, China
Research Center of Aging and Medicine, Shanghai Medical College, Fudan University, Shanghai, China

Grazia D'Onofrio and Antonio Greco
Department of Medical Sciences, Geriatric Unit & Laboratory of Gerontology and Geriatrics, IRCCS "Casa Sollievo della Sofferenza", San Giovanni Rotondo, Foggia, Italy

Beatriz Lardiés-Sánchez and Alejandro Sanz-París
Universitary Hospital Miguel Servet, Zaragoza, Spain

Kotomi Sakai
Department of Rehabilitation, Setagaya Memorial Hospital, Tokyo, Japan
Department of Dysphagia Rehabilitation, Nihon University School of Dentistry, Tokyo, Japan

Kunihiro Sakuma
Institute for Liberal Arts, Environment and Society, Tokyo Institute of Technology, Tokyo, Japan

Raoul Saggini
Department of Medical Sciences, Oral and Biotechnology, "G. d'Annunzio" University, Chieti, Italy

Simona Maria Carmignano, Lucia Cosenza and Tommaso Palermo
School of Specialties in Physical and Rehabilitation Medicine, "G. d'Annunzio" University, Chieti, Italy

Rosa Grazia Bellomo
Department of Medical Sciences, Oral and Biotechnology, "G. d'Annunzio" University, Chieti, Italy

Shinichiro Morishita and Atsuhiro Tsubaki
Institute for Human Movement and Medical Sciences, Niigata University of Health and Welfare, Niigata, Japan

Jack B. Fu
Department of Palliative, Rehabilitation & Integrative Medicine, University of Texas MD Anderson Cancer Center, Houston, TX, USA

Michelle Guan and Andrew E. Hendifar
Samuel Oschin Comprehensive Cancer Center, Cedars Sinai Medical Center, Los Angeles, CA, USA
Department of Medicine, David Geffen School of Medicine, Los Angeles, CA, USA

Arvind M. Shinde
Samuel Oschin Comprehensive Cancer Center, Cedars Sinai Medical Center, Los Angeles, CA, USA

Raoul Saggini
Physical and Rehabilitation Medicine, Department of Medical Oral and Biotechnological Sciences, Director of the School of Specialty in Physical and Rehabilitation Medicine, "Gabriele d'Annunzio" University, National Coordinator of Schools of Specialty in Physical and Rehabilitation Medicine, Chieti-Pescara, Italy

Simona Maria Carmignano, Lucia Cosenza and Tommaso Palermo
School of Specialty in Physical and Rehabilitation Medicine, "Gabriele d'Annunzio" University of Chieti-Pescara, Italy

Rosa Grazia Bellomo
Physical and Rehabilitation Medicine, Department of Medicine and Sciences of Aging, "Gabriele d'Annunzio" University of Chieti-Pescara, Italy

Vinod Chainani, Russell Riehl, Carl J. Lavie and John P. Reilly
Ochsner Health System, John Ochsner Heart and Vascular Institute, Jefferson, Louisiana, USA

Abir Abdo
Louisiana State University Health Sciences Center, New Orleans, Louisiana, USA

Mauricio G. Cohen, Carlos Alfonso and Pedro Martinez-Clark
University of Miami Miller School of Medicine, Miami, Florida, USA

Nidal Abi-Rafeh
Tulane University School of Medicine, New Orleans, Louisiana, USA

Geeta Chainani
Windsor University School of Medicine, Saint kitts, Carribean

Bryon A. Tompkins
The Interdisciplinary Stem Cell Institute, University of Miami Miller School of Medicine, Miami, USA
The Department of Surgery, University of Miami Miller School of Medicine, Miami, USA

Ana Marie Landin, Victoria Florea, Makoto Natsumeda and Angela C.Rieger
The Interdisciplinary Stem Cell Institute, University of Miami Miller School of Medicine, Miami, USA

Wayne Balkan, Ivonne Hernandez Schulman and Joshua M. Hare
Ochsner Health System, John Ochsner Heart and Vascular Institute, Jefferson, Louisiana, USA
University of Miami Miller School of Medicine, Miami, Florida, USA

Nidal Abi-Rafeh
Tulane University School of Medicine, New Orleans, Louisiana, USA

Geeta Chainani
Windsor University School of Medicine, Saint kitts, Carribean

Bryon A. Tompkins
The Interdisciplinary Stem Cell Institute, University of Miami Miller School of Medicine, Miami, USA
The Department of Surgery, University of Miami Miller School of Medicine, Miami, USA

Ana Marie Landin, Victoria Florea, Makoto Natsumeda and Angela C. Rieger
The Interdisciplinary Stem Cell Institute, University of Miami Miller School of Medicine, Miami, USA

Wayne Balkan, Ivonne Hernandez Schulman and Joshua M. Hare
The Interdisciplinary Stem Cell Institute, University of Miami Miller School of Medicine, Miami, USA
The Department of Medicine, University of Miami Miller School of Medicine, Miami, USA

Index

www.ingramcontent.com/pod-product-compliance
Lightning Source LLC
LaVergne TN
LVHW081012210926
848485LV00004B/843